"In the current volume, esteemed clinicians Augustine Meier and Micheline Boivin continue their innovative therapeutic model first published in *Self-in-Relationship Psychotherapy: A Complete Clinical Guide to Theory and Practice* (2022). The unique characteristic of SIRP is the inclusion of core relational (need for emotional connection and autonomy), self (need for significance and competency), and physical intimacy needs (need for sensual contact and sexual intimacy) in its assessment, conceptualization, and treatment of individuals, couples, and children. A rare and exceptionally rich clinical model bridging various schools of thought seamlessly, both conceptually and clinically. A must-read for all practicing clinicians."

Loray Daws, PhD, *clinical psychologist and psychoanalyst, International Masterson Institute, Object Relations Institute for Psychotherapy and Psychoanalysis, New York*

"The chapters that illustrate the application of SIRP with children provide further evidence that play therapy is a useful approach to help ameliorate children's distress. With a clear focus on children's core needs (relational, self, and physical intimacy needs), the authors show how play therapy techniques such as story-telling, puppet play, guided imagery, sand and dollhouse play, and metaphors encourage children to express their thoughts and feelings in a developmentally appropriate way. In addition, the integration of play therapy to advance treatment goals within the context of this promising theory appears to provide a useful way of helping children achieve mastery and resolve a range of intra- and interpersonal behavioral and social-emotional difficulties. I thoroughly enjoyed the well-articulated case conceptualizations, the systemic lens, and the highly specific treatment goals that are advanced using expressive therapies."

Eliana Gil, *PhD, Founder and Partner, GIL Institute for Trauma Recovery and Education, Fairfax, VA*

"To bring about significant and lasting change in your clients, I recommend you not only read *Self-in-Relationship Psychotherapy in Action* but study and apply the profound teachings contained in it. We need to go beyond our common approach to therapy and bring about valuable transformations with individuals, couples, and families. This book will help you achieve transformational success. I highly recommend it. Congratulations."

John Banmen, R. Psych., *co-author, The Satir Model: Family Therapy and Beyond, Director of Training Emeritus, Satir Institute of the Pacific, Professor Emeritus, University of British Columbia, Canada*

Self-in-Relationship Psychotherapy in Action

This book presents a comprehensive guide to applying Meier and Boivin's Self-in-Relationship Psychotherapy model to clinical work with individuals, couples, families and children.

The central theme of the book is that the paradigm of affects, cognitive processes, and behaviors that informs current psychotherapy approaches needs to be broadened to include core self, relational, and physical intimacy needs as motivating factors in psychotherapy. Drawing on multiple influences including relational psychoanalysis, the authors illustrate how to work with core needs when providing therapy to children and adults. They establish that core needs are universal, and their realizations are essential for healthy living and argue that clients achieve the healthiest outcomes by finding a way to balance the self alongside their relations with others. The concept of core self, relational and physical intimacy needs is what binds all the chapters in this book and makes it unique among psychotherapy approaches.

With a clear transtheoretical approach and rich clinical vignettes, this book is core reading for any psychotherapist, psychoanalyst, or practicing psychologist.

Augustine Meier is a certified clinical psychologist; individual, couple, and family psychotherapist; clinical researcher; author; and Professor Emeritus at Saint Paul University, Ottawa, Canada. He is the founder of the Institute for Self-in-Relationship Psychotherapy.

Micheline Boivin is a certified clinical psychologist; child, parent, and family psychotherapist; clinical researcher; and author, and based in Ottawa, Canada. She is a Board Member of the Institute for Self-in-Relationship Psychotherapy.

Self-in-Relationship Psychotherapy in Action

Individual, Couple, Family, and Child Psychotherapy

Augustine Meier and Micheline Boivin

Routledge
Taylor & Francis Group

LONDON AND NEW YORK

Designed cover image: © Getty Images

First published 2025
by Routledge
4 Park Square, Milton Park, Abingdon, Oxon OX14 4RN

and by Routledge
605 Third Avenue, New York, NY 10158

Routledge is an imprint of the Taylor & Francis Group, an informa business

British Library Cataloguing-in-Publication Data
A catalogue record for this book is available from the British Library

ISBN: 9781032655260 (hbk)
ISBN: 9781032678795 (pbk)
ISBN: 9781032655291 (ebk)

DOI: 10.4324/9781032655291

Typeset in Times New Roman
by Newgen Publishing UK

This book is dedicated to
Margaret Mahler and Virginia Satir
who inspired our work.

Contents

Acknowledgments

Many professors, graduate students, supervised mental health workers, and those who sought our professional help, contributed to the development of our therapeutic approach called Self-in-Relationship Psychotherapy (SIRP). It is impossible to acknowledge the contributions of all who have significantly contributed to our thinking and articulation about psychotherapy that led to the development of SIRP and to the publication of this book. We are heartily grateful to all for their insightful questions and comments.

We would like to express our deepest appreciation to Dr. William Barry, psychologist, University of Ottawa, Ontario, who spoke eloquently and comprehensively about the most profound psychological concepts in his classes on psychopathology and psychophysiology. The body and mind relationship were consistent topics in his presentations of human growth and problems.

Appreciation is expressed to Dr. Agatha Sidlauskas (Agota Sidlauskaite), University of Ottawa, for introducing us to a biopsychosocial approach to human development. Her clinical approach to understanding the normal growth of children, the development of their emotional problems, and how these can be carried into adolescence and adulthood was enlightening. It provided an essential component in the development of our psychotherapy approach.

We express our appreciation to Dr. Angelina Celovsky, University of Ottawa, psychologist, for her insight into projective techniques, such as the Rorschach and drawings, and for her clarity in presenting a perceptual theory to understand projective techniques.

It would be amiss not to mention Dr. William Beniskos, University of Ottawa, psychologist, who taught a graduate course on adolescent psychology from a practical and clinical perspective. The insights gained about adolescent development became essential in our clinical practice.

Appreciation is expressed to Dr. Dan Offord and to Dr. James Mullin, psychiatrists, Royal Ottawa Hospital, Ottawa, for their enthusiasm, dedication, and for having freely given of their time in our research on schizophrenia, which culminated in our graduate-level dissertations.

We express our appreciation to the graduate students who participated in our research on psychotherapy, and to the graduate students who attended the training in SIRP and invited us to supervise their clinical practice. Their questions and discussions were stimulating and helpful to define more clearly the constructs of our therapeutic approach.

Appreciation is expressed to the children and their parents, to adolescents and adults, and to the couples and families who sought our services to help them to address their relational and emotional struggles. Our professional work with them helped us refine our approach to couple/family and child psychotherapy and to link theory and research more clearly to their lived experiences.

Lastly, we would like to acknowledge the support of the Senior Editor, Ms. Kate Hawes, at Routledge (England), for her keen and enthusiastic interest in our book and for her help to make it possible. We wish to thank the Assistant Editor, Ms. Aakriti Aggarwal, at Routledge whose expertise, guidance, and dedication helped bring this project to fruition. Appreciation is expressed to Leigh Westerfield, copy editor, for the thoroughness in editing our book manuscript and for the valuable suggestions and ideas. Thanks to Sujeesh Krishna, Project Manager, for patiently coordinating all the aspects that lead to the publication of this book. It has been a great pleasure for us to have worked with the editorial staff.

Introduction

In this volume, Meier and Boivin apply their innovative theory, Self-in-Relationship Psychotherapy (SIRP), to individual, couple, and child psychotherapy. In an earlier book, Meier and Boivin (2022), presented their theory of psychotherapy, identified and described its major constructs, and applied them to the conceptualization, assessment, and treatment of clinical cases.

SIRP is a transtheoretical approach that adopts concepts from developmental psychology and psychodynamic theories and methods, and techniques from psychodynamic, experiential, Gestalt, behavioral, and cognitive approaches. The unique characteristic of SIRP is the inclusion of core relational, self, and physical intimacy needs in its assessment, conceptualization, and treatment of clinical cases. Based on their clinical practice, the authors observed that individuals want to be in a relationship and be part of a community and feel free to contribute to both in their own way; they want to feel that they are valued, significant, and competent to contribute to a relationship and to community; and lastly, they craved sensual contact and sexual intimacy. SIRP condensed these human motives to form a taxonomy of core needs that comprise core relational needs (need for emotional connection and autonomy), core self needs (need for significance and competency), and core physical intimacy needs (need for sensual contact and sexual intimacy). The core needs are universal and are part of human life regardless of age, gender, or skin color; and their realizations are essential for healthy living. The hallmark of SIRP is that it addresses a client's core relational, self, and physical intimacy needs. It is the human needs that provide the energy and the direction for growth and development, and when the human needs are denied, repressed, and/or suppressed, they may lead to emotional problems and to maladaptive behaviors.

The authors contend that emotional and behavioral problems are fundamentally relational in origin. These problems emerge because the individual's core needs, in his infancy, childhood, and/or adolescent years, were not positively responded to. In his failure to achieve these developmental goals, the individual develops negative internal working models (psychic- and self-structures) that impact his perception of self and others and his interactions with others. The goal of therapy, be it in working with children, adolescents, and/or adults, is to modify not only relational and behavioral interactions, but also to transform the internal working model.

DOI: 10.4324/9781032655291-1

In the chapters that follow, Meier and Boivin illustrate how they work with core needs and with internal working models when providing therapy to children and adults in the context of individual, couple, and child psychotherapy. Abstracts of these chapters are presented below.

The book is divided in three parts: Part I: Individual Psychotherapy; Part II: Couple/Family Therapy; and Part III: Child Psychotherapy. The last chapter presents two competing philosophical positions regarding psychotherapy.

Part I, on individual psychotherapy, consists of four chapters. The first chapter consists of three sections that provide a comprehensive overview of SIRP. The sections present: SIRP's fundamental principles and major constructs; the semi-structured interview, the assessment form, and the operational definitions for the SIRP constructs; and the psychotherapy goals, the qualities, and characteristics of an SIRP-oriented therapist, the qualities and characteristics of clients suited for the SIRP approach, and working with core needs.

The case of a middle-aged man, Armand, who struggled with his fourth episode of major depression, is presented in the second chapter. The chapter addresses the themes worked on in his recovery from depression. This was achieved by the client asserting his need for autonomy, which led to a healthy relationship with his partner.

Chapters 3 and 4 present the case of Tania, who struggled with obsessive thoughts and compulsive behaviors (OCD). The third chapter presents Tania's developmental and psychosocial history, her OCD obsessions and compulsions, and the plan for treatment. Chapter 4 presents Tania's recovery from her obsessive thoughts and compulsive behaviors. Thirteen years following therapy, the client continued to effectively manage her obsessive thoughts and compulsive behaviors.

Part II, on couple and family therapy, comprises Chapters 5 and 6. Chapter 5 presents the assumptions, principles, and major constructs of Self-in-Relationship Couple/Family Psychotherapy (SIRCFP). A distinguishing principle is that couple and family negative interaction patterns reflect unmet core relational, self, and/or physical intimacy needs. The heart of couple and family therapy is for the members to become aware of their mutual core needs and to integrate them into their relationships.

The sixth chapter presents the application of SIRCFP to the therapy of a couple. It provides an analysis of their psychosocial histories using the Self-in-Relationship Psychotherapy Assessment Form. The couple's repetitive negative reactional patterns served as the focus for analysis and for treatment. The patterns were treated according to their unmet core needs, which when identified, accepted, and embraced, led to improved communication skills, manner of relating, and coping strategies.

Part III, on child psychotherapy (SIRCP), comprises three chapters. Chapter 7 presents the SIRP core constructs that are pertinent to understanding the development of the child's inner world and how it might play out in the child's problematic behaviors. This is followed by a presentation of play therapy, which includes its definition, change mechanisms, power, techniques, and treatable problems. The last part addresses the therapist's qualities and tasks, therapeutic interventions, and the rationale for including parents in child psychotherapy.

The eighth chapter presents the application of SIRP in working with two boys and their parents. The first case is that of André, 11 years of age, struggling with separation anxiety, which is worked through using puppets and imagery. The second case is that of Louis, nine years of age, dealing with the aftereffects of parental alienation, which he resolves by constructing family scenes in using a playhouse and describing the interactions between the family members and the other characters.

Chapter 9 presents the case of a four-year-old girl, Chantal, to help her become assertive, establish boundaries, and set limits with others. Underlying her difficulties was the failure to develop a secure emotional bond with her caregiver, which led to her lack of confidence to be real and genuine in her relationships. Although it was a goal from the beginning, the focus toward the end of therapy, was on the development of a secure emotional bond with significant others. With the development of a secure emotional bond, the client gained in confidence to be assertive, establish boundaries, and set limits. Four years after therapy was terminated, the gains made in therapy continued.

The last chapter presents two competing epistemologies regarding couple and family therapy. One of the epistemologies comprises modernism, structuralism, and first-order cybernetics, and proposes that there are laws and principals to be discovered. The second epistemology comprises postmodernism, post-structuralism, and second-order cybernetics, and proposes that all human reality is socially constructed. SIRP takes the position that there is objective reality and givens that are shaped by the environment in which they unfold.

The clients presented in this book have given their permission to use the clinical material for training, research, and publication purposes. We have gone to great lengths to protect the privacy of these clients by changing identifying material that includes their names and background information.

To make the text of this book more reader-friendly, the male form of the third-person pronoun is used in the odd-numbered chapters, and the female form of the third-person pronoun is used in the even-numbered chapters.

Reference

Meier, A., & Boivin, M. (2022). *Self-in-relationship psychotherapy: A complete clinical guide to theory and practice*. England, UK: Routledge.

Individual Psychotherapy

Chapter 1

Self-in-Relationship Psychotherapy

A Comprehensive Overview

This chapter presents a comprehensive overview of Self-in-Relationship Psychotherapy (SIRP) that provides the framework for the chapters on individual, couple/family, and child psychotherapy. The chapter is divided into three parts. The first part presents SIRP's fundamental principles and major constructs, the second addresses the assessment procedures, and the third part presents the treatment process. Much of the material for this chapter is taken from Meier and Boivin (2022).

Fundamental Principles and Major SIRP Constructs

Fundamental Principles

Self-in-Relationship Psychotherapy (SIRP) rests on a set of fundamental principles that are derived in part from the authors' clinical practice and in part from their philosophical position regarding psychotherapy, which is presented in the last chapter of this book.

1. Core needs, together with affects and cognitions, form three parallel but inter-dependent systems (Benesh & Weiner, 1982; Lazarus, 1982; Reisenzein & Schonpflug, 1992; Zajonc, 1980). Within this triad, core needs are conceived to be the prime directional motivators of behaviors and relational interactions; feelings are the responses to the satisfaction or to the frustration of unmet core needs; and thoughts pertain to the stylistic ways of processing information, of perceiving reality, of solving problems, and of adapting to reality.
2. The core needs are assumed to be innate and potentially present when life begins (Deci & Ryan, 2000; Kasser, 2002). They are organized according to relational, self, and physical intimacy needs (Meier & Boivin, 2022).
3. A child's core needs evolve and change as he moves from being emotionally bonded with his caregiver to psychologically separating from her, achieving individuation and forming intimate relationships with others (Mahler, Pine & Bergman, 1975). The core needs are reworked each time that the person goes through a major phase in life, such as leaving home to attend higher education.

DOI: 10.4324/9781032655291-3

4. Core needs become the principle around which the person adaptively and/or maladaptively organizes his life. When core needs are consistently unmet, they continue to linger to seek fulfillment, and if unfulfilled, they may lead to emotional, psychological, behavioral, and relationship problems.

Major Theoretical Constructs

The major explanatory constructs that constitute SIRP have been incorporated from psychodynamic theory including psychoanalysis, ego psychology, object relations theory, and self-psychology. The names of the original constructs are kept but are adapted to and interwoven in the SIRP narrative. The constructs are briefly described in this chapter and are illustrated by the cases presented in the following chapters.

Core Relational, Self, and Physical Intimacy Needs

The concept of core needs is foundational to SIRP. The authors arrived at the significance of human core needs from their clinical work with children, adolescents, and adults in the context of individual, couple, and family therapy. SIRP groups core needs according to relational, self, and physical intimacy needs.

Core relational needs

The core relational needs comprise the need for emotional bonding with a significant caregiver and the need to psychologically separate from the caregiver, to individuate and to become autonomous (Mahler et al., 1975). These two relational needs are referred to as the need for emotional bonding and the need for autonomy.

The core need for emotional bonding refers to a need for emotional and psychological closeness that is characterized by affection and trust between people. The core need for autonomy implies the needs for psychological separateness and for individuation. The need for separateness is the need to psychologically separate from one's caregiver and to experience oneself as different from the caregiver. The need for individuation refers to the need to be autonomous, that is, to be the origin of one's own behaviors (Deci & Ryan, 2002); to develop one's own interests, values, and goals in life; and have the freedom to make choices and decisions in matters that concern one.

The quality of the core needs for emotional bonding and for autonomy are dependent upon the infant/child's stage of development. In the early stage of development, the infant/child has not developed a sense of "Me" and "Not me." As well, the need for autonomy is merged with dependency needs at the early stage of development. Thus the definition of the need for emotional bonding and the need for autonomy varies according to the developmental stage achieved (Mahler et al., 1975). The term "emotional bonding" is used to describe the core need of an infant/

child for its caregiver and the term "emotional connection" is used to describe the core need for post-childhood relationships.

Core self needs

The core self needs include the striving to be competent and the striving to be significant. The need for competency refers to the need to experience oneself as effective in one's ongoing interactions with others (relational competency) and to experience opportunities to exercise and express one's capacities (self-competency in relation to oneself) (Deci & Ryan, 2002). The need for significance refers to the need to experience oneself as lovable and important and as being likeable and attractive to others. The child needs the caregiver's admiration and affirmation to foster his sense of competency and to experience that he is a significant and lovable person.

The development of the self needs begins in early childhood. With consistent positive validation, the child gradually develops a sense of competency and significance, and as he develops to become an adolescent and adult, he requires less feedback from others regarding the two self needs. A person who has a good sense of competency and feels significant, is able to maintain these despite negative responses from others.

Core physical intimacy needs

The core physical intimacy needs include the need for sensual contact and the need for sexual intimacy. The need for sensual contact is the urge for contact through physical touch. Sensuality broadens to include sexual intimacy when the infant/child begins to experience pleasure in making physical contact with self by touching erogenous parts of his body and in later years, by sexual intimacy. The need for sexual intimacy refers to the need for physical contact that finds its completion in genital expression. It is to be noted that age, gender, and culture often affect how the need for sensual contact and the need for sexual intimacy are expressed and satiated.

In summary, the relational, self, and physical intimacy needs overlap and affect all aspects of development and growth. When these needs go unmet, problems are apt to occur. It is important to remember that unmet needs do not inevitably lead to emotional problems. One cannot make predictions about the outcome when needs go unmet; rather, one can only trace a problem back to unmet needs and how they were managed.

Internal Representations and Their Linking Affects

In the process of emotional bonding with the parents and then psychologically separating from them and moving toward individuation, the child/infant develops representations of them and of himself, and both the child and the parents develop feelings for each other. Masterson (1976) spoke about these mutual feelings in terms of affects that link the internalized representations of the other and the self. Another aspect regarding representations is how the child felt being brought into his home and living with the parents and other members of the family.

Internal representation of other and of self

In his early experiences with his caregivers, the child forms cognitive-affective representations of them. The representation, which is not the same as a feeling, is a consequence of how he experiences the caregivers responding to his feelings, thoughts, needs, and behaviors. The representations can bear a positive, negative, and/or a mixed positive/negative valence that continues to persist into adolescence and adulthood and impact the quality and nature of future relationships. The representation of a caregiver may correspond to how the person is in real life, or it may deviate from it in some dramatic fashion. An individual's internal representations of his childhood caregivers can give a clue as to which needs were met or unmet. For example, if a client, as a child, experienced his father as being critical and demeaning, this might give a clue as to the client's need to be validated for being a competent person.

From the infant/child's interactions with significant caregivers, he forms an internal representation of himself, which is a cognitive-affective image of self. The mental representation of self is an image and not a feeling about himself. In the formation of the infant/child's first representations of self, he sees himself as his caregivers viewed him and responded to his needs, thoughts, feelings, and behaviors. If the responses were positive, the infant/child thinks of himself as a good person and as having caused the caregiver's positive responses. His self-representations might include seeing himself as lovable, competent, and intelligent. The reverse happens when the caregiver's responses are negative.

Affect linking internalized other and self representations

Masterson (1976) pointed out the importance of considering the mutual feelings that the parent and child have for each other. He described this relationship in terms of the affect that links the internalized representations of the other and the self. This affective linkage refers to the feelings that an infant/child had for a parent and the feeling that the parent had for the infant/child. This is seen through the eyes of the child and reflects his perception of reality but not necessarily objective reality. It is important to differentiate old (familiar) feelings related to past experiences from new feelings that are associated with current experiences of others.

The client's perceived feelings that the parents had toward him when he was a child is referred to as the "affect linking internalized representation of other to self." The feeling is from the perspective of the client, which might or might not correspond to the way things were in reality.

The feelings that the client, as an infant or child, had toward the parents but was not aware of these feelings, is referred to as the "affect linking internalized representation of self to other." The person might experience the same feelings toward his parents today. Again, this is based on the perception of the client.

The feeling when in the presence of primary caregivers

This dimension describes how the person, as a child and teenager, felt when in the presence of and/or living with his parents and with the other members of the family. He might have felt safe, protected, lovable, significant, competent, and fun being part of the family. On the other hand, he might have felt anxious, unprotected, demeaned, tense, and unwanted. These early experiences in being with significant others may continue to influence how the person feels in being with others and how others accept him socially.

In summary, the representations that an infant/child formed of himself and of his parents, the feelings that the members of the family have for each other, and how the infant/child/toddler felt living with other members of the family provide valuable information about the home climate and the quality of parenting. They can provide clues as to the infant/child/toddler's needs that went unmet and provide information that is helpful to understanding how the client's subjective experiences influenced the development of his psychic structure, self-structure, and coping strategies to secure his self and relational needs.

Psychic Structure

The growing child's experiences with significant others and the representations that were formed gradually become organized and take on the quality of a structure. This structure together with the innate biological strivings and the innate adaptive capacities form what has come to be called the psychic structure. The psychic structure is dynamic and impacts all aspects of life and often operates outside of awareness.

The psychic structure, according to Freud (1923), is thought to comprise three parts: the innate energy system (i.e., the id) that embraces the instincts; the acquired social heritage (i.e., the superego) that comprises acceptable behaviors and values by which to live; and the adaptive and creative capacity to think, plan, and act (i.e., the ego). Through the functions of the ego, the needs of the id and the expectations of the superego and of the demands of reality are brought to work together for the benefit of the person

SIRP has modified Freud's (1923) tripartite organization of the psychic structure in the following ways. It has replaced the instincts of the id by the construct of core needs; the *life instinct* by the relational need for emotional bonding and by the physical intimacy needs for sensual contact and sexual intimacy; and the *death instinct*, which is aggression, by the need for autonomy. SIRP does not consider aggression to be innate but an emotional reaction to interference in the pursuit of one's core needs. The need for autonomy, however, is considered to be innate as it refers to the striving to move away from the emotional bond with the caregiver, to psychologically separate and to individuate and become autonomous. The modification of the two instincts is consistent with Freud's (1938) reformulation of the instincts where he wrote,

> The aim of the first of these basic instincts [Eros] is to establish ever greater unities and to preserve them thus – in short, to together; the aim of the second is, on the contrary, to undo connections (and so to destroy things). (p. 148)

The SIRP approach embraces Freud's (1923) concept of the ego, which is innate and potentially present at birth and is described as a "coherent organization of mental processes" (p. 17). The ego's innate characteristics are the capacity for perception, memory, and motility, and its functions include thinking, planning, and action. The functions of the ego can be thought of in terms of adaptive functions and defensive functions. An adaptive ego is flexible, resourceful, and resilient and is capable of managing the challenges of daily living that it faces in a creative, realistic, and rewarding manner. The ego in its defensive mode responds to intrapsychic conflicts and attempts to mediate between the core needs, the prohibitions of the superego, and the demands of reality. In its defensive mode, it protects the person from dangers and threats to one's psychological well-being.

SIRP adopts Freud's concept of superego, which comprises all of that which is socially inherited in terms of acceptable behaviors and in terms of values and ideals to live by. These behaviors and values become part of a person's life through the processes of identification with significant others, which begin at an early age and before the resolution of the Oedipus complex (Jacobson, 1964). Freud (1923) used the term "conscience" to describe socially acceptable and unacceptable behaviors and the term "ego ideal" to describe the values and ideals to live by. The superego can be moderate, severe, or harsh in its function (Jacobson, 1964). A moderate superego is able to integrate the prohibitions without compromising a person's core needs. A severe superego is demanding of self and of others, tends to be perfectionist, feels obligated (rather than responsible), and has a need to control his social environment. A harsh superego is punitive, guilt ridden, and may self-harm and entertain suicidal thoughts.

Self-Structure and Sense of Self

In the early days, weeks, and months of its life, the infant develops an emotional and physical bond with its mother. This bond is the foundation for the development of the self, which is believed to begin as a bodily sense of self (Allport, 1967). Human infants are thought to be born with a self already in place. That is, they have a biologically determined psychological entity (Brinich & Shelley, 2002) and a virtual self (Kohut, 1977).

The potential for a self interacts with caregiver's sense of what is self, and from this interaction and identification with the primary caregiver emerges the infant/child's organization of a cohesive self that is cognitive and affective in nature and is stored as an internal representation of self (Kohut, 1971). The self emerges through the way the infant is physically handled, touched, and embraced (Mahler et al., 1975; Winnicott, 1965). At the beginning of an infant's life, the ego is dominant, but with the development of a self, the "living self" becomes the "organizing center of the ego's activities" (Kohut, 1971, p. 120).

The sense of self is considered to be constituted by three components, which are the need to be competent, the need to be significant, and the capacity to keep the needs for competency and self-esteem in balance and to enable the competencies to turn into achieved goals (Baker & Baker, 1987). These needs are broadly extrapolated from Kohut's (1977) concepts of Nuclear Ambitions, Nuclear Ideals, and Nuclear Talents. With regard to SIRP's taxonomy of core needs, the self needs for competency and significance are included under the construct of the self.

Defense Mechanisms and Coping Strategies

The infant/child develops defense mechanisms and coping strategies to deal with the realities of frustrations, disappointments, and emotional injuries. The earliest of these mechanisms (e.g., dissociation), referred to as primary defense mechanisms, operate at an unconscious and instinctual level, whereas the later coping mechanisms (e.g., displacement), referred to as secondary defense mechanisms, are more learned and cognitive in nature and less unconscious (Kaplan & Sadock, 1991; Sadock, Sadock, & Ruiz, 2014; White & Watt, 1981). Each individual develops a unique system of defense mechanisms, like a coat of armor, based on the nature of issues dealt with and the age at which these were developed. With respect to the SIRP approach that is designed to treat developmental injuries, the significant defense mechanisms include splitting, idealization, projection, introjection, and regression, with splitting being the most significant.

Splitting is a developmental and defensive process of keeping incompatible feelings apart and separate. It refers to dividing external objects into "all good" and "all bad," accompanied by the "abrupt shifting of an object from one extreme category to the other" with possible "sudden and complete reversal of feelings and conceptualization about a person" (Kaplan & Sadock, 1991, p. 183). Splitting is a normal process for a young child as he does not have the capacity to reconcile and synthesize a caregiver's opposite behaviors (e.g., pleasurable, unpleasurable), a capacity that is acquired by the age of two to three (Mahler et al., 1975).

Idealization and devaluation are characteristic of splitting, whether it be by an infant/child, teenager, or adult. Idealization refers to seeing external objects as "all good" and "endowing them with great power," whereas devaluation refers to seeing a person as being flawed, worthless and "all bad" (Kaplan & Sadock, 1991, p. 183).

Projection is an unconscious tendency to attribute one's own unacceptable feelings, thoughts, and impulses to other persons or objects in the external world. It refers to "perceiving and reacting to unacceptable inner impulses and to their derivatives as though they were outside the self" (Kaplan & Sadock, 1991, p. 183).

Introjection has both developmental and defensive functions. Developmentally, introjection is the process of incorporating the characteristics of a person (e.g., kindness of a favorite aunt) unconsciously into one's own psyche with the "goal of establishing closeness to and constant presence of the object" (Kaplan & Sadock, 1991, p. 183). Defensively, introjection can serve the purpose of coping with the anxiety with regard to a lost object or a feared object and in coping with a sense of guilt. For example, with regard to a lost object, an individual deals with the grief by internalizing the positive characteristics of the lost object, thereby nullifying or negating the loss.

Regression refers to returning to a previous stage of development or functioning to avoid the anxieties or hostilities involved in later stages. (Kaplan & Sadock, 1991, p. 183). It refers to reverting to a behavior more appropriate to an earlier stage of development or to reaction patterns long since outgrown.

Quality of the Emotional Bond

This construct refers to the degree to which an infant/child feels emotionally and physically bonded and anchored (Mahler et al., 1975). The two essential components of an emotional bond are that the person feels comfortable, safe, and secure in being with the other (safe anchorage), and that the person expects that his needs will be satisfied (confident expectation) (Mahler & Furer, 1968). The failure to develop a secure emotional bond could be experienced as a longing, emptiness, and a nagging loneliness and take on a compulsive and insatiable quality (Erskine, 1998).

The quality of the emotional bond can be considered according to four categories: being emotionally connected, striving for emotional connection, avoiding emotional connection, and being emotionally disconnected. To be emotionally connected means that the infant/child (later an adolescent, adult) has developed a satisfying, secure, and comfortable emotional connection with the significant other. To seek emotional connection refers to eagerly searching for a meaningful, satisfying, and comfortable emotional relationship with a significant other. Avoiding emotional connection is defined as keeping emotionally distant from significant others, which might happen when the significant other is imposing and does not allow the individual space to be himself. To be emotionally disconnected refers to having limited feelings of affection and empathy for the other and/or to being emotionally cut off from the other.

Characteristic Emotional State

A characteristic emotional state is one that is familiar, was first intensely experienced in the past (e.g., childhood), and is carried into the present. This emotional state is typically brought about by a persistent dissatisfaction in not having core relational, self, and physical intimacy needs met in childhood. The telling sign of a characteristic emotional state is that it is familiar and its expression is disproportionate to a current event or response from another. The emotional state, when carried into adulthood, might manifest itself as a constant underlying emotion of anger, depression, sadness, and/or anxiety, which can become intensified when triggered by experiences resembling those of childhood.

Object Constancy

The development of object constancy is one of the significant achievements of the growing child. Object constancy is a mental representation of a positive libidinally connected person to whom an individual can consistently and reliably turn internally for safety, security, protection, nurturance, love, and self-soothing (Mahler et al., 1975)). Object constancy conjures up pleasant feelings, sensations, and memories of the significant person; it conjures up the feeling of "safe anchorage" and "confident expectations" that its needs will be responded to (Mahler & Furer, 1968).

The achievement of object constancy permits the infant/child to function separately in familiar surroundings despite moderate degrees of tension and discomfort, and acts as an agent to self-comfort (Edward, J., Ruskin, N., & Turrini, 1981). The infant/child has the ability to remain libidinally connected to the loved person whether the person is present or absent and despite internal stress or need.

Having an internalized positive object is essential to good emotional health as it provides a resource to which an individual can turn to gain a perspective on situations, to self-soothe, and to feel uplifted. An individual who lacks object constancy, feels adrift, disconnected from self and others, and struggles to regulate his emotions as he has no internal compass to turn to, to gain perspective on life's problems.

Social Self

An infant/child in his interactions with his caregivers and significant others learns how to relate socially with others. He might learn to organize his life according to his values, interests, ambitions, and dreams that are congruent with his sense of self and self-identity, or he might organize his life around the expectations, demands, and values of others. The former is referred to as living from the "true self" and the latter is referred to as living from the "false self" (Winnicott, 1960, pp. 145–146). The false self begins to emerge during childhood when he complies with the demands of others and puts aside his own needs because he does not have the inner resources to balance the demands from significant others with his own needs. The false self can readily be recognized in an individual who compromises the true self to maintain relationships for fear that if he asserts himself, he might be rejected.

Communication Styles

In his interactions with his caregivers, a child learns how to communicate with them; how to express and assert his thoughts, feelings, needs and preferences; and how to manage disagreements and conflicts. He learns how to verbally and nonverbally "convey information, make meaning with one another, and respond – internally and externally" (Satir, Banmen, Gerber & Gomori, 1991, p. 31).

When communication with others is very difficult and troublesome, the child might learn indirect and dysfunctional ways of communicating. He might learn dysfunctional stances such as placating (i.e., disregarding his own feelings and worth and handing them over to someone else), blaming (i.e., finding faults in others), being super reasonable (e.g., focusing on facts, not feelings), and being irrelevant (e.g., distracting from real issues) (Satir, 1972, 2013; Satir et al., 1991). In every form of communication, there is always an element of one's core needs that is detected in the "words, tone, and quality of expression" (Luthman, 1974, p. 59). A child, adolescent, or adult reveals his inner world in the way he communicates with others.

Projective Identification

Similar to communication styles, a child, adolescent, and adult's inner world is externalized and projected in his relational patterns. An infant/child is born with the innate capacities to form meaningful, satisfying, and enduring interpersonal relationships. In a "good enough" home environment (Winnicott, 1965), the infant/child and adolescent learns to negotiate, compromise, reconcile conflict, problem solve, forgive, repair broken relationships, be empathic toward others, and form meaningful intimate relationships. When the infant/child is exposed to an environment that is not good enough, he might acquire repetitive, compulsive, and ineffective relational patterns that are relentlessly driven by unmet core needs and push for a positive response from others. These repetitive and compulsive interpersonal patterns have been called "projective identifications" (Klein, 1959; Cashdan, 1988).

The common forms of projective identifications are: (a) dependency – the need to be taken care of and feeling dependent on the other; (b) power – portraying himself as being more competent than his partner and wanting to be in charge; (c) ingratiation – laying on guilt trips to get the needed response from the other; and (d) sexuality – using one's sexuality (e.g., flirting) to create sexual arousal in the other so as to get his/her attention (Cashdan, 1988). Projective identifications are driven by unmet core childhood needs.

Developmental Phases

SIRP views the origin of emotional problems and their treatment within the context of human development and its phases. SIRP is particularly interested in the early phases of development, referred to as the pre-oedipal phases, since an individual's personality begins to be formed in these early phases. Failure to negotiate the tasks of the pre-oedipal phases can lead to serious emotional problems in childhood, adolescence, and adulthood.

SIRP has incorporated the phases that Mahler and associates (1968, 1975) identified based on their research and clinical observations. The phases that have significant relevance for SIRP are Symbiosis, Differentiation, Practicing, and Rapprochement.

Symbiotic phase

Symbiosis represents a state of intermittent fusion with the mother, a state of undifferentiation in which the "I" is not yet differentiated from the "not-I" and the inside and outside are only gradually coming to be sensed as different (Mahler et al., 1975, p. 8). The infant is not fused with the mother at all hours since from the beginning they are separate entities with "moments of merger" (Bergman, 1975, p. xvi) in the infant's day when merger or fusion is close to the reality of the infant's experience (Pine, 1975). An example is when the infant, crying ravenously, begins suckling at the breast, achieves satisfaction, and melts drowsily "into the mother's body" (Pine, 1975, p. ix) – this represents fusion.

The major tasks of this phase are the achievement of "safe-anchorage" with the caregiver, the development of "confident expectation" that its needs will be met, the formation of an inner core and bodily self, and the formation of representations of other and self (Mahler & Furer, 1968, p. 17). The infant's inner body experiences contribute to the development of the body ego and body self and form the very core of the self. These experiences are the crystallization point around which a sense of identity will become established (p. 11). The failure to adequately achieve the capacity to merge and to develop a bodily self, can lead to problems such as a lifelong yearning for emotional connection, a disconnection from self and other, and the inability to invest energy externally and find one's path in life.

Differentiation and body image subphase

Differentiation refers to the process of emerging from the "symbiotic state of oneness with the mother, in the intrapsychic sense" (Mahler et al., 1975, p. 290). It is outward and goal directed (p. 54). A major task of this subphase is for the child to separate psychologically from the caregiver and to develop a sense of identity. This refers to the earliest awareness of a sense of being; it is a feeling that includes in part the investment of the body with libidinal energy. Identity is not "a sense of who I am" but a sense "that I am" (p. 8).

The child is helped to differentiate in a timely fashion when its movements toward psychological separation are supported and validated and when the caregiver is available to him when he returns for emotional closeness. It is also important not to burden the child prematurely with adult responsibilities by placing the child in the position of being a caregiver to the parent, or with taking on responsibility for his own life and thereby becoming prematurely self-sufficient and independent. The caregiver provides a balancing act between nurturing the child when needed and nudging the child when ready.

The most serious developmental dangers occur at this phase when the child fails to differentiate or differentiates prematurely. The former may lead to psychoses and the latter is apt to lead to borderline and narcissistic disorders (Mahler et al., 1975). Some of the dangers or disturbances that might occur in this subphase are: (a) delayed differentiation, which refers to the failure to intrapsychically separate from the symbiotic object and to establish the "I" and the "Not I" (p. 58); (b) premature differentiation, which means that the infant moved out of the "safe anchorage" before it was ready (pp. 59–60); (c) premature ego development, which implies that the infant took over functions from his mother or started to do so (Mahler & Furer, 1968, p. 16); (d) development of a false self, which refers to the "as if" personality (p. 16); and (e) narcissistic compensation, where the infant or toddler takes over a function that is not being provided by the mother (Edward et al., 1981, p. 219).

Practicing subphase

The practicing subphase represents the child's movement from the "maternal nest" to exploring the expanding world that lies beyond the relationship with the care-giver; the child begins a "love-affair" with the world (Mahler et al., 1975, p. 70). The child exercises his developing motor capacities (e.g., crawling, walking) and cognitive capacities (e.g., manipulating objects, language), and reality tests his sense of omnipotence. The child feels elated and exhilarated with his own faculties, with the greatness of his own world, and in using his body to explore and master the "other-than-mother" environment and to "escape from fusion with, from engulfment by mother" (Mahler et al., 1975, p. 71).

In being away from the mother for a significant period of time, the toddler develops anxiety. He acquires the capacity to self-soothe, first by internalizing the maternal functions that originally served to soothe, calm, and regulate affect, and later by creating a transitional object (e.g., a blanket) that is invested with the mother's tension-relieving and soothing functions. The transitional object loses its importance when the child begins to perform soothing operations for himself without the need for the external soother (Edward et al., 1981). This subphase leads to the toddler asserting his individuality and to identity formation.

To negotiate this subphase, it is important that the caregiver validate the tod-dler's efforts toward separation and his strivings toward mastery of his world, and be emotionally available when the toddler feels anxious in his separation experiences. Failures to negotiate this subphase could be brought about by the caregiver pushing the toddler too early to psychologically separate and by being critical, rather than validating, of the toddler's efforts to master his environment, resulting in a feeling of inadequacy, low self-esteem, and a fear of risk and of venturing out. The toddler who has failed to become emotionally bonded in the symbiotic phase, might indeed be more preoccupied with the need to be emotionally close to the caregiver rather than to venture out and explore his expanding world. These failures might be carried into adolescence and adulthood.

Rapprochement subphase

This subphase marks a pivotal developmental point in the child's struggle toward establishing his individuality. During the rapprochement subphase, the child continues to strive to: (a) become securely emotionally connected; (b) establish a comfort zone between the "need to be emotionally connected" and the "need to be separated/individuated"; (c) establish physical and psychological boundaries between himself and others (e.g., establishes "what is mine" and "what is yours"); (d) internalize representation of good persons (e.g., object constancy) to whom he can turn mentally to gain perspective on issues, comfort self, and regulate affect; (e) relate to others empathically (e.g., whole-objects); (f) replace splitting with repression; and (g) move toward individuality (Mahler et al., 1975). The two main achievements of this subphase are the establishment of object constancy and individuality.

To help a child to achieve these goals, it is important for the caregiver to be sensitive to the child's emotional needs and to validate self-directed movements toward individuality. Whereas in the previous months, the child was rather oblivious to the caregiver's absence, now being in her presence is vital. The child manifests this by bringing toys and books to the caregiver and invites her to participate in his activities. It is also important for the caregiver to provide a structure to help the child contain his feelings and behaviors and to provide the child with explanations for the limits that are being imposed.

Failure to complete the developmental tasks of this subphase as listed above, can lead to serious emotional problems that are carried into adolescence and adulthood, such as borderline personality disorder. The core unmet need is for emotional bonding, which might be accompanied or triggered by the feeling of abandonment. The goal of therapy is to undo the developmental disturbances by the therapist meeting the client at the level at which the injury occurred.

The Developmental Positions

Klein's (1952) notion of the developmental positions is a useful construct when assessing the degree to which individuals who are intensely angry and express rage, have resolved their love–hate relationships and developed a capacity for relatedness and for empathy. Freud understood development in terms of the maturation of the instinctual energies that manifest themselves in the body and are worked out in the context of relationships. Klein understood and described development in terms of the way an infant deals with love–hate relationships and the different ways he experiences and relates to both internalized and externalized objects.

According to Klein, the infant's basic conflict revolves around constructive (loving) and destructive (hateful) forces or feelings, between a desire to protect those close to the child and the malicious wish to destroy them. This conflict was conceived in terms of "positions," types of interpersonal stances along which the child organizes experiences. Klein (1952a) conceived of two positions, the *paranoid-schizoid* and the *depressive* positions. Each position represents a developmental nodal point along a continuum of love and hate, and describes the manner in which object relations originate and mature (Cashdan, 1988). Klein believed that we do not grow out of these positions and that there remains a continuous tension between the paranoid-schizoid mechanisms and the depressive mechanisms, and that people constantly move from one position to the other (Segal, 2004).

The paranoid-schizoid position is characterized by persecutory anxiety; the dominance of the aggressive instinct; the mechanism of splitting; defenses of projection, introjection, idealization, devaluation, and denial; by relating to part objects; by greed and envy; and by a failure to establish boundaries between self and other. The infant's greatest nightmare is that hate, death, evil, and destruction will overwhelm and destroy the loving libidinal, gratifying, and good aspects of the self and the breast.

The depressive position represents an individual who has developed empathy and fears losing the love of the love object, uses repression rather than splitting, is beginning to see others and self as whole persons, and has established boundaries between self and other. The dominant emotion of this stage is depression for having hurt his mother by the projection of his aggressive impulses and hateful feelings toward her. When the infant/child feels that he has hurt his loved object through his destructive impulses and phantasies directed at her, he gradually re-owns his projected aggression, which leads to feelings of guilt and an urge to "repair, preserve or revive the loved injured object" (Klein, 1952a, p. 74).

Assessment Procedures and Operational Definitions

This part presents the three instruments developed to apply the SIRP approach to psychological assessments. The three instruments are: the Self-in-Relationship Semi-structured Assessment Interview (SIRP-SSAI); the Self-in-Relationship Psychotherapy Assessment Form (SIRP-AF); and the Operational Criteria and Coding Procedures (OCCP). This part concludes by presenting the procedures to formulate a conceptualization using SIRP constructs.

Self-in-Relationship Semi-structured Assessment Interview (SIRP-SSAI)

The therapist uses the SIRP-SSAI (Appendix A) to gather clinical information pertinent to SIRP constructs to permit him to perform an assessment, formulate a conceptualization, and plan treatment. He uses this instrument to collect information regarding the quality of a client's present and past relationships, and his present and past experiences regarding his sense of self and self-identity. The SIRP-SSAI is designed to gather information about a client's family of origin, current and past relationships, physical and mental health, and more. The therapist guides his interview keeping in mind the SIRP constructs.

The SIRP-SSAI is to be used as a guide to gather the relevant information. It is not meant to be used in a rigid way and to proceed from question to question and/or to follow the order of the questions as presented in the SIRP-SSAI. The client might spontaneously offer relevant material and therefore there is no need to ask questions. The order of questioning will often depend on how the client begins the session.

The therapist should use open-ended questions as they require a more elaborate response than closed questions. It might also be necessary to follow up a client response to an open-ended with another open-ended question. This is shown in the following example:

Therapist: What was your relationship with your father like?
Client: Mixed (This question needs to be followed up by another question such as)
Therapist: In what way was it mixed?

Self-in-Relationship Psychotherapy Assessment Form (SIRP-AF)

The SIRP-AF (Appendix B) has been specifically designed to assess a client's psychological state with reference to the SIRP constructs. The form provides two types of data, Descriptive Data and Scaled Data.

The descriptive data provide information about a client's unmet core needs with regard to significant others (e.g., father, mother) and his representations and feelings of himself and of the significant persons of his childhood. The data present a picture of the atmosphere of the home environment in which the client was raised and what it was like to have lived with others in the home of his childhood. It is assumed that the manner in which these experiences were perceived and internalized continue to impact a person's current relationships and day-to-day living.

The Scaled Data are designed to provide a glimpse into the client's inner world that was formed in large part through his infancy and childhood interactions with significant others. The inner world is composed of memories, affects, motives, image, perceptions, and sensations that influence, to a great extent, how the client processes incoming information and shapes his interactions with others and with the world. The constructs that are assessed and are pertinent to the client's inner world include: psychic- and self-structures; living from a true self; coping mechanisms; quality of emotional bond; object constancy; characteristic emotional state; characteristic developmental phase; characteristic position; and projective identification.

It is essential that the psychotherapist who uses this form have an in-depth understanding of the SIRP constructs and how they together form a client's psychological picture. When clinical material is not available to code a specific construct, the psychotherapist may choose to code the construct based on an inference from the clinical material. It is important that the inferred code is consistent with the codes for the other constructs. Research has demonstrated that trained psychotherapists can reliably use the SIRP-AF to code clinical material (Meier & Boivin, 2022).

Operational Criteria and Coding Procedures (OCCP)

To assure consistency in the application of the SIRP-AF, its constructs have been operationally defined and illustrated with examples as presented in the OCCP (Appendix C). This section addresses the operational definitions for the constructs that generate descriptive data and for the constructs that generate scaled data (quantitative data) under separate topics. This is followed by a brief note regarding coding guidelines.

Operational Criteria for Constructs That Generate Descriptive Data

The constructs that generate descriptive data include a description of the client's unmet needs that push for satiation, the client's internal representation of the significant other and the representation of self as seen through the eyes of the other, and the feelings that the client and the other have for each other.

In coding the descriptive data, it is important to clearly distinguish between needs, feelings, and representations, although in real life they overlap and together they influence all behaviors and attitudes. The therapist is asked to describe the unmet needs, mental representations of significant others and of self, the affects linking these representations, and the quality of his/her childhood interactions and experiences with his/her caregivers. The OCCP operationally defines each of these constructs.

The following example illustrates the application of the OCCP to the description of a client's internal representation of significant others. It is to be noted that when identifying a person's internal representations of others, the focus is on the mental and affective image and not on how the person feels about the other or on the way the other is needed. The mental picture of a person may correspond to what the person is like in real life, or it may deviate from this in some dramatic fashion.

Examples:

1. My father was self-centered, controlling; it was always about him and about no one else. He was heartless (Negative internal representation of father).
2. My mother was caring, did crafts with us, took us to the park; she was fair with us and yet she expected that we participate in household chores (Positive internal representation of mother).

Operational Criteria for Constructs That Generate Scaled Data

The second part of the SIRP-AF, the scaled data, comprises the constructs to be coded. The results from the scaled data provide a picture of a client's inner world that was formed in large part through his infancy/childhood interactions with significant others. The inner world that is formed serves as virtual map and/or an internal working model through which to make sense of incoming information and to guide his interactions with others.

More specifically, the scaled data provide information regarding the degree to which the client has integrated external demands with the strivings of his core needs, the structure of the self, his characteristic emotional state, the capacity to self-soothe and regulate affect, and the nature of his strivings for emotional connection. The scaled data also provide information about the coping strategies that the client developed to deal with the stressors and challenges of day-to-day living and how to deal with the anxieties, discouragements, and internal conflicts. Equally important, the scaled data indicate which of the unfinished tasks of a developmental subphase serve as an organizing principle for the client's perception of self and others and for his interactions with others. For example, a client who has not sufficiently achieved the task of emotional separation may fear to venture out, to individuate and to risk, and may, instead, unconsciously choose to remain emotionally dependent on others.

The OCCP provides operational definitions for each of the constructs. In completing the tasks required by the scaled data section of the SIRP-AF, it is important for the assessor to read the directions very carefully. Some of the constructs are rated on a five-point scale (Object Constancy), other constructs are identified and rated according to the degree of their striving (Core Need), while other constructs are checked off with a check mark (Coping Strategies).

The following example illustrates the operational definition and coding guidelines for the construct Social Self. This construct refers to the extent to which a client organizes his life according to that which is integral, genuine, and congruent with his sense of self and self-identity, and the extent to which he lives from the expectations, demands, and values of others. The former is referred to as living from the True Self, and the latter is referred to as living from the False Self. To simplify the coding for this construct, only a value will be given for True Self. This construct is coded on a five-point scale where 1 indicates that the construct is minimally operative and 5 indicates that the construct is strongly operative.

Examples:

1. I just became a pleaser, I aimed to please the people around me, to impress people, and it was easier to do it that way than to speak for myself. I don't like it, I want to get out of it, and I keep slipping back into old patterns (Possible score, True Self = 1.5).

2. I just like to be me and not have to worry about what others think (Possible score, True Self = 4).

Coding guidelines

In using the SIRP-AF and the OCCP to code a client protocol, the examiner is reminded to pay attention to the following guidelines (Meier & Boivin, 2022). First, read the protocol from beginning to end to get a sense of the whole before starting to code the constructs. Second, read the protocol for a second time and underline the parts of the protocol that relate to different constructs. Third, as you read the protocol, imagine being the client and ascertain what this might feel like. The goal is to meet the client as a whole person before working with his symptoms. In coding a construct, compare it to other constructs to assess for consistency of coding. When the information to code a construct is unavailable, make an inference from the available clinical material, keeping in mind to assure consistency in coding.

Formulating a Case Conceptualization

A conceptualization seeks to theoretically explain the client's current symptoms by linking them to predisposing factors (i.e., vulnerabilities), precipitating stressors, perpetuating factors (situations that maintain the symptom), and to protective factors (compensatory behaviors) to minimize the presenting problem. SIRP pays particular attention in the way unmet core needs and predisposing factors are related to the presenting problem.

From the perspective of SIRP, one can consider six steps in formulating a conceptualization. First, identify and clearly describe the problems, symptoms, and concerns and indicate their intensity, extensity, and when they were first experienced. Second, indicate the factors that predispose a client to a specific symptom or to an emotional and a psychological problem. Predisposing factors are areas of personal vulnerability (e.g., childhood rejection) that increase the risk of developing a particular symptom, emotional response, and/or psychological problem. Third, determine the precipitating events or factors that triggered the symptoms, concerns, and/or problem. Fourth, indicate the factors in a person's current life that perpetuate the symptoms. Fifth, indicate the protective factors that minimize the potency of the predisposing, precipitating, and perpetuating factors, such as a client's support system and interests that promote healthy and adaptive living. Sixth, select the theoretical construct that best explains the client's problem and provides direction for treatment.

The Psychotherapy Process

The process of psychotherapy, as presented here, is taken from Meier and Boivin (2022). It begins by presenting its principal and the subsidiary (ancillary) psychotherapy goals. This is followed by a summary of the essential qualities and characteristics of a SIRP-oriented psychotherapist, the qualities and characteristics of clients suited for SIRP, and the uniqueness of the SIRP approach. The last two topics present the main therapeutic techniques used by SIRP and the possible barriers in working with core needs.

Goals of Psychotherapy

The psychotherapeutic goals of SIRP are multiple as they are keyed to its many constructs that define various psychological conditions, such as internal conflicts, low self-esteem, and being critical of oneself, to mention a few. SIRP considers psychotherapy goals according to its principal goal and according to its subsidiary goals.

Principal Psychotherapy Goal

The principal goal of SIRP is to help clients uncover and reclaim their unmet core relational, self, and physical intimacy needs; reorient their lives according to these needs; become agents of their own lives; free themselves from their symptoms; and establish meaningful and wholesome relationships. SIRP pays particular attention to working with unmet core needs, but it does not in the process minimize the importance of working with cognitions and affects. Core needs, however, are conceived to be the prime motivators and give direction to the formation of perceptions of self, other, and the world and to behaviors and interactions. SIRP's task is to help clients link their current psychological and behavioral problems to unmet core needs and to realize that these needs might have been subverted by ineffective coping strategies, relational patterns, and communication styles, and compensated by behaviors such as being a caregiver and/or striving for excellence as an unconscious means to have their core needs partially met.

Subsidiary Psychotherapy Goals

The psychotherapy subsidiary goals are intimately connected to the principal goal and usually present themselves in individual therapy sessions. One can visualize the relationship between the subsidiary goals and the principal goal, similar to the relationship of the spokes of a wheel to its hub. The hub represents the principal goal. All of the spokes lead to the hub. In the same way, the subsidiary goals lead to the principal goal. In addressing subsidiary goals, one often works indirectly with the principal goal.

The subsidiary goals included in this presentation are adopted from object relations psychotherapists and self psychologists who extended and modified psychoanalysis in their work addressing unique psychological problems and with varying populations. Among the subsidiary goals presented, there is not one that is more important than the other; their importance is dependent upon the concern presented by the client.

Gaining awareness of the source of the problem

It is essential that clients gain insight into the source of their problem and its pre-disposing, precipitating, perpetuating, and protective factors. SIRP emphasizes the detection and the uncovering of the predisposing factors and how they impact current problems without negating the importance of the precipitating, perpetuating, and protective factors. Predisposing factors are those that put a person at risk of developing a problem. For example, a client who was harshly criticized as a child might have felt insignificant and incompetent. Thus an adult, when criticized by his supervisor, is predisposed to feeling insignificant and incompetent. Predisposing factors are vulnerabilities due to repeated negative experiences in early childhood and/or adolescence.

Unfreezing earlier emotional failures

Frozen early emotional failures refer to developmental stages that were not worked through at the appropriate age. This may include a failure to individuate and to assert one's feelings, thoughts, and needs (Mahler et al., 1975). A goal of therapy is to "unfreeze the early emotional failure" (Winnicott, 1959–1964, p. 128). This can be accomplished by reliving the aspect of the environment that originally failed, but this time succeeding with the client confidently asserting his feelings, thoughts, and needs and thereby completing the process of individuation. This can be facilitated by controlled regression to the stage of environmental failure. The successful negotiation of a developmental failure serves as a building block for continued growth and development.

Transforming psychic structure and ego building

A good number of clients seek psychotherapy because they are driven to perform and succeed, and feel guilty and are critical of themselves when they do not excel at their expected level or at the level expected of others. In such situations, the psychic structure is skewed in the direction of duties and obligations and to conforming behaviors, with the core needs being repressed, oppressed, and/or compromised. The goal of therapy is to give that part of self, referred to as the inner child, a greater voice and to assert its core needs and to help that part of self that is demanding (superego), to become more kind and empathic toward the inner child. This involves strengthening the ego to bring about a harmonious working together among the core needs, the demanding part of self and reality. To resolve the conflict between the inner child and the demanding part of self, the therapist can engage the two parts in a dialogue using the Gestalt Two-Chair technique (Perls, 1969). The goal is bring about a transformation of the psychic structure so that the core needs, superego, and reality work together for the greater good of the person.

Transforming bad objects

A child who is brought up in a home where he was physically and psychologically abused by a parent might internalize that parent as being a bad person, that is, a bad object. A repressed bad object continues to impact the individual's thoughts, feelings, and behaviors. When the child becomes an adolescent or an adult, he might want to reconcile his relationship with that parent. Fairbairn (1943, 1944) spoke about releasing bad objects. It might be more appropriate to speak about transforming bad objects since in the majority of cases an object is not totally bad but does possess some redeeming qualities. To transform a bad object implies bringing in something new (e.g., seeing the good aspects of the object) and seeing the person as a whole person with strengths and weaknesses.

A therapist can facilitate the transformation of the bad object by having the individual dialogue with the bad object using the Gestalt Two-Chair technique (Meier & Boivin, 2011). Usually the dialogue leads to a resolution, to a transformation of the bad object and to seeing the bad object as a whole person with weaknesses and strengths.

Increasing the capacity for relatedness

Fairbairn (1946) believes that therapeutic change comprises an increased capacity for relatedness, the ability to relate in new ways, and to restore the capacity to make direct and full contact with others. The task of psychotherapy is to help a client increase his capacity for relatedness. This entails drawing the client's attention to his way of relating, to his expectations of the relationships he has, and to what he is ready to give or not to give to the other. It also entails the development of relational skills such as being empathic and having the ability to negotiate, compromise, solve relational conflicts, and repair ruptures in his relationships. Often, these skills are lacking because the client is operating from his own unmet core needs and therefore is blinded to the core needs of the other.

Connecting with one's inner wisdom

A child who is brought up in a home where he was emotionally deprived or oppressed, might repress or suppress his feelings and core needs. The child learns to avoid feelings and thereby loses contact with his body. For such adult clients, SIRP might help them develop the capacity to connect with their bodily felt feelings, thoughts, and needs by the use of Gendlin's (1996) Focusing technique. SIRP believes that a client's direction for personal growth rests on the inner wisdom that is embedded within the bodily felt sense of the problem. Focusing on the bodily felt sense helps the client subjectively resonate with the "deep sense of truth and veracity that lives in the body" and which "makes therapy effective" (van der Kolk, 2014, p. 347). The goal is for the client to be guided by his inner wisdom and accept responsibility for self-growth, to become self-determining, self-oriented, and self-validating (Briere, 1992; Briere & Lanktree, 2012).

Therapist Qualities and Characteristics

It is assumed that a SIRP-oriented psychotherapist embodies the three Rogerian (Rogers, 1957, 1959) core conditions of unconditional positive regard, empathy, and congruence and that he has the ability to collaborate with the client to establish the psychotherapy goals and work toward achieving them (Bordin, 1979; Beck, Rush, Shaw & Emery, 1979), In addition, it is assumed that the therapist is able to provide a safe, secure, and protective environment for the client to access and disclose very private and intimate thoughts, feelings, and needs. The following are additional qualities and characteristics required of psychotherapists who work from the SIRP perspective.

Be Present in the Moment

The SIRP approach requires that the therapist be present in the moment and be focused. The therapist makes all efforts to try to understand the client's moods, feelings, thoughts, behaviors, and needs from the client's frame of reference. The psychotherapist observes the interaction between himself and the client, and makes use of this information to provide a broader context within which to understand the client's presenting concerns and difficulties. The therapist relies on his intuitive sense, in addition to an intellectual understanding, of the client's inner world and real-life struggles.

In order to develop the ability to be present in the moment, it might be helpful for the therapist to set aside some time prior to seeing the client to prepare himself to receive the client. This is particularly true for clients who have developmental injuries and histories of abuse and trauma and who perceive themselves to be flawed and who act out in angry ways.

Be Attuned to the Client's Developmental Needs

For clients who present with feelings of anxiety, anger, and depression, it is important to determine whether the feelings are related to current stressors or whether that are of long standing. It is important to determine whether they are linked to the client's failure to achieve appropriate childhood developmental tasks such as emotional bonding and to become a separate and autonomous person. In such cases, a SIRP-oriented psychotherapist pays particular attention to the developmental needs of the client, identifies the missed stages of development, and provides the necessary conditions for the client to move forward at his own pace (Mahler & Furer, 1968, p. 184).

To help the client reverse the developmental failures, the therapist may offer the client opportunities to re-experience the missed early stage of development, with the therapist serving as an auxiliary ego and performing the necessary healing functions. The therapist acts as a "catalyst" for the client's growth and development, and balances "nurturing" and "nudging" within the therapeutic relationship. This enables the client to go deeper and to reach higher levels of relating (Mahler & Furer, 1968, p. 167).

Have Capacity for Emotional Intimacy

A SIRP-oriented therapist tries to feel what it is like to live in the client's inner world and not to stand outside of it as an observer. To be with a client by identifying with his inner world is an emotionally intimate moment. One can conceive of Kohut's (1977) concept of "empathic immersion" as representing psychotherapist's capacity for emotional intimacy. Empathic immersion entails immersing oneself into the experience of the client, moving around in that experience, living it with the client, and allowing that which is essential to emerge. The big challenge for the therapist is to maintain relational boundaries and not to lose who he is, that is, his identity, when deeply and intimately engaged with the client's emotionally intense narrative.

Possess Capacity to Emotionally Engage with the Client

It is essential that a SIRP-oriented therapist have the capacity to emotionally engage with the client and to meet the client as a person before actively addressing the presenting symptoms. The meeting of the person of the client provides the broad context within which healing is to take place. Clients who present themselves in therapy with histories of developmental injuries, abuse, and trauma often report feelings of being emotionally broken, flawed, and loathing self, and are consumed by feelings of terror, anger, and rage. To help clients heal the experiences from which these feelings derive, it is important for the therapist to emotionally engage with these experiences, to empathically understand them, and to have a bodily felt sense of what it is like be emotionally broken and flawed, for example. It is important for the therapist to know what it "feels like to be a client" (Winnicott, 1963, p. 229) and to bring to these painful places, inner strength, hope, understanding, and care.

Ascertain What Leads to the Client's Health

In meeting the client for the first time, the psychotherapist tries to get to know the person of the client before beginning to address the presenting problems. Unlike medical problems that may affect a specific organ, such as appendicitis, a psychological and/or relational problem affects the whole person and is the product of the whole person. The psychotherapist endeavors to ascertain what it is in the client that needs to be healed so that the client is enabled to move forward in a healthy way. To gain this understanding, the psychotherapist attempts to experience within himself that which needs to be healed in the client to restore healthy living. This task can uncover the core issue that needs to be addressed. Then the psychotherapist uses his awareness of the core issue to guide the therapy process. To approach psychotherapy this way requires limiting the analysis and discussion of the client's anger, anxieties, depressive mood, and unwanted behaviors and paying more attention to that which leads the client to healthy living. This entails that the psychotherapist help the client access the positive energy embedded in his repressed core relational, self, and/or physical intimacy needs. The core needs provide the energy and direction toward healing and toward healthy and purposeful living.

Work with Client Transference

Transference can be defined as a client directing his emotional feelings and wishes toward the therapist as though he were the original object that caused the feelings (Freud, 1938). Included in the notion of transference are "the client's attempts to draw the therapist into assuming different roles such as being a rescuer, caretaker, and sexual partner" (Meier, 2010 p. 52). It is important to differentiate a transference from an expected emotional reaction that transpires in therapy. One can assume that there is transference when the client's emotional response is disproportionate to what the therapist said or did, tries to draw the therapist into unwanted behaviors, and/or idealizes or devalues the therapist. Regardless of the nature of the client's transferences, it is important to address them according to the client's capacity so as to enable him to work through the original conflict (Freud, 1938). It is to be noted that transferences are not unconscious creations of the analyst, as some authors claim (Smith, 2003). Freud (1925) states that transference is not created by analysis; rather, transference is "merely uncovered and isolated by analysis" (p. 42) and that psychoanalytic treatment "merely brings them to light" (Freud, 1905, p. 117).

Manage Countertransference

When confronted with a client's transference, a therapist is bound to have an emotional reaction, which is referred to as countertransference. Freud (1910) defined countertransference as resulting from "the patient's influence on his [psychoanalyst's] unconscious feelings […] [which need] […] to be overcome" (pp. 144–145). This definition maintains that countertransference is unconscious, is located in the psychoanalyst, and is triggered by the patient.

In recent years there have been efforts to broaden the definition of countertransference (Meier, 2010b). The outcome of these discussions differentiates between a therapist's emotional reactions that originate from his own unfinished childhood business, and the emotional reactions that emerge from working with a particular client. The latter type of therapist emotional reaction may be effectively used as part of the therapy process. To manage his countertransference, the therapist can consider the following guidelines: be aware of his countertransference; assess the emotional response and determine what belongs to him; take distance from the feeling; empathize and validate the client's experience; understand the dynamic underlying the emotion; and explore and link the current experience to an earlier experience (Gelso & Hayes, 2001; Briscoe-Dimock, 2010).

Client Qualities and Characteristics

Clients suited for SIRP must possess specific qualities and characteristics. Among these are the capacity for reflection and self-awareness, tolerance for psychologically painful experiences, commitment to growth of self, and the ability to use the therapist as an alter ego.

Capacity for Self-Reflection and Self-Awareness

SIRP promotes behavioral, attitudinal, and relational changes through the transformation of internal structures such as psychic and self-structures. In order to achieve these transformations, it is essential that the client have the capacity to reflect on his subjective experiences (e.g., thoughts, feelings, motives) and become aware how these subjective experiences might act as predisposing factors (vulnerabilities) that influence his current problems. It is also essential that the client become aware of how these subjective experiences were formed, at least in part, by childhood interactions with significant persons in his life, and realize that these subjective experiences have shaped his psychic and self-structures. These structures serve as a mindset, a lens, or a template through which information is processed and acts as a motivator that influences behaviors and relationships.

Tolerance for Psychologically Painful Experiences

Clients who present with developmental injuries and experiences of abuse and trauma often report feeling anxious, flawed, worthless, broken, and insignificant, and painfully fear being abandoned. The client's natural tendency is to avoid these very painful experiences and not to bring them up in therapy. They fear that they might be judged, not be understood, be a burden to the therapist, and/or that the therapist will not be able to go with them into the depth of their painful experiences. To address these psychologically painful feelings, the client must possess the capacity to tolerate them. It is important for the therapist not to encourage the client to open up these painful experiences unless both the client and therapist are ready and able to go to these places. To be with the client in the depth of his painful experiences and help him tolerate them, the therapist must be able to be present in hope, understanding, inner strength, and care, and provide safety, security, and protection.

Commitment to Therapy and Their Self-Growth

SIRP presents a unique challenge to clients to remain committed to therapy and to their self-growth because of its focus on internal transformation (e.g., softening the internalized critic) rather than only on behavior change. When clients experience and observe that their therapy is helping them bring about their desired personal and/or interpersonal changes, they remain committed to the process and to their personal growth despite how painful and difficult it might be. However, for clients whose efforts seem not to bring about the desired changes, and when they come to realize that to bring them about, they need to make changes within themselves, they can become discouraged, impatient, question the value of therapy, and lose motivation. It is easier for clients to remain committed to therapy and self-development when they are able to observe and experience the changes, but it is more difficult for a client who must make internal transformations to remain committed because these transformations are not tangible and immediate changes are difficult to perceive.

Ability to Use the Therapist as an Alter Ego

The client must have the capacity to utilize what is being offered in therapy and use the therapist as an alter ego to develop the necessary skills, understanding, and attitudes to address his issues and move forward in life. In interacting with the therapist, the client might feel understood, accepted, significant, and cared for, and might learn skills of assertiveness, open communication, and of solving conflicts and problems. These therapist qualities might serve as a strong impetus for the client to rethink and modify his own perceptions of self and other, style of communication, and relational patterns. The client uses the therapist as a model for change and transformation.

The Therapeutic Change Process

Three of the characteristics that reflect SIRP's approach to bringing about change include: fostering a self-discovery, insight, and action-oriented approach; focusing on psychotherapeutic themes; and viewing treatment in terms of phases that unfold across space and time. These three characteristics are briefly described.

First, SIRP subscribes to a self-discovery, insight, and action-oriented therapeutic approach. Self-discovery entails asking clients to reflect on their problems and to uncover the sources rather than for the therapist to explain or interpret their sources. This typically leads to an increase in insight and to linking the problem to predisposing factors (vulnerabilities) and to its precipitating factor. The therapeutic process is completed with the client implementing the newly gained insight in new perceptions of self and other, in new ways of interacting and relating with others, and in the management of his emotional state and psychological problems. SIRP assumes that insight and awareness are therapeutically meaningful if they lead to new and more effective actions and behaviors. Equally, SIRP assumes that new actions and behaviors need to be informed by insights and awareness for them to endure.

Second, SIRP approaches the treatment of emotional and behavioral disorders by addressing its constituents, that is, in terms of themes. For example, for a client struggling with major depressive disorder, one might treat feeling obligated, a sense of helplessness, and the need to please; these are referred to as themes. The core theme for the client might be the fear of being true to himself and to others (Meier, Boivin & Meier, 2006). Themes are conceptualized as "being bi-polar with one end of the continuum representing the problematic pole (e.g., being depressed) and the other end representing the [latent positive] pole (e.g., being joyful) toward which to strive" (Meier & Boivin, 2000, p. 59).

Third, SIRP views psychotherapy as a process characterized by significant client moments that are referred to as phases. The phases of the change process have been operationalized to form the Seven-Phase Model of the Change Process (Meier & Boivin, 1998, 2000; Meier, Boivin & Meier, 2006). The seven phases represent a progressive and cyclical forward movement in working through psychotherapeutic themes. The first three phases, Problem Definition, Exploration, and Awareness/ Insight, present the client's problems and concerns and trace them back to their origins, which include the unmet childhood needs, predisposing factors, and the strategies to deal with them. In the fourth and fifth phases, the Commitment/ Decision and Experimentation/Action phases, the client becomes determined to make changes in his perception of self and the other and how he relates to others. In the last two phases, Integration/Consolidation and Termination, the client consolidates his new way of relating to others and his perceptions and prepares himself to live without the support of therapy.

Psychotherapy Techniques

Fundamental to SIRP are the basic interviewing skills (Ivey, Gluckstern & Ivey, 2006) with empathic responding holding a significant place. Empathic responding, however, has been broadened to include all of a client's subjective experiences, including feelings, perceptions, thoughts, meanings, values, needs, determinations, and commitments. SIRP also incorporates advanced techniques such as Experiential Focusing and Ego State therapy, which are used according to SIRP theory. In addition to these techniques, the present authors have developed exercises and/or techniques, such as the Wholesomeness exercise, the Progressive forward exercise, the Modified breathing exercise, and the Track Record Technique. These techniques are described in detail in two publications by Meier and Boivin (2011, 2022) and are briefly presented here.

Experiential Focusing Technique

Experiential Focusing (Gendlin, 1996) is designed to uncover the deeper layers of presenting problems by paying attention to a bodily felt sense of them. The client begins the technique by being asked to clear a psychological space and put aside the worries of the day. As the client creates this space, he gradually arrives at a bodily felt sense of the problem. The crucial point in this technique is the client being asked what is needed to make the bodily felt sense of the problem better. The articulation of the need marks the beginning of accepting the unmet childhood or growth needs and of asserting and integrating them into his daily life.

Ego State Therapy

Ego state therapy (Lawrence, 1999; Watkins & Watkins, 1997) links (i.e., bridges) a chronic current emotional state (e.g., anxiety) to an underlying problematic ego state (e.g., feeling incompetent) that was formed in early childhood and/or at a later age. The client is asked to uncover, to describe, and to re-experience the life situation in which the problematic ego state was formed. This is followed by the client being asked to do what is needed to make the problematic ego state better. The result is the formation of a healthy ego state whereby the person perceives himself differently, such as feeling confident, competent, and courageous. The client is then asked to address the presenting problem through the healthy ego state.

Gestalt Two-Chair Technique

The Gestalt Two-Chair technique (Perls, 1969) was designed to resolve intrapsychic conflicts by engaging the two parts (e.g., Topdog and Underdog) in a meaningful and focused dialogue. The goal is to encourage the Underdog (e.g., inner child) to express its needs and for the Topdog (e.g., demanding parent) to hear and respect them. In presenting and respecting their mutual needs and making compromises, the Topdog and Underdog come to a resolution of their conflict. A significant moment in the resolution is when the Topdog empathically understands the position of the Underdog and states it as such. The resolution of the internal conflict brings with it a transformation of the psychic structure, resulting in greater harmony among its parts (e.g., id, ego, and superego.

Task-Directed Imagery

Task-Directed Imagery (TDI; Meier & Boivin, 2011, 2022) is designed to help a client address and confront a feared situation or problem. TDI begins by empowering and enabling the client by asking him to imagine being in a place where he is himself and feels empowered being there. The client then is asked to hold on to the sense of being empowered and the associated feelings and, at his pace, to face the feared situation such as speaking in public. TDI is a flexible technique that can be used for countless goals and purposes. It has been found to be effective to help clients to self-soothe, let go of excessive control in relationships, and to build trust in intimate relationships (Meier & Boivin, 2010a, 2010b, 2010c).

Regression Therapy

Regression therapy refers to enabling a client to revisit and to re-experience the early missed stages of development and to progress through them with the help of the psychotherapist. Regression therapy is a process of controlled regression to the stage of environmental failure (Winnicott, 1959–1964). The goal of therapy is to undo the early emotional failure by providing a successful experience of empowerment. Regression is facilitated by providing a safe and protective therapeutic relationship and validating the client's relational, self, and physical intimacy needs. It is important that therapy be attuned to the needs of the client, be it a child or an adult (Mahler & Furer, 1968, p. 167, n.3).

Wholesomeness Exercise

The goal of the Wholesomeness exercise is for clients to become aware of their sense of goodness and wholesomeness, and to challenge and replace the negative perceptions and feelings that often mask their sense of goodness and wholesomeness. In this exercise the client is asked to take a comfortable and relaxed position in a chair and let go of his daily worries. He is then asked to name the qualities and traits about himself that he likes. When he has completed naming the qualities that he likes, the therapist asks the client to emphatically restate them. The client is then asked to embrace the qualities and traits that he likes about himself, to have a bodily felt sense of these qualities, and to experience them as being part of him.

Progressive Forward Exercise

Progressive forward exercise refers to helping a client become aware of the extent to which a new feeling, thought, need, and/or experience that emerged in therapy has been part of his life across all ages without his knowing it. The client might on his own state that it is not a new-new experience, thought, or feeling. The client is asked when he first had such an experience. This is followed by asking the client to proceed forward from the age at which he had this experience and determine when he experienced it again. He might have experienced this for the first time at the age of two and again at the age of 11, 18, and 25. He is asked to describe his experience at each age when he had the experience. The purpose is to consolidate the impression that the experience that he had at the age of two was always present.

Deep Breathing, Acceptance, Movement, and Competency to Manage Panic Attacks

In a panic attack, individuals are terrified and feel that they have no control over their thoughts and their emotions. There is the fear that their emotions will overtake them; it is for them hell on earth and they want to jump out of their skin. They fear that they will succumb to the panic attack and that they will never come out of the attack.

A strategy that combines deep breathing, accepting the feeling, movement, and empowerment can help a client calm himself. The tentative strategy to manage a panic attack would proceed as follows.

When an individual senses that a panic attack is coming on, or when he is in the depth of a panic attack, he is to bodily move around, if possible, to neutralizes the intensity of the attack. As he is moving, he is to take deep breaths, pay attention to his breathing, and accept the feeling, not fight it. At the same, he is to think of some difficult situation of past that he faced and overcame. He is to focus on how he overcame it. This sense of competency (empowerment) over something difficult from the past gives him hope and confidence that he will overcome his panic attack and the associated fears and thought processes. In going through this process, the client is to go slowly and at his own pace. The goal is for the person to accept his panic feeling and at the same time turn to something from the past over which he had control. The sense of having dealt with a difficult situation of the past can empower him to deal with the current panic attack.

Track Record Technique

The inspiration for this technique comes from horse racing. The idea is that if a person wants to know how well a horse will do on a race, he need only look at its past track record. A client can apply this technique to events or situations that he repeatedly interprets in a fixed but wrong way. For example, a client might interpret a friend's social unavailability as she rejecting him. However, when the client reviews these incidents, he realizes that there always was a legitimate reason for the unavailability and that after the incident the friend would consistently contact the client. The client came to realize that social unavailability did not mean rejection.

Working with Unmet Core Needs

Working with unmet core needs can be challenging, particularly when it comes to detecting them in the midst of emotional, psychological, relational, and behavioral problems, and when it comes to managing the barriers that stand in the way of the client recognizing and accepting them. This section presents how to detect and uncover unmet core needs and how to manage the barriers that predispose a client to not accepting his core needs. Before addressing these two topics, it is important to point out that unmet childhood and growth core needs persist and push for response because they represent the energy that brings life to the individual, give direction to his life, and lead an individual to living life to its fullest.

Unmet core childhood needs differ from unmet core growth needs. Unmet childhood core needs refer to legitimate needs, such as the need for emotional bonding and autonomy, for which the child was not validated and the child continues to push for their validation. Core growth needs refer to needs that were met in childhood but continue to be essential for continued growth and development in adolescent and in adult relationships. Unmet childhood core needs tend to be insatiable, unreasonable, colored by fantasy and idealism, and tend to have been with the person for as long as he can remember. Unmet core growth needs, on the other hand, are satiable, reasonable, reality based, and are more situational in their origin, such as a partner being away on work assignments for long periods of time.

Detecting and Uncovering Unmet Core Needs

The first task in working with unmet needs is to help a client detect and uncover an unmet core need that often lies outside of his awareness. The uncovering of needs entails helping the client differentiate between feelings, needs, and thoughts. It is important for the client to become aware that how one thinks about something is very different from how one feels about something, and both are very different from what one needs.

How, then, to detect the unmet core needs? Where to look for them? This section will limit itself to demonstrating how analyzing feeling stages, the manner of communicating, and relational patterns, and making sense of one's concerns can serve as avenues to helping an individual detect, uncover, name, and accept unmet needs.

First, an effective way to uncover and access unmet core needs is through an individual's affective system, that is, through his feelings. Feelings are about something, but they are not the something that underlies an individual's concerns and difficulties. One must go deeper than feelings as they are perceived to be responses to either the satisfaction or the frustration of needs. Feelings can lead an individual to his unmet core needs and to connect with them. When a client describes what is bothering him, the therapist carefully listens to his description of a situation with an eye focused on the unmet or threatened core need that generated the feeling.

A second way to detect and uncover core needs is by analyzing the manner of communication. This is easier to observe in couple and family therapy. Communication includes the words spoken and the tone of voice that is given to the words. It includes a client's readiness and ability to articulate his feelings, thoughts, and needs, and his ability to tolerate and respect differences and to work collaboratively (Luthman, 1974; Roberto-Forman, 2008; Satir, 1972; Satir, Banmen, Gerber & Gomori, 1991). When communication becomes conflictual, and partners are not ready to listen to each other and judgmental words are exchanged, one can anticipate that their mutuals needs are not being heard, validated, and responded to. When a therapist has an intuitive understanding of the unmet needs, he might carefully guide the client to uncover them.

A third way to discern unmet core needs is by analyzing a client's relational pattern. There are two elements to a relational pattern, namely, the manner in which an individual relates to others in word and behavior, and how the client expects others to relate to him. Relational patterns may include those such as the placater, blamer, computer, and distracter (Satir, 1972); fusion and distancing (Roberto-Forman, 2008); dependency, power, ingratiation, and sex (Cashdan, 1988); and maladaptive cyclical patterns (Strupp & Binder, 1985). Underlying problematic relational patterns are unmet growth and/or unmet childhood needs. Relational patterns have as their goal, having these needs responded to and satisfied in a particular way. Relational patterns that are driven by unmet childhood needs can best be understood as the externalization and projection onto another of an individual's own internal struggle between his inner child needs and parental demands (Berne, 1961). These internal struggles indicate that the individual has not accepted his own childhood's needs, and similar to his actual parent, the child's internal parent is critical and unaccepting of his childhood needs.

A fourth way to detect unmet core needs is to analyze a client's reaction to an event such as not being invited to a party. The therapist invites the client to express his feelings and to provide the meaning given to being excluded, which often leads to the client stating that his needs and feelings do not matter. In situations such as this, the therapist might ask the client if he felt this way in the past and to give examples. Often such analysis leads the client to become aware of the repeated childhood experiences to his unmet core need to feel significant.

Barriers to Accepting Core Needs

The barriers that stand in the way of a person accepting and expressing his needs and living from them can be thought of in terms of external factors and internal factors. An external factor might include a negative attitude toward needs, and an internal factor might include feeling guilty and selfish in asserting one's needs. The following examples illustrate several barriers to accepting and asserting one's needs.

First, in our Western culture, the acceptable attitude in the workplace, educational institutions, and business establishments is not about relationships and community, but about independence, performance, accomplishment, and success. When the word "need" arises, the thought is about unmet childhood needs and rarely about growth needs. Adults are expected to have outgrown their childhood needs and not have lifelong growth needs. This negative attitude toward needs is a barrier for a person to have his growth needs accepted by others and for the individual to assert his needs for fear of a negative reaction.

A second barrier to the acceptance and assertion of one's needs is the feeling of guilt and selfishness in putting one's needs ahead of those of others. This is particularly characteristic of individuals who have an internalized critic that is prohibitive and idealistic and is not adequately moderated by the internalized adult. To breach the prohibitions and ideals, engenders feelings of guilt and selfishness that stand in the way of living authentically and congruently.

Third, children who are emotionally neglected, maltreated, traumatized, and/ or abused, often develop the sense that they are bad, flawed, and not deserving of having their core needs met and that good things cannot happen to them. These experiences are internalized to form an internal critic that constantly reminds the inner child of its flawed nature and that it is not deserving of an affectionate and loving relationship. These children, as adults, might fear being found out not to be the person that they are thought to be and may also find it very difficult to accept compliments and rewards, thinking that it was a mistake. For this reason they do not risk asking for favors and affection from others.

Fourth, there are situations where it is too painful to address unmet childhood needs. This is particularly true for an adult who as a child, felt emotionally neglected or rejected. As a child, he might have gone out of his way to please his parents but without an appropriate response from them. The child was left emotionally broken and in order to deal with the pain, he disconnected from his feelings. He may avoid his desire to access his feelings and unmet core needs because of the pain that would emerge.

A fifth barrier to accepting one's core needs might be that the client was brought up in an overprotective home where decisions were made for him. Thus the child was not given an opportunity to learn how to assert his needs, feelings, and preferences. On the other hand, the child might have been raised in home where the atmosphere was tense and hostile and one's feelings and needs were either dismissed or criticized. The child managed his feelings and needs by repressing and/or suppressing them. In brief, in both situations the child did not learn how to assert his needs.

Weaning from the Unrealistic Pursuit of Needs

An important step in weaning from the pursuit of needs is to determine when an individual's needs are unrealistic. An individual's needs are deemed unrealistic when they are insatiable and cannot be reasonably satisfied by anyone, and by his experiencing a sense of emptiness when alone and when not being constantly validated for being competent, for example. How to wean from the unrealistic pursuit of needs? It is important for the client to: recognize and accept when a need is unrealistic and insatiable; become aware of the assumption on which the unrealistic needs rests and to challenge the assumption; and resist the impulse to pursue the unrealistic need. It is helpful for the client to observe the consequences in resisting the impulse and pursuing the unrealistic need. This helps form a new perspective on the unrealistic pursuit of needs.

Grieving Unmet Childhood and Loss of Growth Needs

Children whose relational, self, and physical intimacy needs were unmet for a prolonged period of time will enter adolescence and adulthood struggling to recapture what was lost in childhood. They will grieve that which they had a right, as a child, to receive from significant others and recognize that which could have been theirs will never be. Circumstances also arise when one is faced with grieving core growth needs. Every person needs to belong to someone and to feel loved and competent and to grow as a person individually, relationally, intellectually, and spiritually. When a relationship is broken, the individual left behind experiences the loss of that which enriched his life and his sense of being fully alive. With the loss of a loved one, there is also a loss of a sense of part of self and a sense of emptiness.

This chapter presented the major constructs of Self-in-Relationship Psychotherapy and demonstrated how they are applied in assessments and treatment. These constructs and their application provide the framework for the following chapters on individual, couple, family, and parent-child therapy.

References

Allport, G.W. (1967). *Becoming: Basic considerations for a psychology of personality*. New Haven: Yale University Press.

Baker, H.W., & Baker, M.N. (1987). Heinz Kohut's self psychology: An overview. *The American Journal of Psychiatry, 144*(1), 1–9.

Beck, A.T., Rush, A.J., Shaw, B.F., & Emery, G. (1979). *Cognitive therapy of depression*. New York: Guilford Press.

Benesh, M., & Weiner, B. (1982). *On emotion and motivation: From the Notebooks of Fritz. American Psychologist, 35*, 151–175.

Bergman, A. (1975). Introduction. In M. Mahler, F. Pine & A. Bergman (Eds.), *The psychological birth of the human infant* (pp. xv–xix). New York: Basic Books.

Berne, E. (1961) *Transactional analysis in psychotherapy*. New York: Grove Press.

Bordin, E.S. (1979). The generalizablity of the psychoanalytic concept of the working alliance. *Psychotherapy: Theory, Research and Practice, 16*, 252–260.

Briere, J.N. (1992). *Child abuse trauma: Theory and treatment of lasting effects*. New York: Sage Publications.

Briere, J.N., & Lanktree, C.B. (2012). *Treating complex trauma in adolescents and young adults*. New York: Sage Publications.

Brinich, P., & Shelley, C. (2002). *The Self and personality structure: Core concepts in therapy*. Buckingham, England: Open University Press.

Briscoe-Dimock, S. (2010). Working with transference and countertransference in psychotherapy. In A. Meier & M. Rovers (Eds.), *The helping relationship: Healing and change in the community context* (pp. 79–100). Ottawa, Ontario: University of Ottawa Press.

Cashdan, S. (1988). *Object relations therapy: Using the relationship*. New York: W.W. Norton.

Deci, E.L., & Ryan, R.M. (2000). The "what" and "why" of goal pursuits: Human needs and the self-determination of behavior. *Psychological Inquiry, 11*, 227–268.

Deci, E.L., & Ryan, R.M. (2002). *Handbook of self-determination research*. Rochester, New York: University of Rochester Press.

Edward, J., Ruskin, N., & Turrini (1981). *Separation-individuation: Theory and application*. New York: Gardner Press..

Erskine, R.G. (1998). Attunement and involvement: Therapeutic responses to relational needs. *International Journal of Psychotherapy, 3*(3), p. 235-244.

Fairbairn, W.R.D. (1943). The repression and the return of bad objects (with special reference to the "war neuroses." In W.R.D. Fairbairn (Eds.) (1994), *Psychoanalytic studies of personality* (pp. 59–81). New York, NY: Routledge.

Fairbairn, W.R.D. (1944). Endopsychic structure considered in terms of object relationships. In W.R.D. Fairbairn (Ed.), *An object-relations theory of the personality* (pp. 82–136). New York: Basic Books.

Fairbairn, W.R.D. (1946). Object-relationships and dynamic structure. In W.R.D. Fairbairn (Ed.), *Psychoanalytic studies of personality* (pp. 137–161). New York, NY: Basic Books.

Freud, S. (1905). Three essays on the theory of sexuality. *Standard Edition, 7*, 23-243.

Freud, S. (1910). The future prospect of psychoanalytic therapy. *Standard Edition, 11*, 141–151.

Freud, S. (1923). The Ego and the Id, *Standard Edition, 19*, 12–63.

Freud, S. (1925). An autobiographical study. *Standard Edition, 20*, 7–70.

Freud, S. (1938). An outline of psychoanalysis. *Standard Edition, 23*, 144–207.

Gelso, C.J., & Hayes, J.D. (2001). Countertransference management. *Psychotherapy: Theory, Research, Practice, Training, 38*(4), 418–422.

Gendlin, E.T. (1996). *Focusing-oriented psychotherapy: A manual of the experiential method.* New York: Guilford Press.

Ivey, A.E., Gluckstern, N.B., & Ivey, M.B. (2006). *Basic attending skills*, 3rd Edition. North Amherst, Massachusetts: Microtraining Associates.

Jacobson, E. (1964). *The self and the object world.* New York, NY: International Universities press.

Kaplan, H.I., & Sadock, B.J. (1991). *Synopsis of psychiatry: Behavioral sciences clinical psychiatry.* 6th Edition. London: Williams & Wilkins.

Kasser, T. (2002). *The high price of materialism.* London: Bradford Book.

Klein, M. (1952). Some theoretical conclusions regarding the emotional life of the infant. In Melanie Klein (Eds.) (1975), *Envy and gratitude and other works 1946–1963* (pp. 61–93). London: Delcorte Press/Seymour Lawrence.

Klein, M. (1959). Our adult world and its roots in infancy. In M. Klein (Ed.), *Envy and gratitude and other works 1946–1963* (pp. 247–263). New York: Delacorte Press/Seymour Lawrence.

Kohut, H. (1971). *The analysis of the self.* New York: International Universities Press.

Kohut, H. (1977). *The restoration of the self.* New York: International Universities Press.

Lawrence, M.A. (1999). *The use of imagery and ego state therapy in holistic healing.* Paper presented at the annual meeting of the American Association for the Study of Mental Imagery, Orlando, Florida, April.

Lazarus, R.S. (1982). Thoughts on the relations between emotions and cognition. *American Psychologist, 37*, 1019–1027.

Luthman, S. (1974). *The dynamic family.* Palo Alto, California: Science and Behavior Books.

Mahler, M., & Furer, M. (1968). *On human symbiosis and the vicissitudes of individuation.* New York: International Universities Press.

Mahler, M., Pine, F., & Bergman, A. (1975). *The psychological birth of the human infant.* New York: Basic Books.

Masterson, J.F. (1976). *Psychotherapy of the borderline adult: A developmental approach.* New York: Brunner Mazel Publishers.

Meier, A. (2010). Transference and countertransference revisited. In A. Meier & M. Rovers, (Eds.), *The helping relationship: Healing and change in community context* (pp. 47–78). Ottawa, Ontario: University of Ottawa Press.

Meier, A., & Boivin, M. (1998). *The seven-phase model of the change process: Theoretical foundation, definitions, coding guidelines, training procedures, and research data*, 5th Edition. Unpublished manuscript. Ottawa, Ontario: Saint Paul University.

Meier, A., & Boivin, M. (2000). The achievement of greater selfhood: The application of theme-analysis to a case study. *Psychotherapy Research, 10*(1), 60.

Meier, A., Boivin, M., & Meier, M. (2006). The treatment of depression: A case study using theme-analysis. *Counselling and Psychotherapy Research: Linking Research with Practice, 6*(2), 115–125.

Meier, A., & Boivin, M. (2010a). *Task-directed imagery: Its effectiveness to develop ability to self-comfort.* Ottawa, Ontario: Saint Paul Universty. Unpublished paper.

Meier, A., & Boivin, M. (2010b). *Task-directed imagery: Its effectiveness to develop (build) trust in intimate relationships.* Ottawa, Ontario: Saint Paul University. Unpublished paper.

Meier, A., & Boivin, M. (2010c). *The effectiveness of task-directed imagery to develop competency to let-go of excessive control in intimate relationships.* Ottawa, Ontario: Saint Paul University. Unpublished paper.

Meier, A., & Boivin, M. (2011). *Counselling and therapy techniques: Theory and practice.* London, UK: Sage.

Meier, A., & Boivin, M. (2022). *Self-in-relationship psychotherapy: A complete clinical guide to theory and practice.* London: Routledge.

Perls, F.S. (1969). *Gestalt therapy verbatim.* Toronto: Bantam Books.

Pine, F. (1975). Preface. In M. Mahler, F. Pine & A. Bergman (Eds.), *The psychological birth of the human infant* (pp. vii–xiii). New York: Basic Books.

Reisenzein, R., & Schonpflug, W. (1992). Stumpf's cognitive-evaluative theory of emotion. *American Psychologist, 47*(1), 34–45.

Roberto-Forman, L. (2008). Transgenerational couple therapy. In A.S. Gurman (Ed.), *Clinical handbook of couple therapy* (pp. 196–226). New York: Guilford Press.

Rogers, C. (1957) 'The necessary and sufficient conditions of therapeutic personality change', *Journal of Consulting Psychology, 21*(2), 95–103.

Rogers, C. (1959). A theory of therapy, personality and interpersonal relationships as developed in the client-centered framework. In S. Koch (Ed.), *Psychology: A study of a science. Vol. 3: Formulations of the person and the social context.* New York: McGraw Hill.

Sadock, B.J., Sadock, V.A., & Ruiz, P. (2014). *Kaplan and Sadock's synopsis of psychiatry Behavioral sciences clinical psychiatry,* 11th Edition. New York: Walter Kluwer.

Satir, V. (1972). *People making.* Palo Alto, California: Science and Behavior Books.

Satir, V. (2013). The therapist's story. In M. Baldwin (Ed.), *The use of self in therapy,* 3rd Edition (pp. 19–27). New York: Haworth Press.

Satir, V., Banmen, J., Gerber, J., & Gomori, M. (1991). *The Satir model: Family therapy and beyond.* Palo Alto, California: Science and Behavior Books.

Segal, J. (2004). *Melanie Klein,* 2nd Edition. London, England: Sage.

Smith, D.L (2003). *Psychoanalysis in focus.* London: Sage Publications.

Strupp, H.H., & Binder, J.L. (1985). *Psychotherapy in a new key: A guide to time-limited dynamic psychotherapy.* New York: Basic Books.

Van der Kolk, B. (2014). *The body keeps the score: Brain mind and body in the healing of trauma.* New York: Penguin Book.

Watkins, J.G., & Watkins, H.H. (1997). *Ego states: Theory and therapy.* New York: Norton.

White, R., & Watt, N.F. (1981). *The abnormal personality.* Chichester, West Sussex, England: Whiley & Sons.

Winnicott, D. (1959–1964). Classification: Is there a psycho-analytic contribution to psychiatric classification. In D. Winnicott (Ed.) (1965), *The maturational processes and the facilitating environment* (pp. 124–139). New York, NY: International Universities Press.

Winnicott, D. (1960). Ego distortion in terms of true and false self. In D. Winnicott (Ed.) (1965), *The maturational processes and the facilitating environment* (pp. 140–152). New York: International Universities Press.

Winnicott, D. (1963). The mentally ill in your caseload. In D. Winnicott (Ed.) (1965), *The maturational processes and the facilitating environment* (pp. 217–229). New York: International Universities Press.

Winnicott, D. (1965). *The family and individual development*. London: Tavistock Publishers.

Zajonc, R.B. (1980). Feeling and thinking: Preferences need no inferences. *American Psychologist, 35*(2), 151–175.

Chapter 2

Armand

Recovery from Major Depressive Disorder

This chapter presents the case of Armand (pseudonym), who struggled with his fourth episode of major depressive disorder during the past 20 years. The presentation begins with Armand's psychosocial history. This is followed in turn by a diagnosis, an assessment using the Self-in-Relationship Psychotherapy Assessment Form (SIRP-AF), and by a conceptualization of Armand's depressive symptoms. The last part of the chapter presents the treatment process for depression from the perspective of Self-in-Relationship Psychotherapy.

Psychosocial History and Its Contributing Factors

The psychosocial history of Armand is based on the information provided in the assessment interviews. All identifying material has been removed or altered to protect the privacy of the client. Armand provided permission to use the material for the purpose of training, publication, and research.

The psychosocial history provides two types of information. First, it provides information regarding Armand's childhood experiences and how he might have internalized these experiences to form his psychic structure, self-structure, coping strategies, and relational patterns. Second, it provides information on how the internalized structures and relational patterns are re-enacted in his adult relationships.

Armand was in his mid-forties, married, a university graduate, was efficient at work, and was a committed Christian. In the sessions he tended to speak rapidly and shifted from one topic to another. He came across as being sensitive, insecure, and a pleaser. Armand has a younger brother who is married and is a successful businessperson.

Family Background

Armand was raised in a middle-class home in a city in eastern Canada. Armand's father, a college professor, was quiet, laid-back, emotionally absent, and had little influence on Armand's personal, social, and emotional development. Armand

DOI: 10.4324/9781032655291-4

and his father did spend some time together on weekends in outdoor activities. Armand was angry at his father for not having given him life skills and guidance to cope with life's difficulties and conflicts, to deal with emotions, and for not having helped him become a man. Armand was aware that his feelings of anger were a reaction to the loss and sadness that he felt in not having had a father who responded to his needs. When he was older, he spent good times with his father, with whom he spoke mostly about business and politics.

Armand described his mother as anxious, insecure, demanding, manipulative, imposing, and intrusive. When Armand complied with her demands, expectations, and wishes, she showered him with love and affection. When he did not comply with her wishes but asserted his autonomy and independence, she would withdraw her "gracious favor," a "dark cloud" would descend, and he felt that he did something wrong. His mother's criticisms elicited within him feelings of anger, worthlessness, helplessness, guilt, and of being a bad person. Armand felt that his mother did not accept nor respect his self-directed behaviors. He reported that his psychological and personal space were "intruded upon and violated." Armand was pressured by his mother to take music lessons and to participate in sports; she instilled in him a sense of obligation and duty. Performance and achievement were valued, while playfulness and recreational activities were not. Armand did not learn how to confront his mother as he feared that he would end up being hurt by her. He dealt with his conflicts with his parents by tuning them out.

In terms of the relationship between his mother and father, Armand's mother controlled his father in the same way that she controlled her son. His father was not free to express his opinions, feelings, and needs. She would often get angry at him for having his nose stuck in a book or a paper rather than paying attention to her. Armand was angry at his father for being laid-back and not providing a corrective influence to the mother's dysfunctional behaviors and interactions. Armand saw himself as having, in the past, been like his father in that he let the demands of others guide and direct his destiny.

Armand was angry at himself for not having caught on earlier that he was playing the game of satisfying the needs of his mother (and others) and not attending to his own needs. He also regretted that he was not given guidance on how to avoid letting others exploit and abuse him. He felt sad that he was missing the social skills whereby he could assert himself and protect himself without feeling guilty.

Educational Achievements and Work Experience

Armand was a top student throughout high school and university. He obtained two graduate degrees, one in mathematics and physical science and the other in economics. He also earned a diploma in education. He completed all the course requirements for a PhD in economics but did not complete his thesis because of illness in the family. He has regrets not obtaining his PhD. In high school and university, he participated in the seasonal sport activities.

After graduating with a diploma in education, Armand taught physics for two years in high school. He then accepted a position as a researcher with a crown corporation and has been a senior researcher for the past ten years. For one year he assumed the position of manager, which caused him enormous stress as he found it difficult to evaluate the performance of employees. This assignment preceded his current bout with depression. He also struggled with the values of the workplace, which clashed with his own values, particularly the pursuit of profit at the expense of disregarding ethics.

Marital Relationship

Armand, married for 19 years, had a difficult marital relationship. He had trouble being himself and rightfully requesting that his personal and social needs be respected without getting a strong negative response from his wife, Sophia. He tended to be overindulgent toward her and to comply to her needs in order to maintain peace, harmony, and stability. She had her own personal struggles with depression, self-esteem, and social connections. At the most difficult moments in their relationship, Sophia threatened to leave him.

Social Background and Church Involvement

Armand and Sophia were zealous and committed Christians and were actively involved in church activities. They viewed the church community as an extended family that provided them fellowship, emotional and spiritual support, a sense of belonging, and an opportunity to share their faith with others. Despite their desire to be involved with the church, they failed to find a church community in which they felt comfortable, experienced a sense of belonging, and with which they could share their faith. They had church friends; however, these relationships did not last long because Sophia tended to become suspicious of others.

Health History

Armand has been depressed four times in the past 20 years. His first major depression occurred during high school, the second after their marriage, the third about eight years later, and the fourth just recently. Regarding his current major depression, he consulted a psychiatrist, who put him on an antidepressant and referred him to a psychologist (A.M.). Physically, Armand was healthy.

Hobbies and Leisure Pursuits

As a child, Armand was playful and fun loving. However, he lost both qualities in late childhood and early adolescence, which he attributes to being pressured

by his parents, specifically by his mother, to take music lessons and to participate in sports. The parents' subtle message was that he was not allowed to play
nor use his free time the way he wanted to. His parents passed on to Armand a
work ethic and a sense of obligation and responsibility when he was still a child.
These combined experiences created an anticipation that it was wrong for him
to engage in playful activities and if he did, he would be scolded for wasting his
time in play. Performance and achievement were valued. Consequently, as an
adult, Armand did not feel comfortable about asserting his need for autonomy
and to pursue hobbies.

Diagnosis and Assessment

To assess the depth of Armand's depression and his recovery from it, the *Diagnostic
and Statistical Manual of Mental Disorders* (DSM-IV-TR) (American Psychiatric
Association, 1994) and the Minnesota Multiphasic Personality Inventory (MMPI)
(Hathaway and McKinley, 1967) were administered at the beginning of therapy
and again at the termination of therapy. The results from the pretreatment and posttreatment measures are as follows.

The DSM-IV-TR

The DSM-IV-TR presents nine characteristics of a major depressive episode,
which are: (a) depressed mood; (b) diminished interest in usual activities or loss
of pleasure; (c) significant weight change and disturbance of appetite; (d) sleep
disturbance; (e) psychomotor agitation or retardation; (f) fatigue or loss of energy;
(g) feelings of worthlessness and guilt; (h) difficulties in thinking; and (i) recurrent
thoughts of death and suicide (Code 296.3x). Armand met the DSM-IV-TR criteria
for a Major Depressive Disorder (Code 296.3x) at the beginning of therapy, but not
at the termination of therapy. The results from this diagnosis indicate that Armand's
depression diminished.

The MMPI

The MMPI was administered at the beginning of therapy and again at the termination of therapy to assess the depth of his depression and his recovery from it.
The elevation of the MMPI T-scores across the clinical scales is an indication of
the depth of the emotional problems. Prior to therapy, the average T-score for the
clinical scales was 77.40, and following therapy, the average T-score was 58.2.
This represents a drop from the third standard deviation to the first standard
deviation (Mean = 50; Standard deviation = 10). The T-score for depression
dropped from 105 prior to therapy to 69 following therapy, which represents a
shift in score from the third standard deviation to the second standard deviation.
There were similar changes in the report of symptoms, idiosyncratic thinking,
and degree of anxiety. The results from the DSM and the MMPI indicate that

Armand was less depressed following therapy when compared to when he began therapy.

Theme-Analysis (TA)

Armand's progress in therapy was assessed by a research project that analyzed transcripts from his psychotherapy sessions using Theme-Analysis (TA), which combines both a qualitative and a quantitative method of analysis (Meier, Boivin & Meier, 2008). This mixed-method identifies psychotherapeutic themes (i.e., the constituents of depression) and traces how they are worked through across sessions (i.e., time) using as a measure of change the Seven-Phase Model of the Change Process (SPMCP; Meier & Boivin, 1992; Meier, Boivin & Meier, 2010). The assessment entails performing (paired) correlations between Phase and Session for the themes organized according to their target (e.g., self, partner) and themes taken separately or combined. A Pearson r of .57 (rsq = .32) was obtained when the themes were combined; a Pearson r of .78 (rsq = .61) and .68 (rsq = .46) was obtained for the cluster of needs for self and partner, respectively; a Pearson r of .64 (rsq = .41) was obtained for feeling states; and a Pearson r of .74 (rsq = .55) was obtained for actions and behaviors. The strong positive correlations support the notion that themes were worked through in a progressive forward course and that psychotherapy regarding these themes was successful.

The SIRP Assessment Form: Results

The SIRP-AF is designed to code SIRP's constructs by using the material from the psychosocial history. Each of the constructs has been operationally defined (Appendix C). The SIRP-AF has been found to be a reliable instrument to code the constructs (Meier & Boivin, 2022). This section presents the results from the application of the SIRP-AF to the psychosocial history of Armand. The findings on the pertinent SIRP constructs are presented in Table 2.1 and briefly discussed here.

Relational, Self, and Physical Intimacy Needs

Armand's unmet core childhood needs comprised the need for autonomy and the need for significance. These two needs pressed for positive responses from others throughout his life. His first experience in not having these needs met was with his mother, who affirmed him for complying with her wishes and withdrew her love and affection when Armand attempted to assert his need for autonomy. When Armand asserted his need for autonomy, he felt unloved by his mother and perceived himself to be a bad and unlovable person. His mother maneuvered to have her needs met and to have Armand compromise his needs by eliciting in Armand feelings of guilt and of being a bad person when he pursued his need for

Table 2.1 SIRP Assessment Form for Self-in-Relationship Psychotherapy constructs

Part I. Descriptive Data: For each of the dimensions presented below, provide descriptive material for the persons (e.g., mother, father) entered in the top row of the table. If there are other persons who were or are important to the client's life (e.g., partner, grandfather), additional columns can be created and assessed for each topic under Dimension.

Dimension	Father	Mother	Wife
1. The striving of self, relational, and physical intimacy needs relative to:	(Validation for) competency	(Validation for) autonomy and lovability	(Validation for) autonomy
2. Internal representation of:	Weak, socially inept	Insecure, controlling, intrusive	Emotionally broken, with limited resources
3. Internal representations of self relative to: (How I view myself when with)	Powerless, helpless, inadequate to get the parenting needed	Controlled, powerless, unlovable	Powerless, trapped
4. Affect linking representation of other to self: (How I felt my father, mother, etc. felt about me)	Indifferent; helpless, Caring passively,	Mixture of caring when complying and angry when asserting himself	Angry, fearful
5. Affect linking representation of self to other: (How I felt about my father, mother, etc.)	Sad and angry	Trapped, angry, ambivalent, not good enough, guilty	Inadequate, not good enough
6. How I felt/feel when in the presence of:	Not responded to, unfulfilled	Anxious, trapped	Anxious, conflicted
7. Quality or degree of good enough parenting:	Inadequate, emotionally unavailable	Inadequate, emotionally unavailable	

Part II. Scaled data: Rate dimensions 1, 4, 7, and 11 on a five-point scale. For dimensions 2 and 3, indicate the strength of each component using a five-point scale with 1 = barely and 5 = greatly. For dimension 10, indicate the characteristic phase and indicate the strength of its presence using the five-point scale indicated above. For the remainder dimensions, check off those that are relevant. See Operational Criteria for more precise instructions. If the dimension is not relevant, leave the space blank. PO = part object; WO = whole object; PSP = paranoid/schizoid position; DP = depressive position; EB = need for emotional bonding; SC = need for sensual contact; AU = need for autonomy; SI = need for sexual intimacy.

| 1. Manner of relating to | Father: | 1 (PO) | 2 | 3 | 4 | 5 (WO) |
| | Mother: | 1 | 2 | 3 | 4 | 5 |

| 2. Psychic structure | Core Needs: ___ EB   3.5 AU
___ SC   ___ SI | 3 Ego | 3.5 Superego |

| 3. Self-structure | 3.5 striving for significance | 3.5 striving for competency | 2.5 capacity to secure sense of significance and competency |

| 4. True self
(Living from) | 1
Minimally | 2 | 3 | 4 | 5
Strongly |

| 5. Coping mechanisms | X repression
___ denial
___ dissociation | ___ splitting
X introjection
___ projection | ___ regression
___ sublimation
___ idealization | ___ devaluation
X Suppression
X Reaction formation |

6. Quality of emotional bond	— emotionally connected	X striving for emotional connection	— avoiding emotional connection	— emotionally disconnected
7. Object constancy	1 Not Formed	2	X ___ Partially Formed	3	4	5 Fully Formed

8. Characteristic emotional state	2 angry / abandoned	— anxious / smothered	1 depressed / oppressed	3 sad / Other
9. Projective identifications	X dependency / other	— power	— ingratiation	— sex
10. Characteristic phase	— Symbiosis	3 Differentiation	— Practicing	1 Rapproche- ment / Consolid- ation

11. Characteristic position	1 (PSP)	2	3	4	5 (DP)
12. Level of personality organization	X higher	— inter-mediate	— lower	

autonomy rather than responded to her needs. Armand also felt that his need for autonomy was not validated at his place of work and in his relationship with his wife. His need to be significant to others continued to be a strong striving force into his adult life. The feeling of guilt when he attempted to pursue his own needs rather than to respond to others was a strong barrier to Armand pursuing his need for autonomy.

Representations of Other and Self

In his infancy/childhood relationships with his parents, Armand began to form representations of them and of himself (Klein, 1948/1975). His representation of his mother was that she was controlling and intrusive; she was emotionally available only when he conformed to her needs. When he attempted to pursue his need for autonomy, she undermined his efforts through her messages that Armand was a bad person by placing his needs ahead of hers. His sense of guilt and feeling selfish motivated him to compromise his needs and respond to those of his mother. Relative to his mother, Armand perceived himself to be trapped, in a bind, controlled, and powerless. He was the caretaker of his mother; he was a parentified child.

Armand perceived his father as weak and socially inept. His father was not able to counter the controlling and intrusive behaviors of his wife; rather, he complied with them. Equally, his father did not provide Armand with the social, relational, and coping skills to challenge his mother's controlling and intrusive behaviors and demands. Armand perceived himself to be like his father, weak, socially inept, and helpless to assert his needs. In brief, Armand perceived his parents as being either domineering and controlling, or weak or inept relative to responding to his own needs. He perceived himself to be powerless and helpless in having them respond to his legitimate needs.

Psychic Structure

Armand's psychic structure (Freud, 1923, 1938) reflected his actual lived childhood relationship with his mother and father. That is, he internalized the demands and expectations of his mother and the message that it is wrong to assert his needs, which, when taken together, formed his superego that kept his internalized child in check and under control. Armand's ego was impoverished due to not experiencing the father as having the capacity to provide a corrective influence to the mother's behaviors toward Armand and not helping him develop relational and coping skills to deal with his mother's intrusive, domineering, and controlling behaviors. From his childhood experiences with his parents, Armand formed a psychic structure where the ego aligned itself with the superego that undermined his core needs. Thus, Armand in his significant relationships was influenced by his superego, which is reflected by his putting aside his own needs, feeling obligated to satisfy the needs of others, and feeling guilty and selfish when he asserted his needs.

Self-Structure

Armand's self-structure is characterized by a striving for significance and competency in his relationships and at his place of work. His low sense of feeling significant and important is reflected in Armand's thinking that his feelings, thoughts, and needs do not matter. He came to believe that the needs and feelings of others were more important than his own. His sense of ineptitude is reflected in his inability to influence his mother and wife to respect and respond to his needs as indeed he responded to theirs. His sense of inadequacy also prevented him from venturing out and taking risks for fear that his self-directed behaviors would be received with rejection and criticism. Armand did not have the inner resources to build and maintain a healthy sense of self and a sense of competency.

From the perspective of a social self, Armand's behaviors, attitudes, and interactions were influenced by what he thought others expected of him. His decisions and choices did not emanate strongly from his sense of self, that is, they were not primarily self-directed but other-directed. He was not true to himself and authentic in his responses (Jourard, 1971); he lived more from a false self than from a true self (Winnicott, 1960/1965).

Coping Mechanisms

Armand's unconscious coping strategies appear to comprise repression, introjection, projection, and reaction formation, and his conscious coping strategy appears to be suppression. He repressed his own needs and feelings in order to avoid childhood conflicts with his mother; he internalized (i.e., introjected) the expectations, demands, and mores of his parents without seriously scrutinizing them; and he was outwardly pleasant and caring but internally he was frustrated and angry (i.e., reaction formation). He consciously suppressed his feelings, preferences, needs, and choices to placate his parents.

Quality of Emotional Bond

Armand sought a relationship where he experienced "safe anchorage" and a "confident expectation" that his needs would be responded to (Mahler, Pine & Bergman, 1975). He did not experience this with his mother; thus, he was left with the lifelong pursuit to emotionally bond with a significant other. Since he did not experience a safe, protective, and secure emotional bond with his mother, he was not able to ascertain when such a bond was achieved. Although he might have thought to have found this in his relationship with his wife, he entered a relationship with her that was like that of his mother; he became a caregiver. Armand continued to strive for a relationship wherein he felt emotionally safe, secure, and protected and his need for autonomy and significance were respected.

Object Constancy

Armand's four episodes with major depressive disorder are strong indicators that he did not develop object constancy, which would have helped him gain a perspective on relational or self-issues and to regulate his affective response to them (Mahler, Pine, & Bergman, 1975). Object constancy is correlated with ego capacity and a sense of self, which, for Armand, were impoverished.

Characteristic Emotional State

Armand's prevailing (i.e., familiar) emotion was that of depression, which appears to be due to his need for autonomy, competency, and significance not being validated. He was trapped in the sense that if he pursued his autonomy, his mother withdrew her love and affection, and if he complied with her wishes, he compromised his sense of self and his pursuit of autonomy (Mahler et al., 1975). Neither of these two situations was life giving. He lived the life of another; he did not live his own life and this was depressing and dead-ending. Armand experienced sadness in that his father did not provide him with the tools needed for daily living. Rather than turn his anger outward toward the appropriate person, Armand turned his feelings of anger inward to avoid, it appears, interpersonal conflict and the loss of the love from his mother; he suppressed his feeling of anger to maintain peace and harmony with his mother. It appears that feelings of guilt in pursuing his own needs rather than responding to the needs of others, prevented him from assertively pursuing his needs, particularly for autonomy.

Projective Identification

The term "projective identification" refers to a relational dynamic by which a person tries to draw a significant other into their way of relating (Cashdan, 1988). Underlying a projective identification is an unmet childhood need that a person attempts to have the other satisfy. In his relationship with his parents and with Sophia, Armand assumed the role of the dependent person, while both the parents and Sophia asserted their needs. That is, he was being drawn into their way of relating and thereby commanding the nature of the relationship. He accepted that they led the way in their relationships to maintain peace and harmony.

From another perspective, Armand related to meaningful others in terms of how he needed them to be in his life and how they needed him to be in their lives, that is, as part objects and part-self (Klein, 1948/1975). That is, he did not relate to others as persons with their own needs, feelings, and preferences. He related to them in terms how he wanted them to be present for him.

Characteristic Developmental Phase

In terms of the separation and individuation continuum (Mahler et al., 1975), Armand was pressured to remain emotionally bonded to his mother and not to move toward individuation and autonomy. He failed to establish an emotional maternal bond wherein he felt "safe anchorage" and a "confident expectation" that he could count on his mother to respond favorably to his needs, particularly for significance and the pursuit of autonomy. When he attempted to assert his need for autonomy, he was reprimanded and he felt guilty and angry in having his needs rejected. He was not helped by either his father or his mother with how to deal with his anger and set limits and boundaries. Since Armand did not have the opportunity to pursue his interests and to assert his needs and feelings and to establish his personal goals, he did not develop social skills (e.g., setting limits and boundaries), relational skills (e.g., empathy), and self-skills (e.g., comforting, and soothing self). That is, he did not develop self-directed and autonomous behaviors.

In summary, it seems that Armand's relational interactions and subjective experiences are characterized by the differentiation subphase as he was not validated to pursue psychological separation and autonomy. His relational interactions and subjective experiences appear to be characterized by the rapprochement phase as he did not achieve object constancy, establish boundaries, and acquire skills to self-comfort and self-soothe. His challenge was to establish "safe anchorage" with a meaningful person and learn how to assert his needs within the context of the relationship and move toward autonomy.

Characteristic Developmental Position

Characteristic developmental position refers to the way the infant/child deals with love-hate relationships and to the different ways she experiences and relates to both internalized and externalized objects (Klein, 1935/1975, p. 276, note; 1952). The infant/child and mother relationship is thought of in terms of two positions (i.e., types of interpersonal stances), the paranoid-schizoid position and the depressive position. The former is characterized by destructive (hateful) forces or feelings and the latter by constructive (loving) forces or feelings. The infant/child's basic conflict revolves around the forces of these two positions, that is, between a desire to protect those close to the child and the malicious wish to destroy them. The infant/child organizes her experiences around these positions. The characteristic that marks a movement toward the depressive stance is empathy and the infant/child's fear of losing the love of the love object. The way the development positions are worked through affects our adult life (Klein, 1959/1975).

Given the above, it can be stated that Armand fluctuates between the paranoid-schizoid and depressive positions. This is based on the observation that Armand is torn between love and hate toward his mother and wife for keeping him dependent on them, that is, being a reluctant caregiver to both. The paranoid-schizoid position is manifested in his feelings of anger toward his mother and in his bout with depression. The depressive position is manifested in his feelings of empathy for his wife.

Conceptualization

The conceptualization of Armand's depression and relational struggles is based on the psychosocial history, the SIRP constructs, and on the results from the assessment using the SIRP-AF. The conceptualization is organized according to symptoms, predisposing childhood experiences, pertinent internalizations, and precipitating factors and reenactments.

Symptoms: At the beginning of therapy, Armand reported feeling depressed, anxious, and fearful of expressing his needs for autonomy, setting limits to his giving, and establishing boundaries. In his intimate and significant relationships, he felt obligated to put the needs of others ahead of his needs and if he did not, he would feel guilty, think of himself as being selfish and a bad person, and risk being rejected and/or fired from the workplace.

Predisposing childhood experiences: Armand as a child was affirmed and rewarded for compliant behavior and was reprimanded and made to feel guilty for his autonomous strivings. To maintain a good relationship with his mother, Armand did not risk behaving contrary to her wishes and demands, but complied with them. He felt obligated to make her happy. Consequently, Armand was predisposed to put his needs aside and respond to those of others, and if he did not, he felt guilty and thought of himself as a bad person. At his young age, Armand was in a vulnerable position to counteract the negative responses to his natural strivings for significance and autonomy, and his ambivalent feelings remained unexpressed. He did not acquire the skills to assert his own needs, particularly for autonomy, without feeling guilty and selfish. He was predisposed not to assert his needs and to feeling depressed when his legitimate needs were ignored and dismissed.

Pertinent internalizations: Armand internalized the childhood interactions with his parents to form his psychic structure, self-structure, coping strategies, perceptions of self and other, relational dynamics, and behaviors, which influenced his future relational interactions. The internalizations paralleled and reflected the real-life experiences of his interactions with his parents. That is, he developed a psychic structure that was skewed toward being hard on himself, having high expectations and demands, feeling obligated to respond to the needs of others (i.e., superego), and not accepting his core needs and feelings. At the same time, he lacked the ability (e.g., ego strength) to mediate the demands and expectations of the superego and his core needs and feelings. Thus, Armand's need for autonomy was not validated and was left unmet, which underlay his relational frustrations and depression.

Precipitating factors and re-enactments: The internalized psychic structure and self-structure, relational dynamics, perceptions of self and other, and coping strategies were activated and re-enacted in his current relationships including his wife and coworkers. He hesitated to assert his need for autonomy for fear that he would be rejected or that he would create a situation over which he would have no control. His sense of obligation, desire to avoid feeling guilty, and the need to please contributed to his compliant behavior and to his fear of asserting his need for autonomy and being his own person. Due to his psychic structure being skewed toward denying his own core needs, he was left frustrated, angry, sad, and depressed. Armand's depression, therefore, appears to be related to not having his need for autonomy and significance respected and validated and to his living a life ruled by obligations that left him empty and questioning the purpose of living.

In summary, Armand's inner world was characterized by a sense of obligation and duty and the suppression of his core needs for autonomy and significance. The ensuing conflict between these two forces was dealt with by compromising his core needs in favor of having relationships with significant others. The continued frustration of his needs for autonomy and connection eroded his self-esteem and eventually led to his depression.

Treatment: Goals, Process, Orientation, and Therapeutic Relationship

The treatment of Armand's depression is presented in terms of its goals, description of the therapy process, therapist orientation, and the therapeutic relationship. The results from the DSM-IV-TR, MMPI, the research, and a five-year follow-up indicate that Armand recovered from his depression.

Goals of Treatment

The treatment goals were grouped according to a principal goal and to subsidiary goals (Meier & Boivin, 2022). The principal goal was to help Armand uncover and reclaim his unmet core needs for significance and autonomy, reorient his life according to these needs, be the agent of his own life, free himself from the depressive symptoms, and establish genuine relationships. The task was to help Armand link his current depressive state to his unmet core needs for significance and autonomy and to realize that these needs were subverted by ineffective coping strategies, relational patterns, and communication styles and disguised in compensatory behaviors such as being a caregiver as an unconscious means to have his core needs partially met.

The subsidiary goals that are intimately connected to the principal goal include: (1) increasing self-esteem and self-worth; (2) bringing about greater harmony within his psychic structure by empowering the ego and to give greater voice to his inner child; (3) directing the anger turned inward to the appropriate external targets; (4) establishing limits and boundaries in his intimate and significant relationships; and (5) fostering self-directed decisions, behaviors, and interactions. These themes were reworked simultaneously within the context of his intimate and significant relationships. The assumption was that since Armand's psychic and self-structures and coping strategies originated in "not good enough" relationships (i.e., parenting), they would be transformed within the context of his current "good enough" relationships.

Description of Therapy Process

Armand was seen for 32 one-hour psychotherapy sessions over a one-year period. The psychotherapy was guided by constructs from SIRP, the SPMCP (Meier & Boivin, 1992), the Self-discovery Approach to Counselling (Meier & Boivin, 1987), and by using techniques from various theoretical orientations (See Chapter 1).

The process of therapy was also studied in terms of the themes (e.g., constituents of depression) that emerged and how they evolved across the sessions. The evolution of the themes was investigated according to the SPMCP, of which the major phases were exploration, insight/awareness, experimentation/action, and integration/consolidation.

Therapist Orientation

The therapist (A.M.), male, Canadian, was a doctoral-level trained and experienced developmental, psychodynamic, and humanistic-oriented psychotherapist who worked full-time in a university graduate counseling and psychotherapy program and had a part-time private practice. The therapist used attending and focusing skills, empathic responses, and summarized the client's implicit and explicit messages (Ivey, 1983). As well, he used "linking" statements to connect various facets of the client's current experiences (e.g., cognitions, affects, and motives) and behaviors, and current patterns of behavior and those of years past (Meier & Boivin, 2000, p. 61). The therapist also used advanced techniques, which had specific goals in mind. For example, Experiential Focusing (Gendlin,1996) was used to uncover unmet childhood needs; the Gestalt Two-Chair technique (Perls, 1969b) was used to help the client to attend to and express his feelings, thoughts, and needs/wants, to reformulate some of his assumptions and expectations; and Task-Directed Imagery (Meier & Boivin, 2011) was used to help the client become empowered and competent to assertive his core needs.

The therapist worked in the "here-and-now" as opposed to "there-and-then" (Joyce & Sills, 2007, pp. 27sq), was actively engaged in therapeutic dialogue, and constantly checked back with the client to assess what he was experiencing and processing, particularly when he demonstrated changes in behavior, tone of voice, and mood (Meier & Boivin, 2000). The goal of therapy was to engage the client in experiential learning, to better understand himself and the nature of his relationships, to become skilled and empowered, to take ownership of his own life, and to become an agent of his own person within the context of his intimate and significant relationships.

Therapeutic Relationship

The therapeutic relationship was characterized by collaboration, the client's responsiveness to the therapist's interventions, a strong motivation to change, and a solid therapeutic bond. In the initial three to four sessions, Armand tended to be anxious, spoke rapidly, was performance bound, and found it difficult to stay with his feelings. He was very concerned about his ability to overcome his depression and return to work, for which he sought reassurance from the therapist. As therapy progressed, Armand became more reflective and attended to his inner experiences, particularly with his ambivalent feelings, assumptions, and aspirations and began to express them. In the process, Armand accepted more responsibility to search for answers to his depression and to do something about it. In the last half of therapy, Armand became more poised, focused, reflective, and upbeat; was more at peace with himself; and manifested greater self-confidence.

Recovery from Major Depressive Disorder

The origin of Armand's depression, in large part, was relational in nature and had its roots in his relationship with his parents, particularly with his mother, where he felt obligated to attend to her needs and to neglect his own needs particularly for significance and autonomy. He felt burdened, helpless, angry, and worthless and depressed for not being able to pursue his autonomy and be his own person.

Armand carried his "unfinished business" (Perls, Hefferline & Goodman, 1951, p. 30) with his mother into his relationships with his wife, Sophia, where he initially felt obligated to take care of her and put his own needs aside, but eventually learned how to set limits to his giving and to assert his needs. The goal of psychotherapy was to transform his psychic structure and self-structure and to acquire the necessary skills to relate to Sophia as adult-to-adult rather than from the position of an angry, neglected, and emotionally deprived child with unmet needs to a demanding and critical internalized parent.

This section on Armand's recovery from his depression presents his work in improving his relations with his wife. The presentation is based on the therapist's clinical notes of the 32 one-hour therapy sessions and on 18 transcripts from the 32 therapy sessions. The presentation is thematic, not chronological, in nature. The numbers in brackets refer to session and line numbers. The numbers to the left of the colon represent session numbers, and the numbers to the right of the colon represent line numbers. When there is a single number, it refers to the session number.

The first part of this section presents the roots and experience of Armand's depression and its management. The second part presents the reworking of themes associated with depression.

Roots and Experience of Depression and Its Management

Roots of depression

Armand linked his depression to feeling obligated (precipitating factor) to take care of Sophia, who was going through her own struggle with depression. He felt burdened by her and angry at having to give of himself and angry at her for not respecting his need for his space, to have time for himself and to exercise his autonomy. Yet he felt guilty in feeling angry toward her and was angry at himself for not catching on to the game that she was playing (7, 8, and 27).

He felt that his depression was his way of saying that he could not respond to his wife's needs and that he has giving as much as he could. He stated that "my depression was indeed a cry of desperation saying that I've done all I can. And I think mixed in with that is a sense that I've done all I can and it's not acceptable" to her (16: 485–509).

Linked to his inability to help Sophia recover from her depression, Armand felt that he was a failure, which eroded his self-esteem and self-worth. "The deepest root of sadness was that I thought I had failed her badly. I wasn't able to be there much as a husband" (19: 38). He also feared that he would lose her, or she would just walk away from him. The deepest "roots of my depression were the fear of being rejected and being alone" (15: 413–430).

In some ways, Sophia's depression was a double-edged sword. When asked what it would be like if he did not feel obligated toward Sophia and if she were more autonomous, he responded:

> There's the fear that if that was the case, then maybe she wouldn't need me at all. I wrestle with it in my mind. But if she was more autonomous, I'd be able to find more fulfilment in life elsewhere. And maybe she would just leave. (15: 413–430)

Regarding his recurrent depression, Armand attributed it to being given the cold shoulder by people that he relied on. He stated that "when I sunk into that depression and felt the cold shoulder by other people, it was a double hurt" and that it was a "really deep wound and took a long time to get over that" (3: 386–396).

From a conceptual perspective, Armand's depression is a function of a severe superego overriding the legitimate core needs and a weak ego that was not able to mediate the two forces. This skewedness on part of the superego kept Armand from becoming autonomous, which resulted in feelings of anger, frustration, and depression.

The experience of depression and its devastating effects

For Armand, the experience of depression was "frightening and potentially life-destroying in the sense that you can really fall apart and can't piece it back together very easily. Depression can wreck your life" (15: 93–94, 114). He added that when you are in a state of depression,

> you are in some sense in darkness. All your feelers are wrong or your senses are giving you the wrong data and your perceptions about yourself and others are distorted. And it's frightening and it's been difficult for me to learn, not to trust [myself]. (25: 135–140)

When he was in his state of depression, Armand stated that "it feels like your whole life is falling apart and there's this big void in front of you. You don't know where you're going, where you're going to land. It's very frightening" (19: 530–540). When in a depression, he found it "hard to know what makes sense" and wrestled with guilt and with meeting the legitimate needs of self and others and feeling free to express his own needs without being manipulated (22: 593–614).

In his description of his depression, Armand said that

I feel like I'm hanging onto this log in a raging river and I'm trying to swim upstream against the river to keep from being swept up under the falls. I felt that I was constantly having to fight upstream against this current that was threatening to wash me away. (20: 441–457)

Armand was constantly afraid that his depression would return but with an awareness that there was no sure way to avoid another bout of depression. He added that

I'm sure there's no sure-fire way of avoiding it. The knocks of life simply happen. You have to adjust. But I need to know what I have to do to find myself from lapsing into another one. I need to have a preventative package. (15: 93–114)

Practical ways of dealing with depression

Armand and Sophia were constantly searching for practical ways to deal with their respective depressions. Initially, Armand lacked the enthusiasm to become engaged in anything outside of him, including his relationship. He did not experience any sense of liveliness and had no hobbies in which he could lose himself. But he was motivated to become engaged in different activities. He and Sophia began to play Scrabble, watched videos, and walked the dog (17: 57–69); stopped watching depressive news (15: 149–150; 16: 396–398); and Armand enjoyed reading and he took up jogging (16: 44–45).

In addition to doing things together, Armand realized that he needed something else to do on his own such as meeting people and having a hobby that occupied his interests (17: 71–80). He rearranged his priorities and attended to his wellness, both physical and emotional, and to the development of friendships and to connecting deeply with people (13: 81). This need for connection was probably driven by his unmet need for a connection with his parents that he never experienced as a child.

On a broader scale, Armand rediscovered playfulness, which he had lost in childhood and adolescence and after marriage. He had replaced playfulness with obligations (17). He summarized his inability to play this way: "I can see that if you're always tense or worried about whether you're doing the right thing or whether you're going to be accepted or rejected, it makes it difficult to have a playful attitude and to be playful" (17: 455–460). Armand rediscovered the pleasure of play by walking his dog and by throwing bones for it to chase. He stated that

it's rejuvenating to play with the dog. I'm able to play with the dog, but playing with other people is still difficult [but] the sense of playfulness is coming back slowly, but it's still hard to lose myself to something, to be really immersed in it and enjoy it. (17: 350–380)

In bringing play back into his life and validating it, Armand was, conceptually, transforming his psychic structure by moderating the voice of the superego and validating and respecting the voice of the inner child that needs to have fun and play. This endeavor was a forward move toward a harmonious psychic structure and the lifting of depression since his core needs began to be gratified.

The Process of Recovery from Major Depression with Regard to Its Themes

The treatment of a major depressive disorder is not achieved by focusing directly on the depression, but by focusing on the cluster of interrelated feelings, thoughts, behaviors, and unmet needs that constitute depression (Meier, Boivin & Meier, 2006). Three of the constituents, referred to as themes, that emerged from the analysis of the case notes and the transcripts of the therapy sessions include: feeling obligated to take care of others; having difficulty setting limits; and failing to identify and assert his needs.

All the themes are related, in one way or another, to the quality of Armand's psychic structure (e.g., superego vs. inner childhood needs), self-structure (e.g., feeling competent, significant), relational dynamics (i.e., projective identification), and to his coping strategies. This section focuses on the reworking of three themes according to the phases of the SPMCP (Meier & Boivin, 2000). The reworking begins with a statement of the problem and exploration of the underlying dynamicsm and then moves to gaining awareness/insight and finally to commitment, action, and consolidation. The words in italics refer to a phase of the SPMCP. The phases are worked through cyclically, not linearly.

From obligation to responsibility

Obligations differ from responsibilities. Obligations have an element of duty and of owing something to others, whereas responsibilities have an element of freedom to choose and accept. The sense of obligation emanates from a demanding, controlling, and judgmental internal parent (i.e., superego) that prevents the inner child from pursuing his autonomy. Responsibility emanates from the internal adult (i.e., ego) that mediates the demands of the superego and the needs of the inner child. Obligations are more fear based, whereas responsibilities are more caring and love based.

Armand's psychic structure was skewed toward the superego from which derived his feelings of obligation toward others, feeling like a failure if he was not able to make them happy, and feeling selfish and guilty if he pursued his needs. Armand saw a similarity between his mother and Sophia. Both rewarded him when complying with their demands but were angry when he was not responsive to them, which led to his feeling selfish and guilty and like he was a bad person who did something wrong (29).

Problem definition phase: At the beginning of therapy, Armand expressed how he felt obligated to take care of Sophia and to make her happy, which he resented because it took up so much of his energy, time, and space (2, 7, and 8). Yet, he felt selfish when putting his needs ahead of her needs and felt guilty about resenting having to cater to her. Despite Armand being available to Sophia, she constantly criticized him. He felt enmeshed, which prevented him from growing as an individual (12). He resented himself for being drawn into her demands and for compromising his own needs (i.e., projective identification) (16).

Armand spoke of how he has been "wrestling with the issues of guilt and meeting legitimate needs of other people and feeling free to express [his] own needs and opinions without being manipulated" (22: 593–614). He felt that Sophia was taking up his space, imposing herself on him, and constraining him. He stated that she constantly demanded his time and attention "but without it being explicitly stated, and without my explicitly assenting to it" (29: 89–107).

Awareness/insight phase: Armand became aware that being there for others out of a sense of obligation was not benefiting him since when he needed others, they were not there for him. He said,

> I've given so much of myself because of a sense of obligation, and now I've realized, that you can give yourself for others and they're not there for you when you need them. So. I am withdrawing to build up my own strength again, and I'm simply saying no for now. (28: 265–282)

Experimentation/action phase: Armand began gradually to accept, without feeling guilty, that he was not obliged to make Sophia happy. He stated:

> I'm not going to allow myself to continue to believe that I'm responsible for her happiness. I've done the best I can to deal with the problems that she's raised but I'm not going to twist myself out of shape again to continue to satisfy her. I'm going to be somewhat firm about saying no, I'm sorry, I've had enough. If she gets frustrated with that, fine. (27: 199–214)

In a later session, Armand repeated that he was not obliged to make Sophia happy. He added that "it's up to me to be a loving husband, but that doesn't mean that I either have to do everything she wants, or feel bad and guilty because she happens to be out of sorts or not happy" 33:515–526). However, he accepted that he was responsible for providing security and love, but not her happiness, thinking that this was beyond the capability of any mortal.

He sensed that his refusal to be obligated to make his wife happy was having a positive effect in their relationship. Sophia began to respect his need for space, and both became better at negotiating their needs (31: 222–239). He also recognized that Sophia was home alone all day and needed to talk when he came home from work. He made that a priority, but at the same time made sure that "some of my own needs are being met" (27: 275–281).

Consolidation/integration phase: Armand learned how to be responsible to Sophia without compromising his own needs. In achieving this, he said, "the world is not on my shoulders, which is a strange feeling. I think there's a better sense of perspective in what's important and what isn't". (19: 445–450). When called upon to comply with the demands of another, he learned, when possible, not to respond immediately to the demands of others, which gave him time to think about it and decide to accept or reject these demands (29).

Armand's most significant learning was not to hold onto things that are of value to him with "clenched fists"; it is better to hold them "with open hands." At the same time, he realized that he was not responsible for the happiness or success of others, including Sophia, and if they were upset with his behavior, that was not a reason for him to comply. He acknowledged that in the past he had been too compliant with the needs of others and that if he did not comply, they might withdraw their affection, love, and support. He articulated his new way of thinking thus:

> Now with a sense of letting go or at least holding with open hands, there's a sense of saying: yes, I value these things but I'm not prepared to hold onto them at any cost. I won't sacrifice what I believe to be ultimately important. And I'm certainly not going to drive myself into the ground where I fall apart emotionally and physically again. (27: 152–167)

With this new frame of mine, Armand became more relaxed and content, lived more in the here and now, and let go of things over which he had no control. At the same time, he believed it was necessary for him to do what was correct for him, be respected for setting limits, and feel rewarded for asserting himself (30).

Setting limits to his availability and giving of self

Armand recognized that his depression was, in part, due to his not setting limits on his emotional availability to others and to overinvesting himself in doing things for others. Being able to set limits is a function of the ego, which mediates the demands of the superego and the needs of the inner child (i.e., core needs). Setting limits has less to do with controlling the behaviors of others and more to do with conserving energy and time to do the things that one wants to do. The goal of therapy was to empower the ego so that it was not swayed by the demands of the superego or by the needs of the inner child. Setting limits implies giving voice to the inner child and respecting its voice. This theme was a topic in 15 of the 32 therapy sessions.

Problem Definition: Very early in therapy, Armand expressed a wish to set limits at work and with Sophia, to establish priorities and to have a good relationship with

Sophia (4). He was tired of being everything for others and a loser for himself. In a Gestalt Empty-Chair exercise with Sophia, Armand expressed being tired of taking care of her and wanting her to take responsibility for her own happiness (11).

Commitment phase: Armand took the position that he would be there for his wife in a limited way and after that she would have to take care of herself (13). He committed himself "to be there for Sophia and try to be a good husband but it doesn't mean that I'm doing everything that she wants" (16: 215). He realized that setting limits with Sophia was more delicate than setting limits at the workplace. He stated:

> With my wife, it's more delicate. I'm going to have to withdraw and say: I'm not responsible for her happiness and I'm not going to feel that I'm the one who has to come up with things that will keep her happy. I'll be there to support her but I don't think that I have to be there all the time. I need to take some time for myself and I'm going to do that. (16: 500–505)

Armand was strongly determined to take ownership of his life and say no to unreasonable demands from others. He wanted to learn ways "of saying no gracefully, not offending other people, but at the same time not allowing them to infringe [upon him] and say yes" (16: 594–600).

Experiment/action phase: Armand began to set limits with Sophia in terms of time spent with her and in not taking responsibility for her happiness. He did not give in to her demands, and he resigned himself to accepting her where she was and yet encouraged her to organize her life and to be her own person (24, 25). With regard to setting limits with Sophia, Armand stated:

> I can't let her reactions control my reactions. And if I feel that it's important for me to do this, then I'm going to do it. I think I'm coming more to see what's important in my life, that I do have freedom of action. I don't have to be governed by other people's reactions. I think I've been very easily manipulated and made to feel guilty if I'm not doing what others want. And I think I'm much better now to pick up things like that on the spot and say it. (24: 131–138)

In the past when his wife would go into a dark mood, he would feel down, anxious, and depressed and think that it was his fault. He feels differently now. He reported:

> this time I'm surprisingly unphased. I feel badly for her but I don't feel that there's a lot more that I can do other than to just love her and let her know that I'm there, put my arm around her, encourage her to do what is helpful. (19: 51–59)

He also came to the realization it is likely not possible for a husband to give her more than what he did (17: 142–152).

Armand resisted taking blame for what she lacked in her life. He said that some of her complaints might be legitimate, but he was convinced that

> she's not taking the bull by the horns and taking actions that she could. And I'm not going to push her but at the same time, I have a couple of times said: well Sophia, there's nothing I can do about that; this is up to you. (24: 278–297)

Yet he did not want to push her away too quickly for fear that she would be hurt. For him it was "a matter of knowing how to do it" (21: 333–343). Armand began to see that Sophia could be manipulative in the same manner that his mother was manipulative. However, in the past he did not see it and found it hard to accept it now (24: 278–297).

Integration/consolidation phase: Armand was able to reconcile and integrate being responsive to Sophia's needs, setting limits to his giving, and taking care of himself. At the same time, Sophia became more sensitive to Armand's need for time for himself. In this regard, Armand stated that Sophia

> is becoming more sensitive towards my needs. Quite often I'll say: I just need to be quiet now, and she'll say o.k. She'll go off and do something else and let me be, which is nice because then I don't feel that I'm weighed down and I can experience peace and calm. (16: 77–83)

In the process of learning how to set limits and assert his needs with Sophia, Armand said that he is

> more flexible with my wife. She makes demands on me and you say: well o.k., that's part of marriage. But even with my friends, I'm having to find polite ways to say no, and if they don't like it, then that's too bad. I have my own agenda. (13: 137–147)

As Armand began to set limits, he also began to feel a bit more selfish and added that "I'm not going to give them [people at the workplace] everything. I have to set my priorities" (16: 494–497).

It was a new experience for Armand to be able to integrate being available to others and at the same time to set limits to their demands and take care of himself. In his own words:

> I'm having to deal with feelings of guilt, standing up for myself whether it's selfish, asserting myself in a legitimate way in the various areas of my life, whether it's work or marriage. It's new for me. I think my past behavior got me into trouble probably because I didn't know how to look after my legitimate interests, and I ended up giving myself away, and other people would take advantage of that. Why did I do that? It's because I felt that I had to have the

approval or good favor of other people, and I felt that I was somehow wrong if someone was angry with me or if we had a disagreement [...] that somehow, I was at fault. And I know that probably comes from childhood. (22: 528–539)

In the past Armand mentioned that he tended to be reactive rather than proactive. That is, he responded to the demands and needs of other people rather than pursued his needs and interests. In having learned to set limits, he has become more proactive. He summarized this experience this way:

I was feeling whip-sawed between the demands from my wife and feeling that there was no room left for me to exercise my own aspirations. I have a life for myself, and live out of my own sense of beliefs. I have always been at the beck and call to the demands of other people. And my role was only to be reactive and to structure these demands in such a way that I am not overwhelmed. And now I'm becoming more proactive and saying: well, it's not only other people who have demands and aspirations. I do too. I can negotiate these. And that takes some risks and some real growth. (32: 400–416)

Identifying, asserting, and negotiating his needs

The topic of asserting and negotiating his needs with Sophia was addressed in 14 of the 32 sessions. The major work on asserting his needs took place in the later therapy sessions. This is consistent with Meier and Boivin's (2006) research on the resolution of intrapsychic conflicts where clients began the process of resolution of their conflicts by expressing negative affects and being judgmental but ended the process by expressing their mutual needs.

Problem definition phase: Armand began to address the issue of asserting his needs by expressing his difficulty in being his own person and in asserting his needs (2) and as no longer wanting to compromise himself for others but to live his life (4). Yet he wanted a balance between taking care of his wife and attending to his own needs. He described his relationship with his wife as being "pulled in by her depression; like walking on a tight rope; having to walk carefully so as not to give her the impression that he is ignoring her" (18) (i.e., resisted giving in to her projective identification). He strove to have greater space for both himself and his wife (21–22). Armand described his difficulty to do things for himself this way:

It's a fight to get the space and the time I need to do what I want to do. I do feel that when I'm at home my wife demands my attention in various ways. Even when I say I need half an hour, it's sort of grudgingly given [...] I need to be at one with myself and I need to have some mental space. It feels like somebody is nailing my mind to the ground. I'm not free to think and to have my own thoughts. Somebody else is demanding my attention and my concentration all the time. (28: 362–379)

Armand expressed his desire to restore the physical intimacy that he had with Sophia but which had been damaged and lost. He also had the desire to get in touch with his artistic side in terms of music, writing, and art and to "begin to experience pleasure again" (13: 322–338).

Exploration and insight phases: In exploring his relational difficulties with Sophia, Armand began to sort out his own values and preferences and to resist living out the agendas of others. He was better able to identify his needs and to make choices. He came to the realization that it is best to do "what you believe to be important, structure that into your life, make sure there's some flexibility. Take into account the needs of other people, but don't allow yourself to be exploited. Have the self-respect and value your own person" (32: 379–391). He prioritized his life so as not to fall back into depression (24, 25). He was convinced that he would not fall back into depression if he lived according to his values, goals, and need for autonomy (15).

Commitment phase: As therapy progressed, Armand became more and more determined to assert his needs in his relationship with Sophia. He made a commitment to himself to live by his values, priorities, and needs, even at the risk of losing his relationship, and to deal with his feelings of guilt, selfishness, and potential loss (14). He also indicated that she "can't bend me out of shape continually because she is unhappy. I have to live for myself and love her the best that I can, but ultimately, it's her decision to make and if she leaves, I'll adjust to it". Having come to this position brought him real freedom (32: 379–391).

Experiment/action phase: Having identified his need for wanting to be his own person (i.e., to assert his autonomy) and having committed himself to this task, Armand proceeded to be more assertive of his needs with Sophia. He searched for means and ways to assert his need without alienating her (9, 14). He began asserting his needs by asking Sophia for time for himself when he came home from work (27, 28). Initially this was a struggle as his wife felt pushed out by his request because her need for time together was equally as strong (27). He stated that

> I would like not necessarily go home, but go do something else. But I have difficulty trying to express that to my wife. We've talked about the need for me to go through a transition time of some sort. It's actually proving to be quite difficult to get that. (27: 25–34)

Another time in therapy, Armand stated, "I do crave some time to myself which I'm finding still difficult to get and to take the time to do that" (21: 333–343). Despite the difficulty of obtaining time for himself, Armand remained convinced that he had "a legitimate need to unwind and to spend time on my own for my own emotional and physical well-being" (27: 120–121). Armand indicated that he is learning "how to give myself breathing space" (28: 52–67).

Consolidation/integration phase: As Armand became more graced in asserting and negotiating his needs, Sophia became more responsive to them. He became more relaxed and content, lived more in the here and now, let go of things over which he had no control, did what was correct for him, and felt respected and rewarded for asserting himself (30). He also noted that he was becoming more organized (i.e., integrated) based on his values, wishes, needs, and on taking ownership and charge of his life. He stated:

> It's my values and goals that I'm shifting toward. But the way I was living before, I had elements of compulsiveness and obsessiveness. And now I'm coming more to the place where I'm saying: I'm going to live more by my goals and values and they require a bit more attention so that I'm clearer on what they are. But they still require discipline and persistence. I don't want to get back into the mindset of thinking that because I'm slipping in terms of progress, that somehow, I'm unworthy and I've failed. I have to change that mindset and say: well, o.k., maybe the goal wasn't worth the effort or the cost of whatever was involved with it. Maybe I have to be prepared to change those goals and values and not be hard on myself. (21: 51–163)

Learning the skill to negotiate his needs brought Armand a sense of lightness, the shedding of a heavy load, and an acceptance of his own needs (31). He also became more responsive to Sophia's needs and to her less orderly and structured lifestyle, which for him "opened up new realms of spontaneity" (32: 93, 120, 130–135). He was better able to let go of his need for structure and respond to Sophia's spontaneous, and at times, impulsive behaviors.

Lifting of depression and staying out of it

Several times during therapy, Armand reported that his depression was lifting. His first sense of the depression lifting was his statement that "I don't know if I am out of the depression, but I am out of the worst of it" (15: 65–70). Later he said, "I would say that the depression is lifting, or at least I've been considerably raised out of it" (20: 246–256), and "I think that I am coming out of this depression, I certainly feel a lot better about my life" (22: 563–567).

As indicators that his depression was lifting, Armand stated that "I am able to laugh and cry again" (15: 65–70), "I'm finding that I'm joking more and laughing with people at work" (21: 65–67), "I'm calm. I don't feel particularly troubled in my soul in any respect, which is a strange place to be" (21: 515–516), and "I don't feel that the world is on my shoulders which is a strange feeling" (19: 445–450). Another indicator was that he enjoyed playing with his dog. Regarding his pleasure in playing with the dog, the therapist suggested that he carry with him the sense of playfulness and fun that he had in walking and playing with his dog, to his workplace and in his relationship with Sophia (20: 246–256; 21: 46–50). This suggestion stayed with Armand.

Armand compared his life before depression to his life after depression. Before his depression, he stated there was a "sense of striving," whereas after his depression lifted, there was more a "sense of being settled and less a sense of having to prove himself" and to "fight for causes" (32: 197–205). For Armand, there was a "sense of settledness and internal peace that comes with it" (33: 39–42). He found that his home was becoming a safe haven, a place to go to for emotional nourishment and for self and other-comforting.

Summary and Conclusion

This chapter presented the case of a middle-aged man, Armand, struggling with a fourth episode of major depressive disorder. The main part of the chapter addressed his recovery from depression by focusing on three themes (e.g., obligations, setting limits, and asserting unmet needs) relative to one person, namely his wife. The main task was reworking the psychic structure and self-structure, and replacing the coping strategies with more effective coping strategies. He reworked these within the context of his relationship with his wife who resembled his own mother. Armand transformed his psychic structure by identifying and asserting his unmet childhood needs for autonomy and significance, by giving voice to the inner child, empowering the ego, and moderating the demands of the superego. This transformation led to the lifting of the depression and to a healthy relationship with his wife and to personal satisfaction and happiness.

References

American Psychiatric Association (1994). *Diagnostic and statistical manual of mental disorders (DSM-IV)*. Washington, DC: Author.

Cashdan, S. (1988). *Object relations therapy: Using the relationship*. New York: W.W. Norton & Company.

Freud, S. (1923). The Ego and the Id. *Standard Edition, 19*, 12–63.

Freud, S. (1938). An Outline of Psychoanalysis. *Standard Edition, 23*, 1953, 144–207.

Gendlin, E.T. (1996). *Focusing-oriented psychotherapy: A manual of the experiential method*. New York: Guilford Press.

Hathaway, S.R., & McKinley, J.C. (1967). *Minnesota multiphasic personality inventory*. New York: Psychological Corporation.

Ivey, A.E. (1983). *Intentional interviewing and counseling*. Monterey: CA: Brooks/Cole.

Jourard, S.M. (1971). *The transparent self*. New York: D. Van Nostrand Company.

Joyce, P., & Sills, C. (2007). *Skills in Gestalt counselling psychotherapy*. London: Sage.

Klein, M. (1935/1975). A contribution to the psychogenesis of manic-depressive states. In M. Klein (Ed.), *Love, guilt and reparation and other works, 1921–1945* (pp. 262–289). New York: Delacorte.

Klein, M. (1948/1975). On the theory of anxiety and guilt. In *Envy and gratitude and other works 1946–1963* (pp. 25–42). New York: Delacorte.

Klein, M. (1952/1975). The mutual influences in the development of the ego and id. In M. Klein (Ed.), *Envy and gratitude and other works 1946–1963* (pp. 57–60). London: Hogarth Press.

Klein, M. (1959/1975). Our adult world and its roots in infancy. In M. Klein (Ed.), *Envy and gratitude and other works 1946–1963* (pp. 247–263). New York: Delacorte.

Mahler, M., Pine, F., & Bergman, A. (1975). *The psychological birth of the human infant.* New York: Basic Books.

Meier, A., & Boivin, M. (1987). Self-discovery approach to counseling. *Pastoral Sciences, 7,* 145–168.

Meier, A., & Boivin, M. (1992). A Seven phase model of the change process and its clinical applications. Paper presented at the 8th Annual Conference of the Society for the Exploration of Psychotherapy Integration, San Diego, California, April 3.

Meier, A., & Boivin, M. (2000). The achievement of greater selfhood: The application of Theme-Analysis to a case study. *Psychotherapy Research, 10*(1), 60.

Meier, A., & Boivin, M. (2006). Intrapsychic conflicts, their formation, underlying dynamics, and resolution: An object relations perspective. In A. Meier & M. Rovers (Eds.), *Through conflict to reconciliation* (pp. 295–328). Toronto: Novalis.

Meier, A., & Boivin, M. (2011). *Counselling and therapy techniques: Theory and practice.* London, England: Sage Publishers.

Meier, A., & Boivin, M. (2022). *Self-in-relationship-psychotherapy: A complete clinical guide to theory and practice.* London: Routledge

Meier, A., Boivin, M., & Meier, M. (2006). The treatment of depression: A case study using theme-analysis. *Counselling and Psychotherapy Research, 6*(2), 115–125.

Meier, A., Boivin, M., & Meier, M. (2008). Theme-analysis: Procedures and applications for psychotherapy research. *Qualitative Research in Psychology, 5,* 289–310.

Perls, F. (1969b). *Gestalt therapy verbatim.* Toronto: Bantam Books.

Perls, F., Hefferline, R.F., & Goodman, P. (1951). *Gestalt therapy: Excitement and growth in the human personality.* New York: Delta.

Winnicott, D. (1960/1965). Ego distortion in terms of true and false self. In D. Winnicott (Ed.), *The maturational processes and the facilitating environment* (pp. 140–152). New York: International Universities Press.

Chapter 3

Tania

Obsessions and Compulsions: Assessment and Conceptualization

This chapter presents Tania (pseudonym), who struggled with obsessive-compulsive disorder (OCD) for many years prior to seeking help in therapy. Her determination and efforts to free herself from this disorder generated a lot of useful and rich clinical material and insights. For this reason, it was decided to present the therapy of Tania in two chapters. The first of the two chapters presents the assessment and conceptualization of the symptoms associated with OCD and the second chapter (Chapter 4) presents the treatment of the disorder.

This chapter begins with a brief description of the essential features of OCD. This is followed by Tania's psychosocial history and the factors that contributed to the origin of OCD. The chapter concludes with a diagnosis, a psychological assessment using the Self-in-Relationship Psychotherapy Assessment Form (SIRP-AF), and by a conceptualization of Tania's symptoms.

The numbers in brackets refer to the session number and line numbers. The number to the left of a colon represent the session numbers and the numbers to the right of a colon represent the line numbers. When there is only one number, it refers to the session number.

Obsessive-Compulsive Disorder

OCD is a chronic and long-lasting disorder in which an individual has reoccurring and uncontrollable thoughts (i.e., obsessions), behaviors (compulsions), and/or rituals that he feels the urge to repeat. The *Diagnostic and Statistical Manual of Mental Disorders* (DSM-5) (American Psychiatric Association; APA, 2013) defines the essential features of OCD to comprise recurrent obsessions, compulsions, or both and rituals (Code: 300.3).

Obsessions are described as "recurrent and persistent thoughts, urges or images that are experienced, at some time during the disturbance as intrusive and unwanted, and that in most individuals cause marked anxiety or distress," and "the individual tries to ignore or suppress such thoughts, urges, or images, or to neutralize them with some other thought or action (i.e., by performing a compulsion" (APA, 2013, p. 237). Obsessions are involuntary and are seemingly uncontrollable thoughts,

DOI: 10.4324/9781032655291-5

images, or impulses that intrude into one's mind and cause a great deal of anxiety or discomfort.

Compulsions are "repetitive behaviors (e.g., handwashing, ordering, checking) or mental acts (e.g., praying, counting, repeating words silently) that the individual feels driven to perform in response to an obsession or according to rules that must be applied rigidly," and "the behaviors or mental acts are aimed at preventing some dreaded event or situation, however, these behaviors or mental acts are not connected in a realistic way with what they are designed to neutralize or prevent, or are clearly excessive" (APA, 2013, p. 237). Compulsions are usually performed with the intent of making obsessions go away, such as being afraid of contamination, but the relief never lasts.

A compulsive ritual is a series of acts that a person feels must be carried out even though the person recognizes that the behavior is seen to be useless and inappropriate. When the ritual is interrupted, the person feels compelled to return to the beginning of the ritual and start anew. Failure to complete the acts leads to extreme tension or anxiety (O'Toole, 2022).

Associated features of OCD are those of cleaning (contamination obsessions and cleaning compulsions), symmetry (repeating, ordering, and counting obsessions), forbidden or taboo thoughts (e.g., aggressive, sexual, or religious obsessions and related compulsions), and harm (e.g., fears of harm to oneself or others and checking compulsions) (APA, 2013, pp. 238–239).

Most persons with OCD fall into one of the following categories: (1) washers – fear contamination and usually have hand-washing compulsions; (2) checkers – repeatedly check things, such as doors, that are associated with harm or danger; (3) doubters or sinners – fear that if everything is not done just right or is not perfect, they will be punished or something terrible will happen; (4) counters and arrangers – are obsessed with order and symmetry and might have superstitions about certain numbers; and (5) hoarders – fear that if they throw anything away, something bad will happen (Robinson, Smith & Segal, 2016).

Psychosocial History and Its Contributing Factors

Tania, single, mid-thirties, and of European and Canadian origin, requested therapy to address her obsessive thoughts and compulsive behaviors, which greatly tormented her. She felt immobilized, trapped, encaged, depressed, and hopeless. She devalued herself, and was angry at others for having contributed to her obsessions and compulsions. Tania was disillusioned with life, mistrusted others, and was plagued by intense internal conflicts.

Tania was brought up in a very religious, moralistic, and conservative family and a conservative social environment from which she could not break free (409). Tania's parents, teachers, and church ministers played a significant role in her emotional, social, and religious development. The general message for her was to constantly strive to be perfect and to be on guard not to cause harm morally and psychologically to others without her knowing what this meant.

Tania's relation with her father was ambivalent at best. When Tania was young, her father suffered a back injury at work. He was asked not to continue with the same line of work but continued nevertheless, contrary to doctor's orders (217: 118–120; 400). He could not tolerate noise, became irritable, angry, and critical, and said that his children would drive him crazy. Tania, at her young age, did not know what it meant to drive him crazy. He was constantly sick and had two episodes of depression. She feared that she might have contributed to his illness (217: 110–130; 259). She was angry at him but felt that she had no right to express her anger as her mother stated that her father could not help the way he was. She felt guilty in being angry at her father as he was good to her and to the family by providing generously for them. These mixed experiences resulted in Tania's repressing her feelings of anger and in developing ambivalent feelings – those of love and hate – directed especially toward her father.

Tania describes her mother as a person who was very devoted to the activities of the church and readily responded to the requests of church officials (e.g., the clergy) and put aside her own needs in order to serve the church (400). She resented her mother for "jumping each time the church said jump." She described her mother as having imposed her ideas and wishes, was overprotective, and was preoccupied with safety by keeping dangerous objects (e.g., knives) out of the reach of everyone.

When Tania was growing up, her mother impressed upon her to be a good example to others and not to morally harm anyone (344: 260). She started out by being a good example to the younger siblings in the family and then to the children in the school (344: 217–219). This was later extended to avoiding harm to others by picking up broken glass and nails from the street to avoid accidents and causing harm to others. By assuming responsibility for being a good example, she was "trying to control [her] circumstances" (344: 227).

Tania idealized her younger sister, who was full of energy, did interesting things, and always got her way. Tania realized that she could not be like her younger sister. As for her older sister, Tania felt inferior to her as she could do everything that Tania would like to have done. Her older sister was very disciplined (309) and as a teenager, she was not afraid to say what she felt.

Tania was brought up in a school system staffed by women of a religious community. In her primary school religion classes, she was given the impression that God was a judge watching over all her behaviors and actions. The teachers presented sex as something that was forbidden and that "the girls were the bad ones" and were told to be careful how they dressed so as not to tempt the boys (226: 250–254). Because of the attitude that she developed toward sex, she became preoccupied with books containing pictures of a sexual nature and would either remove the books or destroy them (226: 285–294). At the age of 14, she attended a boarding school and then at 16 she entered a convent where she enjoyed the structured life, although she left it because she had become very compulsive in her behaviors.

Tania was brought up in a church that had very conservative views about adolescence and young women's proper dress and behavior (400). At a retreat, when she was about six or seven years of age, a clergyman, quoting from scripture, preached that "if you are a scandal to one of these little ones (e.g., children), it is better to have a millstone hung around your neck and dropped into the sea rather than to be alive" (157; 228: 52; 247: 425). This experience made her fearful to express her thoughts and behave inappropriately lest she scandalize someone and be judged and dropped to the bottom of the sea. She was careful not to scandalize anyone younger than herself and she assumed that when others were doing something wrong, it was her responsibility to correct them. (228: 47–54). She was taught not "to think critically, [as] everything came from above, the church said it, you do it, no questions were asked, everything was black and white" (344: 91–92).

Tania felt that she was taught to think and behave in ways that were contrary to her natural inclinations. Tania mentioned that she became more and more afraid that she would make a mistake and, consequently, became "more and more paralyzed" (344: 96). She was angry at the church but felt that she had no right to express her feelings as the church meant well. She internalized the church and clergy messages to form a severe, demanding, and critical superego that oppressed her core needs. Tania, in her teenage years, began to experience a conflict between her strivings to be her own person and the restrictions placed on her by her parents, teachers, and clergy. Tania was on guard not to be the cause of moral and physical harm to others (260).

Before the age of five, Tania spent time alone, daydreamed, and created stories in her head (259). She was in her private world for most of her life. She described herself as a nonconforming child who threw temper tantrums and did mischievous things (259; 409). As a teenager, she was shy, felt alone, did not mix well with others, followed the crowd, and could not do the things that she wanted to do. Her teenage years were a source of torment for her (90). Tania was not clued in about sex until she was about 17 years of age (260).

At the age of 20 she was madly in love with a man, had a romantic relationship, but knew that there was no possibility of a long-term relationship. They broke up after four years. She was terrified of sex because of the negative education that she received from her parents and the church (90; 208). Following high school, she completed a diploma in legal secretary and then took a position in a law firm as legal secretary, an occupation that she enjoyed and excelled in.

In brief, her interactions with the family, church, school, and the community had an enormous impact on Tania's perception of others and her world and on her feelings toward them and toward herself. The experiences from these interactions instilled in her a sense of obligation to protect others from harm and inhibited her from expressing her legitimate feelings toward others. She was uncertain as to where the boundary was between morally and psychologically harming and not harming children and the vulnerable. These experiences significantly contributed to the development of her obsessions and compulsions.

Diagnosis and Assessment

To assess for the presence and/or intensity of Tania's obsessions and compulsions and the recovery from them, the *Diagnostic and Statistical Manual of Mental Disorders* (DSM-III-R) (American Psychiatric Association; APA, 1987), the Obsessive-Compulsive Scale (OCS), and the Compulsive Inventory (CI) were administered at the beginning of therapy and again at the termination of therapy. The results from the pretreatment and posttreatment measures are as follows.

DSM-III-R

Based on her psychosocial history, it was apparent that Tania struggled with OCD. To be diagnosed with OCD, the individual must meet four criteria, which are: (a) presence of obsessions, compulsions, or both, (b) the obsessions and compulsions are time consuming or cause clinically significant distress, (c) the obsessive and compulsive symptoms are not attributable to the physiological effects of a substance, and (d) the symptoms are not better explained by another mental disorder (APA, 1987, Code: 300.30).

To assess for the presence of OCD, the DSM-III-R was administered at the beginning of therapy and again at the termination of therapy. Prior to therapy, Tania met the criteria for OCD but did not meet the criteria following therapy. She did not meet the criteria for any of the other DSM-III-R diagnostic categories prior to nor following therapy. On the Global Assessment of Functioning Scale of the DSM-III-R, her score at the beginning of psychotherapy and at its termination were 50 and 80, respectively.

Obsessive-Compulsive Scale

The Obsessive-Compulsive Scale (OCS; Gibb, Bailey, Best & Lambirth, 1983) was administered before and after therapy. The OCS is a 20-item instrument that measures the general tendency toward obsessive thoughts and compulsive behaviors. The instrument has evidence of internal consistency and concurrent validity. It provides normative data for college students with means of 11.15 and 11.24 for males and females, respectively. The OCS provides one single score (Corcoran & Fisher, 1987).

The OCS scores for pretreatment and posttreatment are presented in Table 3.1. Tania's OCS score prior to treatment was 16 and following treatment, it was 3, which indicates a significant decrease in obsessive thoughts and compulsive behaviors. Her pretreatment score was well above the mean for college students. The max score refers to the maximum score that one can achieve on this measure.

The Compulsiveness Inventory

To assess for compulsive behaviors, the Compulsiveness Inventory (CI; Kagan & Squires, 1985) was administered before and after therapy. The CI is an 11-item

Table 3.1 Results from the Compulsiveness Inventory and the Obsessive-Compulsive Scale

	Pretreatment	Posttreatment	Max Score
Obsessive-Compulsive Scale (OCS) (M: F = 11.24; M = 11.15)	16	3	20
The Compulsiveness Inventory (CI)			
Indecision & Double Checking (IDC)	5	0	5
Order & Regularity (OR)	2	1	4
Detail & Perfection (DP)	2	1	2
Total Score (CI)	9	2	11

scale designed to measure compulsive behaviors that are common in the normal population. Pathological compulsiveness is defined in terms of extreme preoccupation with thoughts or activities, a tendency toward overorganization and difficulty making decisions. The CI focuses specifically on an overconcern with decisions and tasks to be performed perfectly according to rigid and well-established norms (Corcoran & Fisher, 1987, p.130). The CI measures three aspects of compulsivity: indecision and double-checking (IDC), detail and perfection (DP), and order and regularity (OR). The CI produced excellent internal consistency scores for each of the subscales and very good validity results. No normative data are available in the primary reference.

The scores for pretreatment and posttreatment are presented in Table 3.1. When compared to the pretreatment scores, there was a decrease on all the scores for IDC and the total score, which suggests that there was a decrease in compulsive behaviors, particularly checking.

In summary, the results from the DSM-III-R, OCS, and CI suggest that Tania struggled with obsessions and compulsions prior to treatment but not following treatment. Based on these measures, it can be said that treatment was successful.

Assessment Using the SIRP-AF

The Self-in-Relationship Psychotherapy Assessment Form (SIRP-AF; Appendix B) assesses a client on SIRP's constructs by using the material from the psychosocial history. Each of the constructs has been conceptually and operationally defined (Appendix C). The SIRP-AF has been found to be a reliable instrument to code the constructs (Meier & Boivin, 2022). This section presents the results from the application of the SIRP-AF to Tania's psychosocial history. The task was to assess these constructs, where possible, relative to Tania's childhood experiences. The findings for the SIRP constructs are presented in Table 3.2 and the rationales for the codes are briefly explained.

Table 3.2 SIRP Assessment Form for Self-in-Relationship Psychotherapy constructs

Part I. Descriptive Data: For each of the dimensions presented below, provide descriptive material for the persons (e.g., mother, father) entered in the top row of the table. If there are other persons who were or are important to the client's life (e.g., grandmother, stepfather), additional columns can be created and assessed for each topic under Dimension.

Dimension	Father	Mother
1. Organizing unmet self, relational, and physical intimacy needs relative to:	For emotional connection; that she matters to him	Autonomy in her thinking and expressing of feelings; that she matters; liked for self-expression; feel secure and safe; connected
2. Internal representation of:	Angry and irritable person; incapable, yet loving, caring	Controlling, imposing, inhibiting, overprotective
3. Internal representations of self relative to: (How I view myself when with)	Unimportant	Not good enough; inadequate; doing things in the wrong way
4. Affect linking representation of other to self: (How I felt my father, mother, etc. felt about me)	Irritable and impatient; caring	Impatient, not satisfied, and pleased
5. Affect linking representation of self to other: (How I felt toward my)	Ambivalent – angry vs. caring	Anger; being imposed upon
6. How I felt/feel when in the presence of:	Conflicted, unsure	Anxious, insecure, avoidant, inadequate, helpless; rejected
7. Quality or degree of good enough parenting:	Loving and caring when young, and impatient and irritable after accident	Characterized by compliance with mother's wishes, anxiety about doing wrong, and obligated to protect others from harm

Part II. Scaled Data: Rate dimensions 1, 4, 7, and 11 on a five-point scale. For dimensions 2 and 3, indicate the strength of each component using a five-point scale with 1 = barely and 5 = greatly. For the dimension 10, indicate the characteristic phase and indicate the strength of its presence using the five-point scale indicated above. For the remainder dimensions check off those that are relevant. See Operational Criteria for more precise instructions. If the dimension is not relevant, leave the space blank. PO = part object; WO = whole object; PSP = paranoid/schizoid; DP = depressive position; EB = need for emotional bonding; SC = need for sensual contact; AU = need for autonomy; SI = need for sexual intimacy.

1. Manner of relating to	1	2	3	4	5
Father:	_1_ (PO)				_ (WO)_
Mother:	_1_	X			_5_

2. Psychic structure				
Core Needs:	__ EB	3.5 AU	2.5 Ego	3.5 Superego
	__ SC	__ SI		

3. Self-structure		
3.5 striving for significance	3.5 striving for competency	2.5 capacity to secure sense of significance and competency

4. True self (Living from)	1 Minimally Strongly	2	3	4	5

5. Coping mechanisms				
X repression	__ splitting	__ regression	__ devaluation
X Undoing	X introjection	__ sublimation	X Suppression
X Avoidance	X projection	__ idealization	X Reaction formation

6. Quality of emotional bond			
__ emotionally connected	X striving for emotional connection	__ avoiding emotional connection	__ emotionally disconnected

7. Object constancy	1 Not Formed	2	3 Partially Formed	4	5 Fully Formed

8. Characteristic emotional state	2 angry — abandoned	1 anxious — smothered	3 depressed 4 oppressed	— sad Other —
9. Projective identifications	X dependency — other	— power	— ingratiation	— sex
10. Characteristic phase	— Symbiosis	1 Differentiation	2 Practicing	3 Rapprochement
				Consolidation

| 11. Characteristic position | 1 (PSP) | 2 | X 3 | 4 | 5 (DP) |
| 12. Level of personality organization | X higher | | inter-mediate | lower | |

Relational, Self, and Physical Intimacy Needs

At the beginning of therapy, Tania's preoccupation was to free herself from her obsessions and compulsions. She had no sense of her unmet core relational, self, and physical intimacy needs. She was constricted and fearful to be herself lest she psychologically or morally harm others. Because of her preoccupation not to cause harm to others, Tania invested minimal energy in the development of herself psychologically and socially.

Although not explicitly stated, one can infer Tania's core relational and self needs from her behaviors and from the behaviors of others toward her. Tania wanted more from her father than he was able to give because of his injury. She craved a loving and carefree relationship with him and a closer emotional connection with him. From her mother, Tania yearned for the freedom and autonomy to express her feelings, needs, and ideas and be validated for them. She wanted the freedom to be herself, be autonomous, and be liked for being herself and to feel safe rather than to comply with the mother's restrictions and inhibitions. Tania felt burdened by the obligation to protect others from moral and psychological harm.

In short, as a child, Tania's core needs for emotional bonding, significance, and autonomy were not positively responded to. Since they were left unfulfilled, they continued to push for satiation. In this chapter, emotional bonding is used to refer to the mother–infant/child relationship, and emotional connection is used when referring to post infant/child relationships.

Representations of Other and Self

Through her relationships with her parents, Tania began to form representations of them and of herself (Klein, 1948/1975). Her representation of her father was mixed. She perceived him to be an angry, irritable, and incapable person, and yet he was loving and caring. As for her mother, she perceived her to be an imposing, controlling, inhibiting, and overprotective and yet a dependent person. Her mother passed on to her not to have a mind of her own, which is inferred from her "jumping when the clergy asked her to jump." It is assumed that the mother did not pass on to Tania the ability to assert her needs and feelings. The father was not able to provide a check on Tania's mother's demands, expectations, and behaviors. With regard to representations of herself, Tania viewed herself as being insignificant, inadequate, and not good enough. She struggled all her life to transform these images of herself.

Psychic Structure

Tania's psychic structure (Freud, 1923, 1938) reflects her actual lived childhood relationship with her mother, father, teachers, and church officials in that it is skewed toward the superego, repressed core needs, and an impoverished ego. She internalized the demands and expectations (i.e., obligations) of her mother, which were reinforced by teachers in elementary and junior high school and by messages from the clergy. She received the message that she was not to entertain and express her core needs and feelings, particularly those of autonomy and anger, although she might have had a legitimate reason to do so. At the same time, she felt obligated not to harm others, particularly children. Thus, her superego was characterized by feeling obligated toward others, being moralistic, and having unrealistic expectations and ideals of self and of others.

Her inner child was characterized by a striving for autonomy, to be respected for her thoughts and feelings and motives. These had not been validated and were pushing for release and expression. They had been inhibited for fear that they would lead her to unacceptable social behaviors and interactions for which she would be punished. Her ego was enfeebled by fear and was not able to reconcile, in an adaptive way, the superego demands and expectations, her core needs and feelings, and reality. The nature of Tania's psychic structure acted as a barrier for her to relate to others in an open, trusting, safe, free, and loving way, and it incapacitated her ability to discriminate between duty/obligation and responsibility.

Self-Structure

Tania's self-structure was characterized by a yearning that her thoughts, feelings, and motives matter to others and be accepted as being significant. It was also characterized by the yearning to be competent to manage her anxieties and conflicts, and particularly, to manage her obsessions and compulsions. She was plagued by the fear that through her negligence or lack of mindfulness, others might get hurt and she would be held morally and psychologically responsible. Her sense of incompetency is reflected in her lack of ability to evaluate her own actions and to conclude that what she was doing was to the best of her ability and correct for her. She lacked the ability to influence her parents to love and accept her unconditionally and to respond positively to her needs.

As for her social self, Tania's behaviors, attitudes, and interactions were influenced by what she thought others expected of her. She was more reactive than proactive. Her decisions and choices did not emanate from her true self. That is, they were not primarily self-directed but other-directed. She was not true to herself and authentic in her responses; she lived more from a false self than from a true self (Winnicott, 1960/1965).

Coping Strategies

Tania dealt with her anxieties and internal conflicts by the defense mechanisms of repression, avoidance, reaction-formation, undoing, and projection and by her coping strategy of suppression. Her coping strategies tended to be nonadaptive and defensive in nature rather than adaptive (Sadock, Sadock & Ruiz, 2014). The latter is characterized by their repetitive and rigid use to defend against anxiety and to protect her from being judged to be a bad person and found to be at fault in hurting others.

Quality of Emotional Bond

Tania feared that she would not live up to the expectations of significant others (e.g., mother, father, clergy), which inhibited her from forming close, warm, caring, intimate, and trusting relationships. Tania's "intimate" relationships were fraught with fear and characterized by avoidance. Without being aware of it, Tania sought "safe anchorage" and a "confident expectation" that her needs would be respected, validated, and responded to (Mahler, Pine & Bergman, 1975). One can assume that these attributes were missing in her early relationship with her mother, who was overly concerned about safety, security, and compliance, which left Tania with a lifelong pursuit for emotional bonding (e.g., connection) with a significant other and at the same time craving to be thought of as a good person.

Object Constancy

Object constancy refers to the internalization of positive representations of significant people who, when one thinks of them, bring about positive feelings of self, provide a perspective on life's challenges, offer a direction for how to deal with them, and provide a capacity to self-comfort and self-soothe. Object constancy is formed by having good significant people in one's life by whom we are loved, admired, and cherished. Through the experience of being loved, admired, and cherished, one begins to love, admire, and cherish oneself, which leads to object constancy. Object constancy provides an "internal grounding," by which an individual can gain a perspective on relational or self-issues and can regulate one's affective response to them (Mahler, Pine & Bergman, 1975). Object constancy is correlated with adaptive ego capacity. Tania lacked object constancy, which is demonstrated by her inability to manage her feelings of depression, inadequacy, and self-worth and by her obsessions and compulsions. A person with object constancy can recover from negative experiences, whereas a person lacking it is not able to recover.

Characteristic Emotional State

A characteristic emotional state refers to a familiar emotion that one has had for a long time, perhaps since childhood, and carried into adolescence and adulthood. Tania's characteristic emotional state was an intense fear that she might cause psychological and moral harm to others, be negatively judged for being responsible for the harm, and be thought of as a bad person. She put an enormous amount of effort into assuring herself that she was a morally good person by removing material from billboards that could psychologically or morally harm others. She strove to be a good person in the eyes of her parents, the church (i.e., clergy), and "God" to avoid being to be scolded or condemned by them. Her compulsions and obsessions served as armor to protect her from being found at fault and scolded. A deeper lying emotion is that of anger, which manifested itself in her resentment toward her mother for believing what the clergy told her and in her resentment toward the church and God. It was also reflected in her childhood temper tantrums and in her adolescence nonconforming and mischievous behaviors.

Projective Identification

Projective identification refers to a relational dynamic by which a person repeatedly tries to draw a significant other into their unique way of relating (Cashdan, 1988). Often underlying a projective identification is an unmet childhood need that an individual pressures another to meet. Using Cashdan's (1988) classification of projective identifications, it can be said that Tania's projective identification was that of dependency. She depended on others to validate and reassure her that she was doing what was morally and socially correct. Tania's unmet need was to be seen as a good person and be loved for her actions and behaviors. She tried to achieve this by going out of her way to assure that others were not psychologically and morally harmed. Tania also craved emotional connection with significant others, which she attempted to achieve by her compulsive (i.e., compensatory) behaviors that were attempts to act correctly. Because she lacked object constancy, Tania was not able to self-validate when confronted with conflicts and anxieties and instead turned to others for validation and reassurance.

From another prospective, Tania related to significant others in terms of how she wanted them to relate to her and from her needy part, not from herself as a whole person. This type of relating to the other has been referred to as relating in terms of part-object and part-self (Klein, 1948/1975) and as self objects (Kohut, 1977). That is, Tania did not relate to others as whole person with her own needs, feelings, and preferences but as she wanted and needed them to be present for her.

Characteristic Developmental Phase

In terms of the separation and individuation process, Tania failed to secure "safe anchorage" and to develop "confident expectation" (Mahler, Pine & Bergman, 1975) that significant others would positively respond to and validate her needs and feelings. That is, she did not complete the essential tasks of the differentiation subphase and to psychologically separate from the significant other. It can be assumed that her sense of insecurity as a child prevented her from exploring the "not-mother" world, acquiring realistic coping skills (e.g., an adaptive ego), and developing a sense of competency. Rather, her antenna was attuned to the danger to be avoided and/or from which to protect herself and others.

In Mahler and associates' terminology (1975), Tania failed to adequately negotiate the tasks associated with the practicing subphase, which are to invest energy in the "not-mother" world, to test her newly developed cognitive and motor skills, and to acquire tolerance in being separated from the significant other. Tania failed, as well, to negotiate the tasks that are associated with the rapprochement subphase

(Mahler, et al., 1975). The tasks of this subphase include developing object constancy and the ability to regulate affect, establishing boundaries between the "not-me" and the "me," and relating to others in a real way, that is, in terms of both the other and self being whole persons. In brief, Tania's subjective experiences and relational interactions were characterized by failures to complete the developmental tasks of three subphases, namely, differentiation, practicing, and rapprochement. It was essential that treatment address these subphases beginning with the differentiation subphase.

Characteristic Developmental Position

Unlike Freud (1905), who postulated progressive forward-moving stages of human development, Klein proposed two developmental positions with an individual moving back and forth between these two positions. She described a developmental position as a state of psychological growth characterized by the way the infant/child deals with love-hate relationships and how he relates to both internalized and externalized objects (Klein, 1935/1975, p. 276). The names given to the two developmental positions (i.e., types of interpersonal stances), are the paranoid-schizoid position and the depressive position. The paranoid-schizoid position is characterized by destructive (hateful) instincts and feelings, and the depressive position is characterized by constructive (loving) instincts or feelings. The infant/child's basic conflict revolves around the instincts of these two positions, that is, between a malicious wish to destroy those close to the child and the desire to protect them. The infant/child organizes his experiences around these positions. The characteristic that marks a movement away from the paranoid-schizoid position and toward the depressive stance is that the infant/child becomes empathic toward the love object and fears losing the love of the love object. The way the development positions are worked through affects an individual's adult life (Klein, 1959/1975).

Given the above, it can be stated that Tania was more closely aligned with the paranoid-schizoid position than with the depressive position. This was manifested by her anger toward her mother, the church, and God who, she felt, judged her, and held her to high standards and obligated her to do no harm to others, particularly to the innocent and weak.

Conceptualization

Two of the main problems that Tania reported in the first couple of sessions were her obsessions and compulsions. The conceptualization, for this chapter, focuses on Tania's obsessions and compulsions. The conceptualization is based on information gathered at the assessment interviews and on the analysis and assessment of the SIRP constructs. The conceptualization is organized according to symptoms, predisposing childhood experiences, pertinent internalizations, precipitating factors, and reenactments.

Symptoms: At the beginning of therapy, Tania presented a host of symptoms, which were previously reported in a published article and a paper presentation (Meier, 1986; Meier & Boivin, 1998). However, her two main complaints were her obsessive thoughts and compulsive behaviors. She obsessed about: harmful objects, such as broken glass lying on streets or sidewalks that could potentially hurt others; helpless worms on sidewalks where they could be killed by cyclists; and about seeing posters on bulletin boards with messages that could morally or psychologically harm the less informed person. Her compulsions included: repetitive handwashing; repeatedly checking burners and doors before going to work; removing posters from bulletin boards perceived to be harmful; separating secular garbage from sacred garbage; and removing harmful objects and worms from sidewalks and streets.

Predisposing childhood experiences: Tania was brought up in an environment dominated by oppression, fear, and anger. At a very young age, Tania was warned about "scandalizing" the young and the vulnerable. She was given the message that to scandalize them would be despicable. Tania's father had fluctuating moments of depression, intense anger, and irritability and of love and care for her. His anger dominated the mood of the home.

Family relationships were dominated by compliance and obligations with limited allowance for individualized thoughts, feelings, and behaviors. Compliance with church teachings was communicated by Tania's teachers, church officials, and by her mother's adherence to the messages from church officials. The sense of obligation to protect the young and weak from moral and psychological harm was imposed upon Tania by her teachers, clergy, and mother. In a sense, Tania became a "parental child" (Minuchin & Fishman, 1981, p. 54). That is, she assumed the role of a protective parent to the "less strong" at a very young age.

In brief, she became preoccupied (i.e., predisposed) to live correctly for others, felt guilty when she failed to live up to these standards, and felt obligated to protect the young and weak from moral and psychological harm. She complied with the social expectations and restrictions. Her needs as a child and adolescent were not respected nor validated.

Pertinent internalizations: Tania internalized her childhood interactions with parents, teachers, and church officials, to form her psychic structure, self-structure, quality of emotional bonding, the nature of her coping strategies, the quality of object constancy, and relational dynamics and patterns. The internalizations paralleled and reflected her experiences of her interactions with parents, teachers, and church officials. These internalizations and behaviors were shaped by the way Tania's childhood relational, self, and physical intimacy needs were not validated and responded to.

Regarding her psychic structure, it was skewed toward having unrealistic expectations of self, being prematurely obligated to protect others from moral and psychological harm, being hard on herself, being prone to guilt feelings when failing to meet others' and self-imposed standards (e.g., superego), negating her own needs so as to be accepted as being a good person and receive the favors of authoritative figures, and coping with conflicts between the demands of others and her own needs by complying with and engaging in the use of ineffective coping strategies. Her psychic structure can be characterized as being overly harsh (Edward, Ruskin & Turrini, 1993) and punitive (Kernberg, 1976) because of imposed standards and behaviors by which to live.

Her self-structure was characterized by Tania thinking that her feelings and needs did not matter (i.e., feeling insignificant), feeling incompetent to deal with her anxieties, and an inability maintain a positive sense of feeling significant and competent. She struggled not to be at fault for causing moral and psychological harm to others, for which, when it happened, she would feel guilty, blame herself, and think that she was a bad person.

Tania failed to form an emotional bond (i.e., emotional anchorage) with her mother that resulted in her being in a state of anxiety and failing to develop a good representation of the relationship to form "object constancy." That is, she did not adequately experience being cherished, admired, and unconditionally loved that would normally lead to Tania cherishing, loving, and admiring herself, which are the foundation of object constancy and self-constancy. Without object and self-constancy, it was difficult for Tania to conjure up a new perspective on an issue and to soothe herself when troubled, emotionally hurt, and anxious.

Her relationships were characterized by dependency and avoidance. She relied on others to reassure her that she was a good person based on her cleansing and checking behaviors. She was inhibited in her relationships and mistrusting of others; she kept her distance. She avoided intimacy and closeness in relationships. She felt intruded upon, which interfered with her own ongoing growth and development, and felt threatened by it. She resented others, to the point of revenge, for constraining her behaviors and imposing their ideas and expectations, which interfered with her developing adaptive behaviors. Such impingements are experienced as threats that can lead to revenge (Guntrip, 1992).

Her unmet childhood needs consisted of a need for safe "emotional anchorage" (i.e., emotional bonding) and "confident expectation" that her needs would be validated and responded to, autonomy to think for herself, competency to deal with life issues and problems, and a sense of significance in having her feelings, thoughts, and needs accepted. Her natural tendency toward developing these competencies (Winnicott, 1965/1981) was not nurtured, validated, and supported.

Precipitating factors and reenactments: Tania was predisposed from childhood to obsess about avoiding to be found at fault by morally and psychologically harming others through bad example and behaviors. When Tania moved from the country to the city, her fear of morally and psychologically harming self and others was intensified and extended to her fear of being responsible for avoiding physical harm to others. In the city, she observed nails and broken glass lying on streets and on bicycle/pedestrian paths. This observation exacerbated her fear of being at fault for any harm that might occur by not removing the nails and broken glass. She proceeded compulsively to remove such dangerous items. It appears that her harsh superego with its obligations to protect others from harm, turned into obsessions and compulsions.

In summary, Tania's inner world was characterized by a strong sense of obligation to protect others from harm and to protect herself from being found at fault for the harm. She was prone to guilt feelings, which diminished her self-esteem by thinking that she was a bad person. Her need for emotional connection, significance, and autonomy, of which she was barely aware, were suppressed. She tried, through her compulsive behaviors, to protect herself from being found at fault. These factors contributed to the development of her OCD.

The following chapter presents the treatment of the Tania's OCD. The treatment, which extended over an eight-year period, shifted its focus four times, beginning with her subjective experiences and obsessions and compulsions, and then terminating with her developing real relationships.

References

American Psychiatric Association (1987). *Diagnostic and statistical manual of mental disorders (Third edition revised) (DSM-III-R)*. Washington D.C.

American Psychiatric Association (2013). *Diagnostic and statistical manual of mental disorders (Fifth edition) (DSM-5)*. Washington D.C.

Cashdan, S. (1988). *Object relations therapy: Using the relationship*. New York: W.W. Norton.

Corcoran, K., & Fisher, J. (1987). *Measures for clinical practice: A sourcebook*. New York: Free Press.

Edward, J., Ruskin, N., & Turrini, P. (1993). *Separation-Individuation: Theory and application*. New York: Brunner/Mazel.

Freud, S. (1905). Three essays on the theory of sexuality. *Standard Edition*, *7*, 125–245.

Freud, S. (1923). The Ego and the Id. *Standard Edition*, *19*, 12–63.

Freud, S. (1938). An outline of Psychoanalysis. *Standard Edition*, *23*, 1953, 144–207.

Gibb, G.D., Bailey, J.R., Best, R.H., & Lambirth, T.T. (1983). The measurement of the obsessive-compulsive personality. *Educational and Psychological Measurement, 43*, 1233–1237.

Guntrip, H. (1992). *Schizoid phenomena, object-relations and the self*. New York: International Universities Press.

Kagan, D.M., & Squires, R.L. (1985). Measuring non-pathological compulsiveness. *Psychological Reports, 57*, 559–563.

Kernberg, O. (1976). *Object relations theory and clinical psychoanalysis*. New York: Aronson.

Klein, M. (1935/1975). A contribution to the psychogenesis of manic-depressive states. In M. Klein (Ed.), *Love, guilt and reparation and other works, 1921–1945* (pp. 262–289). New York: Delacorte.

Klein, M. (1948/1975). On the theory of anxiety and guilt. In *Envy and gratitude and other works 1946–1963* (pp. 25–42). New York: Delacorte.

Klein, M. (1959/1975). Our adult world and its roots in infancy. In M. Klein (Ed.), *Envy and gratitude and other works 1946–1963* (pp. 247–263). New York: Delacorte.

Kohut, H. (1977). *The restoration of the self*. New York: International Universities Press.

Mahler, M.S., Pine, F., & Bergman, A, (1975). *Psychological birth of the human infant.* New York: Basic Books.

Meier, A. (1986). Phobic avoidance of confession: Symptomatology, psychological factors, and treatment. In R. Chagnon & M. Viau (Eds.), *Études pastorals: Pratiques et communauté* (pp. 167–191). Montreal: Les Editions Bellermin.

Meier, A., & Boivin, M. (1998). *Treatment changes to compulsive behaviors in obsessive compulsive disorders: A case study using theme-analysis.* Paper presented at the 29th annual meeting of the Society for Psychotherapy Research, Snowbird, Utah, June 24–28.

Meier, A., & Boivin, M. (2022). *Self-in-relationship psychotherapy: A complete clinical guide to theory and practice.* London, UK: Routledge

Minuchin, S., & Fishman, H.C. (1981). *Family therapy techniques.* Cambridge, Mass: Harvard University Press.

O'Toole, M.T. (Ed.) (2022). *Mosby's dictionary of medicine, nursing, and health professionals.* St. Louis Missouri: Mosby imprint of Elsevier.

Robinson, L., Smith, M., & Segal, J. (2016). Obsessive compulsive disorder: Symptoms and treatment of compulsive behavior and obsessive thoughts. Retrieved from www.helpguide.org/articles/anxiety/obssessive-compulsive-disorder-ocd.htm, February, 2016.

Sadock, B.J., Sadock, V.A., & Ruiz. P. (2014). *Kaplan and Sadock's synopsis of psychiatry: Behavioral sciences/clinical psychiatry paperback.* New York: Wolters Kluver.

Winnicott, D. (1960/1965). Ego distortion in terms of true and false self. In D. Winnicott (Ed.), *The maturational processes and the facilitating environment.* New York: International Universities Press, 140–152.

Winnicott, D. (1965/1981). *The family and individual development.* London, UK: Tavistock Publishers.

Chapter 4

Tania

Obsessions and Compulsions: Treatment

The previous chapter presented Tania's psychosocial history and the assessment and conceptualization of her obsessions and compulsive behaviors. The assessment identified Tania's unmet core needs as including the needs for autonomy and significance and as having an emotional connection with a significant other. This chapter presents the treatment of Tania's obsessions and compulsions from the perspective of Self-in-Relationship Psychotherapy (SIRP). Treatment extended over eight years, with six-week breaks for the summers and two-week breaks for Christmas and comprised 400 one-hour audio-taped psychotherapy sessions. The psychotherapy sessions that pertain to obsessions and compulsions, 75 in number, were transcribed and, together with the case notes, provide the material for this chapter.

The therapeutic work was often interrupted by other adversities in her life such as the death of her mother, the separation and divorce of her brother, the suicide of a friend, and a conflict with her employer. The management of these events necessitated temporarily putting on hold the work in uncovering, gaining insight into, and transforming the underlying psychological mechanisms of her obsessions and compulsions, and in developing coping strategies to deal with them more effectively and to relate in a new way with others.

Tania's recovery from her obsessive thoughts and compulsive behaviors began by her accessing and accepting her feelings and core needs, which were repressed. This was followed in turn by reworking her representations of others and her psychic- and self-structures, developing effective coping strategies and assertive skills. With these changes and gains in her inner resources, Tania began to address her compulsive behavior.

This chapter is divided in two parts. The first part focuses on the goal, orientation, and therapeutic relationship and the second part addresses the recovery from obsessions and compulsions, which constitutes the major part of this chapter.

DOI: 10.4324/9781032655291-6

Goals and Orientation of Treatment and Therapeutic Relationship

Goals of Treatment

The treatment comprised principal and subsidiary goals (Meier & Boivin, 2022). The principal goal was to help Tania uncover and reclaim her unmet core needs for autonomy, significance, and emotional connection; reorient her life according to these needs; be the agent of her own life; free herself from her obsessions and compulsions; and establish genuine and meaningful relationships. The task for Tania was to link her current obsessions and compulsions to her unmet core needs for autonomy, significance, and emotional connection and realize that these needs were subverted by ineffective defense mechanisms, coping strategies, and relational patterns, and were disguised by her defensive behaviors to prevent psychological and moral harm to the young and vulnerable.

The subsidiary goals, which were keyed to the principal goal, comprised the following: (a) to access, name, and accept her bodily felt experiences and to identify and accept her unmet core childhood and growth needs; (b) to rework her psychic structure to bring about greater harmony among its agencies by empowering the ego, giving more voice to the inner child, and softening the demands and expectations of the internal critic; (c) to develop object constancy to which she could turn to gain new perspectives and regulate her feelings and needs; (d) to distinguish between obligations and responsibilities and to live more from responsibilities than from obligations; (e) to develop self-directed behaviors and become autonomous in her thinking and decisions; (f) to develop relational skills that foster mutual respect, trust, care, and acceptance; and (g) to develop the skill and courage to assert her needs, feelings, and thoughts.

An assumption of SIRP is that to treat long-standing emotional problems, it is necessary to bring about transformation of the person's "internal working model" (Bowlby, 1988), that is, to transform the psychic- and self-structures, which together with external factors, influence all behaviors and interactions. These internal transformations generally lead to new interactions and behaviors. However, some might need help in translating the transformations into a new way of being. A second assumption of SIRP is that persistent psychological and behavioral problems represent compensatory and/or defensive behaviors that partially secure the core needs not met in childhood. To resolve the emotional problems, it is necessary to access the unmet core needs and find ways to have them realized. These transformations and behavioral changes are accomplished through the exploration of the problem, through gaining insight, and through translating insight into new behaviors and interactions (Meier & Boivin, 1984, 1987b, 1992).

Therapist Orientation and Techniques

The therapist (A.M.), male, European Canadian, a doctoral-level trained clinical psychologist and psychotherapist, worked full-time at a university graduate psychotherapy department, and had a part-time private clinical practice. His psychotherapy was guided by constructs from SIRP, a Self-Discovery Approach to Counselling (Meier & Boivin, 1987a), the Seven-Phase Model of the Change Process (SPMCP; Meier & Boivin, 1992), and by techniques from selected theoretical orientations.

The therapist used the basic attending skills, empathic responses, and summaries to address the client's implicit and explicit messages (Ivey, 1983), and "linking" statements to connect various facets of the client's current experiences (e.g., cognitions, affects, and motives), behaviors, and relational patterns to the client's past experiences (Meier & Boivin, 2000, p. 61). The therapist used advanced techniques such as Experiential Focusing (Gendlin, 1996) to help Tania uncover her deeper lying feelings and needs; Gestalt Two-Chair (Perls, 1969) to resolve intrapsychic conflicts; and Task-Directed Imagery (TDI; Meier & Boivin, 2011) to engage her in new behaviors, and bodily awareness exercises to conjure up psychological material for therapy. TDI, which became the primary technique used in therapy, allowed Tania to access and address her feelings and developmental injuries according to her capacity to tolerate them.

Therapeutic Relationship

The therapist was actively engaged in the therapeutic process, worked in the "here and now," and constantly checked back with the client to assess what she was experiencing and processing, particularly when she became silent and demonstrated changes in behavior, tone of voice, and mood (Meier & Boivin, 2000). He provided a safe and secure environment to help Tania access and express her inner experiences. He balanced nudging and nurturing the client (Mahler et al., 1975).

Tania's expectation in coming to therapy was for her to talk to the therapist and for him to "fix" her as one fixes a broken arm. During the first 100 sessions, Tania was reticent to address and talk about her subjective experiences, which she wanted to talk about but could not. When she left the therapy sessions, she would be frustrated and angry with herself for saying nothing and for making it difficult for the therapist, who tried to have her talk (316: 358). However, the therapeutic relationship changed after the first 100 sessions and was characterized by collaboration, responsiveness to the therapist's interventions, and by the client's increased motivation to change.

Path to Recovery from Obsessions and Compulsions

Since Tania began therapy highly constricted and reticent to disclose her inner experiences, the first phase of therapy focused on helping Tania access, own, and express her private feelings, thoughts, and needs. The second overlapping phase focused on transforming her internal representations of self and other. This was followed by reworking her psychic structure and identifying and accepting her unmet core needs. Fourth, Tania was helped to develop more effective coping strategies and assertive skills. These changes prepared Tania to work through her obsessions and compulsions and to express her thoughts, feelings, and needs assertively and genuinely in her relationships.

This part of the chapter addresses three major aspects of the therapy, which are Tania getting in touch with her inner experiences; transforming her inner world; and developing more effective coping and assertive skills. The numbers in brackets refer to session numbers and line numbers. The numbers to the left of the colon represent the session numbers, and the number(s) to the right represent the line numbers. When only one number is given, it represents the session. When the range in line numbers is great (e.g., 25–37), it indicates that the material was taken from that section.

Accessing, Accepting, and Validating Inner Experiences

At the beginning of therapy, Tania was not in touch with her inner life that included her feelings, thoughts, and her core needs. In order to achieve any success in overcoming her obsessions and compulsions, it was deemed necessary to help Tania identify and work through the barriers that kept her from freely accessing her inner life, beginning with her feelings. At first, she dismissed her feelings, then after some nudging, she began to accept them and considered them to be part of life.

Accessing her inner experiences

During the first year, therapy was labored as Tania was constricted, fearful, and reticent to offer psychological material to work with. She experienced great difficulty in accessing her feelings and expressing them, particularly her feelings of anger toward parents, school, and church officials who she felt had contributed to her problems (16:187). She felt like a captive in her own feelings that had a choking grip on her (17: 115, 153). She presented with a psychic structure that was skewed toward an overly harsh and demanding internalized parent, a fearful and needy inner child, and an inability to integrate the demands of the internalized parent and the needs of the inner child.

Feeling vulnerable and fearing to be exposed and judged (33), Tania was reticent to describe her compulsive behaviors. She felt that what she had to say "seemed stupid and silly" (2: 105) and that her fears inhibited her from doing what she wanted (2: 171).

A major therapeutic goal was to help Tania pay attention to her inner experiences, bring them to light, and to accept them, particularly her feelings, thoughts, and needs. This process met with long periods of silence during the first year, with some periods of silence accounting for 45 minutes of the one-hour sessions.

To help Tania access her inner experiences, the therapist used exercises such as "bodily awareness" and Experiential Focusing (Gendlin, 1996). The subject matter for these exercises was Tania's difficult interactions that she experienced during that week. In the therapy sessions, she was asked to replay an actual conversation that took place earlier in the week with a coworker or friend using the Gestalt Two-Chair technique and to experiment with responses that reflected her true feelings, thoughts, and needs (5: 222–225). These exercises generated material for therapeutic work and facilitated the transition from bodily awareness to psychological awareness.

Struggle to accept and express feelings

After many sessions using "bodily awareness" exercises, Experiential Focusing, and the Gestalt Two-Chair technique, Tania became more keenly aware of her feelings and core needs, but she continued to struggle to accept and express them. Her demanding and harsh internalized critic strongly devalued and prohibited the expression of feelings, thoughts, and needs. The goal of therapy at this point was to break the alliance between her internalized demanding and overly harsh internalized critic and the enfeebled ego, and to help her accept the fact that feelings and needs are part of being human. She continued to fight against their acceptance.

Regarding the difficulty of accepting and expressing her feelings, she tended to dismiss them, making statements such as "I want to be angry but I tell myself: you can't be angry, so forget about it" (5: 31–32); "it won't make any difference whether I'm angry or not. It still won't solve the problem so I might as well not get angry" (5: 47–48); and again, "there was nothing gained in being angry and blaming others, it's a waste of time, just get rid of the problem" (4: 208, 217, 235). She was angry at her parents, the school, and the church that imposed their rules on her and contributed to her obsessions (16:187). She felt that all of them came from the same system "with a million rules and regulations. All lived for security. There was nothing else" (3: 182–183). At times she felt like "slamming" her fist through something (3:140), and at the same time felt that she had no right to express her anger as they meant well and were probably right (3:177; 4: 151).

With regard to expressing her feelings, Tania feared that if she were to express them, she would be judged and thought to be crazy (7: 101). She decided that it was useless to express her feelings and therefore it was best to forget about them (7: 25; 16: 187). When nudged as to what she wanted to say to that which was keeping her from expressing her feelings, her response was mixed. On the one hand she would say, "leave me alone, and then talk about what I want to talk about. But forget it, because I can't. I just can't (7: 38–42), and on the other hand she felt that she "Would start to improve. They couldn't get any worse; they have to improve but it still doesn't make any difference" (7: 89–92). She continued with her internal struggle, saying that one cannot "do anything about feelings, if something happens, then you react to it" (5: 61–64), but one can "do something about our emotional reactions" (5: 67–68). Guilt was an added factor that kept Tania from expressing her feelings, such as anger, as she feared that she might hurt someone (22: 177; 39: 187–194; 247: 325–327). The fear of being judged and her guilt kept her locked in a psychological cage (5: 258–261; 265).

Tania did not learn in her childhood how to deal effectively with anger. She learned to deal with her anger by sulking when she did not get what she wanted (247: 340–341). It was her way to let the others know that she was angry and to get back at them (40: 187–197).

After much work about the role of feelings in one's life, Tania came to realize and accept that feelings do matter (5: 270; 22: 35–37), that feelings "have a place of their own" (22: 51–52) and are more natural and relaxing when integrated (22: 64–68). She experienced at the same time how a "little built-in voice" was telling her how she should behave and not behave (228: 156). She sensed a shift in that the "objective self (i.e., ego) was getting a little stronger" (226: 165) although the other voice (i.e., superego) continued to pressure her to be like others, particularly her parents. Toward the end of therapy, Tania summarized how, at the beginning of therapy, she was not "able to acknowledge [her] feelings at all" and "knew that they were there" but she "did not know how to name them," and she believed that "her feelings did not matter and had no bearing on anything" (344: 51–55).

Transforming Internal Representations of Others and Self

In her interactions with the members of her family and church officials (i.e., clergy), Tania, as a child, pre-adolescent, and adolescent, developed cognitive and affective representations of them and of herself. Tania's initial representation of these authority figures was that they judged her and imposed self-made rules, which were to be followed (43; 44). During therapy, Tania's representations of mother, church, and God changed from idealizing and fearing them, to seeing them as persons with their own feelings, needs, thoughts, and struggles (Klein, 1959). The internalized representations served two functions, namely, as a schema through which information was processed and as agents that influenced her interaction with others and self.

Representation of her mother

Tania was brought up to believe that her mother and her family "were all saints" and perfect (4: 287). Her mother looked at the good side of others' characters and avoided looking at their negative qualities; she made them out to be someone who they were not. Tania wanted her mother to see her as she was and not as someone she was not (140). Both as a child and as an adult, Tania was not able to maintain her sense of self when with her mother, but regressed to the earlier infantile and estranged state and felt cut off and alone (142).

Although she wanted her mother to be perfect, she resented her for being perfect (73). She found it "difficult to live up to [her] standard" of perfection (4: 297). Even when Tania held the same thought as her mother, Tania could not agree with her because she did not want her mother to impose her ideas on her (140). Tania wanted to have a better relationship with her mother by being more open and real, but realized that it was her negative attitude toward the mother's black and white thinking that kept this from happening (136).

During therapy, Tania was delighted to gradually discover that her mother and her mother's family were not saints and not perfect and that they could stand being corrected (4: 287; 74). Tania became aware that the representation that she developed of her mother derived from the way she processed information which did not correspond to reality (74). Knowing that her mother was not perfect, brought about a sense of relief and softened her black and white thinking (73).

Representation of church and its officials

Tania's childhood impression of church officials, an impression that continued into adolescence and adulthood, greatly influenced the development of Tania's obsessions and compulsions. She viewed church officials as being conservative, dictatorial, punitive, and oppressive and focused on fear and demon presence (324). She particularly resented church officials for telling women how to dress (256) and saying that men were superior to women (263). She resented them for taking away her autonomy and her right to have her own thoughts and to express them freely (299).

Tania was also angry at the church because it stood in the way of her having a relationship with God. To help Tania express her resentment toward the church and to arrange for her to have a relationship with God without going through the church, the therapist designed a monologue exercise where she was asked to express her feelings toward the church. The therapist placed three chairs in a straight line, with Tania sitting in the first chair (nearest to the therapist), the church in the middle chair, and God in the far chair. Tania was asked how she felt with the church blocking her from having direct contact with God and what she could do about it. She responded that she could not change the church. She felt stuck in knowing what to do. The therapist then asked Tania to move her chair to the right to bypass seeing the church and to make direct contact with God, which she did. She felt bad in bypassing the church in order to have what she wanted.

During therapy, she became more tolerant of the narrow thinking of the clergy (324) and gradually developed the freedom to express her own ideas, although the experiences of the past tended to hold her back (300). As her "objective self [became] stronger" and as the "little built-in voice" that told her how to behave diminished, she began to change her representation of the church and of church officials (226: 165; 228: 156). She also became aware that the representations that she formed of the church and its officials was a product of how she took in the information rather than how they might have been (74). This awareness brought with it a sense of relief and a change in her black and white thinking (73).

Representation of God

Tania was brought up to view God as an old, stern, gray-haired, and demanding man wearing glasses so that He could better see His records of each person's faults (92; 238). He was someone who was perfect, demanding, exacting, and saw things in black and white. She felt cold toward Him and thought that He was revengeful toward her (83). She feared that God would scold her, be against her, and demand that she report all her faults accurately (95). In not conforming to His wishes, she feared that she would be judged and punished (194). She felt that she had no right to be angry at Him as He meant well and when bad things happened, it was not His fault (40: 172–175).

Despite her negative view of God, Tania wanted to think of God as being generous, friendly, loving her unconditionally, and accepting her for who she was (95). It was difficult for her to believe that His love was without conditions (96). She felt that she and God were caught in an unresolvable situation because she and God wanted different things and she could not give up her need to do her own thing and to let go of her ideas and manner of doing things. Her challenge was how to reconcile a loving and caring God with her freedom to be herself. She felt pressured to conform to His way even if He was loving and caring.

Tania, however, expressed her sincere wish to change her image of God. She had two views of God, one who judges and one who cares. To help her reconcile the two images, the therapist designed a three-chair exercise, with one God in a chair to her right and a second God in a chair directly in front of Tania, who was in the third chair. Tania was asked to describe her images of the two Gods. She described the God to her right as the One who watches and judges her and becomes displeased and angry when asked questions. This image of God represents the rules, sayings, and teachings given to her by others. The God directly in front of her, watched her but was caring and compassionate. When asked what she wanted to do with the God on her right, she said she wanted to discard Him, which she did by pushing away the chair and turning her back to it. Following the exercise, she mentioned that she felt relieved and comfortable with her new perception of God (101).

In addition to the imagery work, Tania's encounter with nature was also instrumental in changing her image of God. Being an outdoor person, she appreciated her sense of oneness with nature and associated God with this experience. She knew that God was the author of nature and of her. Since God is the author of nature and of her, and since nature is good, she perceived herself to be good as well (101). This awareness changed not only her view of God but also her view of herself and of others. This changed image of God brought about a bodily felt sense of relief, she had more energy, became more tolerant of others, and was more hopeful about herself. She experienced this "newness" as something "sacred," permanent but fragile, and that helped her connect with a genuine part of herself which had been cut off (100).

Tania observed that as her image of God was changing, she found it "very hard to shake" the old image of God, which was based on fear (229: 48). To help Tania solidify her new image of God, the therapist asked her to take a moment and get in touch with her experience of the new image of God and allow the old image of God to fade away (229: 58–61). After sitting with the exercise for a few minutes, Tania was able to experience God as someone who was present, caring, treated her fairly, embraced her (238), was on her side, and was not all that "complicated" 239). This permitted her to let go of her way of doing things and brought a readiness to compromise. However, in the back of her mind she humorously had the belief that if "you don't behave, God will get you" (228: 117). With regard to the experience of herself, Tania felt relaxed, strong, solid, harmonious, and at peace. This experience represented a significant transformation of her image of God and of herself (102).

Representation of self

At the beginning of therapy, Tania's representation of self was a mixture of feeling helpless, powerless, incompetent, inferior, inefficient, and not as intelligent as others, including her siblings (224). With regard to an image of her sense of being helpless, she saw herself in an open field, hands and feet tied with a rope, and trapped. She felt helpless to untie the rope and set herself free (30). She was brought up to be competitive and felt best when she was at the head of the pack (258).

Another image was that, everywhere that Tania turned, she saw her self being at a dead end, which she compared to being at the bottom of a well. The therapist designed an exercise using as an image being at the bottom of a well, and asked Tania to find her way out. Her first response was that she did not deserve to get out of the well. The therapist, nevertheless, nudged her to find a way out of the well. By bracing her back against the wall of the well and using her feet and hands, she gradually pushed herself to the top of the well.

In succeeding in coming out of the well, Tania felt a sense of relief, and realized that she was able to do it and was responsible for making changes (90). She added that she wanted to stop fearing fear and wanted to spend more energy on doing with confidence what she wanted to do (89). This success and changed view of herself helped her accept herself and others as they were (90). She stopped thinking that everything had to be perfect; she became more tolerant and empathic of others and less depressed. She also learned that taking time for herself was not a waste of time (55: 157–163; 237).

In summary, Tania attributed her initial difficulty to seeing others, God, and self objectively as a "little built-in voice" that informed her how she should behave (228: 156). However, with progress in therapy, the "objective self [i.e., ego] was getting a little stronger" (226: 165), although the other voice (i.e., superego) continued to pressure her to think differently. In due time Tania began to see her mother, the church and its officials, and God as they were and related to them accordingly. She transformed her representations of them.

Reworking the Psychic Structure

The representations that Tania formed of others, the world, and of herself in her relational interactions, became the building blocks for the formation of her psychic- and self-structures and the development of her coping strategies and interpersonal pattens. She struggled to conform to external demands and pressures that diametrically opposed her natural way of being. Her inner world became a reflection of that which occurred between herself and the real outer world, and she was left with the same struggles in her inner world that she experienced in the real world. This section summarizes the origin and nature of the psychic structure, her internal struggles and conflicts, the pressure to be perfect, and the tendency to procrastinate, downsize the superego, and integrate internal demands and core needs.

Origin and nature of the psychic structure

Tania was brought up in a very conservative and restrictive milieu where she learned to shape her life according to the rules, demands, and expectations of others and to put aside her own developmental and growth needs. As a youngster, her mother impressed upon her to be a good example to her siblings, to the kids at school, and later to the community at large (344: 217–219). From her father she received the message that not to work was to be lazy (309). At a church retreat, the clergyman impressed upon her how horrible it is to scandalize and harm the young (191). The concern not to morally and psychologically harm others extended to the compulsion to pick up broken glass and nails from the street so that she would not be responsible if a car drove over them and got into an accident and someone got hurt. The compulsions included removing worms from sidewalks and placing them on the grass adjacent to the sidewalk (344: 227). Tania took on a life that was controlled by rules rather than by a life freely lived (191). Being young, she assumed that life was meant to be that way.

These demands and expectations were internalized to form her psychic- and self-structures. Her psychic structure was characterized by a sense of duty and obligation and the fear of expressing and asserting her feelings, thoughts, and needs that opposed her perceived duties and obligations. In terms of SIRP concepts, Tania's psychic structure was characterized by a dominant and overbearing superego, a terrified and deprived inner child, and an impoverished and an enfeebled ego.

Internal struggles and conflicts

Tania described her internal struggles and conflicts in various terms, such as being pulled in two directions, being of two minds, being torn by two competing inner forces, and as being caught between what she was brought up to believe as being right and what she felt to be correct (260). Regarding the competing inner forces, Tania felt that there was an inner voice (i.e., superego) that was pushing her to act and behave in a way that went against her grain. For example, there was a bossy, controlling, and impinging part (i.e., superego) (10: 151) that pushed her to check the stove over and over (10: 101) and to repetitively wash her hands (10: 30–31), which she knew to be foolish ,but she could not stop herself from washing them (10: 77–78). There was also a part that resisted the pushes (i.e., inner child), but the controlling part was overwhelming and imposing. She experienced the internal fight and tried to convince herself that it was foolish to give in to the compulsions but to no avail (10: 177). For Tania, it was "easier to go along with the compulsion and then forget it [rather] than to have it bugging [her] in the back of [her] mind" (10: 193–194). In complying with the irrational force, she was able to forget it for a few minutes and have a sense of relief (10: 27; 193–194).

Pressure to be perfect

Part of Tania's internal struggle was pushing herself to be perfect and to do worthwhile activities. When she engaged in pleasurable activities, she felt guilty and neutralized them by engaging in meaningful activities. She was not able to balance work and play (251). She felt pressured to be organized and do things according to a proper order, which she resented as she wished to become more spontaneous and go with the flow and rhythm of life (125). She resented her internal pressures as they brought about feelings of being scattered, overwhelmed, irritable, and depressed (127). Although she struggled with the internal pressures, she came to the realization that it was not important to be perfect in everything, particularly if it is going to create tension and keep one in a rut and "feel[ing] like a tin soldier" (55 142–146). Rather than feeling pressured to do things, Tania was determined to learn and make every effort to live each moment as it presented itself (322).

Tendency to procrastinate

Another aspect of her internal struggle was striving for an ideal only to discover that she could not live up to the ideal. Failure to live up to the ideal was followed by engaging in procrastination, feeling guilty, and being depressed. Tania's procrastination began when she was in junior high school and resisted doing her homework until the last minute. She hated schoolwork (230: 239). She sensed that she was telling the "inner kid" to do the homework, but the child resisted (230: 292). Tania linked her tendency to procrastinate to being torn between her internal demands and her needs, and with her following the least desired path, which was to do her homework. Tania became aware of her rebellion against doing things, which was a revelation to her and which she had denied in the past. In becoming aware of her rebellious attitude, Tania added that "it's amazing, it's a great relief" (230: 374; 231).

Downsizing the superego

During therapy, many attempts were made to downsize the strength of the demanding and internalized critical parent and give greater voice to the inner child. Initially these attempts were not successful since the internal parent was so dominant and imposing. In one such failed exercise using the Gestalt Two-Chair technique, Tania named one part the Bully Part and the other the Weak Part. The two attitudes were at loggerheads and refused to budge (29).

In an imagery exercise, Tania was asked to externalize her internal dialogue, which was between what she called the reasonable one and the dictator. Tania experienced two different sets of feelings depending on whether she spoke from the position of the reasonable one or from the position of the dictator. The dictator did not want to be pushed out and felt that the reasonable one did not want her around anymore, which the reasonable one confirmed to be the case. The dictator offered to share control, but the reasonable one declined, fearing that those were only words. The two sides remained locked in a black and white battle (164). In a second imagery exercise, Tania felt an enormous inner struggle, with her being cut off by a "stone wall" (11:107) that she could not get around, crawl over, or circumvent. The stone wall was saying to her, "I gotcha" (11: 123) and "why don't you give up, you'll 'never get to the other side'" (11:144). Metaphorically, the wall represented the demanding internal parent, and the other side represented the inner child. At this moment, she did not have the ego resources to resolve the conflict and integrate the differences.

Harmonizing core needs and internal demands

As Tania strove to bring about harmony between the internal forces, she expressed sadness in being taught things that she no longer believed in but that continued to influence her feelings and thoughts. After reflecting on the things that she no longer believed in, she stated that she would like to throw the following into a barrel: (1) the thought that the human body is bad; (2) the idea that sex is evil; (3) the thought that women are responsible for men's sexual temptations; and (4) the idea that God is out to get her. She considered the last as the main wrong idea that she was taught (212). According to Tania, these beliefs, which went against her nature and from which she tried to liberate herself, were taught by a church that was punitive and authoritarian (263).

She attributed her difficulty to seeing things objectively to a "little built-in voice" that said how she should and should not behave (228: 156). However, the "objective self [became] a little stronger" (226: 165), even though the other voice continued to pressure her to comply with the expectations of others (228: 192, 204, 260). As Tania progressed in therapy, she became more determined to bring about harmony between the external demands and the core needs. Whereas in the past she had felt torn and stressed because of the conflicts between her demands and core needs, she gradually became more focused and pursued one direction. She stated, "before I would be so stressed out that I'd be trying to do one thing but my mind would be somewhere else" (264: 187). Her thinking shifted to her believing that she was "not responsible for everything anymore" (344: 271–274) as she could not "possibly control everything" (344: 282). She gradually let go of feeling obligated without feeling guilty (264: 275). Tania found it helpful to talk about her inner struggle as she "had to think about it" (344: 288); she stopped having things "going around in her head"; and at the same time "it was out there, it was not totally inside anymore" (344: 297). Gradually Tania toned down the unrealistic expectations that she had of herself (301). An important experience for Tania was her reflecting on her inner conflict and on its ensuing awareness, which she described this way: "I got in touch with me, sort of as if I was a child and I got in touch with what this little person wanted" (316: 318). This experience made a big difference for her and it brought things into a "sharp focus" (316: 322).

Identifying and Accepting Unmet Childhood Needs

Tania indicated that in becoming aware of what she wanted, she was helped to resolve her internal conflict. Beginning around the 75th session, Tania began to recognize and to accept her unmet childhood needs, which were the need for emotional connection, the need for competency, and the need for personal space. As indicated earlier, unmet core childhood needs differ from unmet growth needs. The former represent needs that were not satisfied during childhood and continue to yearn for satisfaction, whereas the latter represent needs that were met in childhood but are not being met in adult relationships.

Need for emotional connection and inclusion

At the beginning of therapy, Tania struggled to acknowledge and to accept her need for emotional connection, with one part (i.e., superego) discounting her needs and urges, and another part (i.e., inner child) craving to be taken care of (8: 79, 84). To help her to understand her need to be taken care of, the therapist asked her for an image to illustrate this need. She responded, "I would like to be five years old forever; then I wouldn't have to do anything. I wouldn't have to think. I wouldn't have any responsibilities. I would be free" (8: 94–100); "I could do what I want within reason, have no worries, don't have to make any decisions; everything would be done for me" (8: 104–105). Tania acknowledged that she was not able to return to the state of a five-year old, but she wanted some kind of compromise between wanting "somebody else to give [her] all the answers so [she didn't] have to do any thinking at all and feel responsible for everything" (8: 203–204). In being taken care of, she would feel at home, safe, and comfortable (320). But she immediately discounted it, saying that it was not possible (8:205).

Much later in therapy, Tania acknowledged her need for acceptance and inclusion. She stated, "I would like to accept myself and be able to feel that others would accept me like I am without always having to feel that I have to change" (77: 90–92). She was tired of "being on guard" and "afraid to let people know who [she was]" (77: 97–98).

Gradually Tania began to acknowledge her need for close and intimate relationships and to be more demonstrative of her feelings (206). In the past she had felt content to do things with friends, but this changed to her wanting to have friends with whom to share intimate feelings, needs, and ideas. She wished to be able to live with someone (246).

As Tania developed close relationships, she became concerned as to whether she was "expecting too much out of some relationships" and added why it was that she couldn't "just let things be?" (316: 74–75). When Tania felt stressed in a relationship, it was related to her not saying what she wanted to say. When she was "more centered" and "more in tune" with herself, relationship issues were not a major concern (316: 78–80). Regardless of the situation, Tania found it risky to get close to others for fear that they would get to know her and reject her (234). Nevertheless, Tania wanted to be able to anticipate relational difficulties to prepare herself to deal with them (319).

Tania became aware that not only did she have a craving for a close relationship with others, but she also had a craving to be present to herself and to feel at home with herself. She brought it around that when she was in her apartment, she would feel at home with herself (268).

Need for competency

Tania struggled with feelings of inadequacy and incompetency. She felt that she was less adequate than others in coping with stress, anxiety, and depression (235). When with others socially, she did not know what to talk about and felt inferior to them, inadequate, and less intelligent. She related her feeling of being inferior to a grade seven experience in thinking that her teacher and mother found her to be stupid as she had difficulty with mathematics (393).

Tania expressed her desire to live more from her thoughts, feelings, and needs and to break away from the deeply ingrained habit of listening to others. When in a meditative state, Tania sensed that others were just as insecure as she was and that they were influenced by the outside in the same way that she was. This helped her see herself as an equal to others (137). Tania gradually learned to believe that she was as competent as others. She observed that when she accepted roles of responsibility, she did succeed. She realized how her belief that she was incompetent affected how she felt about herself and her actions (224).

Need for personal space

In the past, Tania had compromised her need for psychological and physical space and privacy. When she lacked the required psychological and physical space, she felt "boxed in" (265: 95) and resentful, which she repressed, reasoning that she did the right thing in not asserting her needs, although her heart fought against it. The resentment was expressed in her obstinacy and desire to retaliate (289).

For a good part of her life, Tania had been living an ideal given to her early in life, and she came to realize that the ideal was impossible to achieve. In trying to achieve the ideal, her life narrowed in on her and she became burdened and lost the space to grow. She rediscovered herself and wanted to be more real. In being herself, she felt unburdened and that life was open for her to live. She needed the space to grow and expand her energies (114).

Toward the end of therapy, Tania summarized her dilemma in taking care of the needs of others and taking care of her needs. On the one hand, she felt obligated to take care of the needs of others and felt selfish if she did not attend to their needs, and felt guilty if she attended to her needs before the needs of others. On the other hand, she felt resentful in giving up her needs and attending to those of others (176). Tania realized that in taking care of her own needs, she felt content, at peace, liberated, creative, and more in touch with herself and had more to give to others (349).

Developing Effective Coping Strategies

Tania's strategies to cope with internal and external conflicts included avoidance, rationalization, undoing, displacement, and acting-out behaviors. She mentioned that if there was something that upset her, she would put it aside. She described it this way: "I decided not to think about it; granted you can't push it out of your mind forever, but there's times when I can't do anything about it, but I would be thinking about it all the time" (40: 20–22). She realized that pushing it out of her mind served no purpose for her (12:132–133).

Another way that she dealt with problems was to look at them rationally and undo the feeling from the problem. She thought that "there must be a rational way, a way that you can do this in your head without getting involved" (12: 65). When Tania got upset, she felt guilty and it seemed to her like "kicking up a fuss about nothing which seemed like a waste of time" (12: 152–155). Thus, it was better to keep it rational (12: 167).

Prior to psychotherapy, when she felt frustrated or was emotionally hurt by another person, she tended not to express her feelings toward that person but would displace them onto another person or object. For example, she attended a presentation where the presenter mentioned that no one has a right to be angry at God. This angered her, and the following day she released (i.e., displaced) her anger onto her boss (153).

Rebelling was another coping strategy. When Tania was young and did not get her way, she would kick up a fuss. When she got her way, she would not accept it as it was her way to rebel against her mother. She continued to feel the same way today. That is, if she fought hard to have something, she does not want it (12: 200–210).

To take revenge for the bad things that happened to her, Tania secretly took delight when bad things happened to good people. For example, in the case of her coworker who lost her spacious office to a senior worker, Tania was able to "empathize with her and at the same time she was glad that she lost her [office]" (77: 19–20).

During therapy, Tania became aware of her coping strategies, which were characterized by her not being honest with herself and not being open, direct, and honest with others. This awareness came as a shock to her and upset her, and at the same time she experienced a sense of freedom in knowing it. She recognized the origin of her difficulty in being true to herself and to others and expressing her thoughts, feelings, and needs. This discovery helped her be more open to others' opinions and freed her to express her own. She preferred to be wrong in an honest way than to go along with something that she did not believe in (67).

Development of Assertive Behaviors and Competencies

A significant component of SIRP is to help clients develop the competencies and social skills to integrate their newly gained insights, transformations (e.g., psychic structure; representation), and identified core needs into their daily living (Meier & Boivin 1998; 2011). To provide Tania with opportunities to achieve these goals, the therapist designed several imagery exercises. These exercises brought to light the hidden difficulties in asserting herself and at the same time provided opportunities for Tania to assert herself and to experience herself in a new way. This therapeutic work took place, in part, in conjunction with addressing her obsessive thoughts and compulsive behaviors. The topics of this section are: facing barriers to asserting herself; creating opportunities to feel empowered; and being assertive with others.

Barriers to self-assertiveness

Within the context of verbal psychotherapy and the results from the imagery exercises, Tania reported several barriers that stood in the way of her being assertive. First, Tania feared to venture out, to leave that which was comfortable, and to pursue her autonomy and independence. In an imagery exercise, she pictured herself as sitting on a mound and not wanting to leave for fear of getting hurt and drifting afoot (31). A part of her said, "I can't do it; what will happen if?" (32: 82–83).

Second, Tania did not trust her own feelings and opinions and overly relied on the opinions of others. She wanted to "have someone tell her what to do, to look after her and tell her that she does not have to worry about anything" (54: 85–87). Tania tended to trust the opinions of others even if she did not agree with them (54: 190).

Third, Tania had a need to please others even when this went against her nature (131), which was a revelation to her (291). She became aware of a set of assumptions that influenced her: (a) that good girls and good people do not say no to others when asked to do something; (b) that saying no to someone is not being a good person; and (c) that if one is nice to others, one will be liked. To put her needs ahead of those of others engendered feelings of guilt (210).

Fourth, Tania lacked courage to assert herself. In an imagery exercise she was asked to imagine being stuck and then freeing herself from it. In freeing herself, she became aware that it was her lack of courage that kept her stuck. When she became unstuck, she sensed that a load had been lifted from her shoulders and she experienced a mastery of her situation (138).

Fifth, Tania felt inferior to others and intimidated by them. Tania was asked to imagine being with a friend and feeling equal to the person. She visualized herself feeling free in an open space in front of an ocean and being equal to her friend (352). Tania was asked to accept and internalize this experience.

Creating opportunities to feel empowered and be assertive

At given points in therapy, the therapist created opportunities for Tania to acquire the ability to deal with her internal struggles and burdens that enslaved her. Two of the exercises are summarized here.

THROWING AWAY THE CRUTCHES

The first imagery exercise had as its goal for Tania to experience what it was like to be freed from her sense of obligations and dependency on others and to experience her sense of autonomy and independence. Knowing that Tania enjoyed the outdoors, he asked her to imagine walking in a park with a pair of crutches (which symbolized being burdened by external demands). She was asked to walk a distance and then to stop and "throw away" the crutches and experience what it was like not to have the crutches to lean on (54: 270–305). Her first response was that she needed the security of the crutches, but then she challenged the idea, saying that "the security is not worth it. It is too confining" (54: 324). The therapist encouraged her to continue to walk and to repeat to herself that the security was not worth it and at the same to attend to her feelings. To her surprise, she

> felt a lot freer, could breathe easier, felt more confident of herself, had more energy, felt more in control, felt that she can do what she wanted to do even if people did not agree with her, she could be more assertive, and was more open-minded to what others say. (54: 318–359)

The tossing aside of the crutches had an enormous impact on Tania. First, it "dawned on her" (55: 397) that her subjective experiences (e.g., feelings) mattered and with this came a "burst of energy," an experience that she owned. Second, the tossing aside of the crutches was a confidence builder and an enabler. In the past she feared to do something new as it might go wrong, which she could not handle. Following this exercise, she stated that "maybe the outcome is opposite to what I want, but I can't live like that; I have to take a chance" (55: 225–226). She then told herself, "Well, if things turn out not the way I wanted them to, I can still handle the situation and there is no point in getting all steamed up" (55: 229–230).

For Tania, the crutches represented authority (i.e., superego demands) that was bigger than herself. Without wanting to admit it, she saw authority not as helping her but as oppressing her. She could not say that the church was oppressive because this would mean that she was disloyal to the church (55: 435–442). Tania began to think that perhaps it was not the church that was oppressing her, but it was her attitude that was oppressing her. In tossing aside the crutches, Tania "destroyed" her idea that the church was out to destroy; she began to see things differently (55: 464–469).

PUSHING HERSELF OUT OF A WELL

The goal of a second imagery exercise was to offer Tania the opportunity to experience herself being enabled and competent. Tania began the session stating that she felt that she met dead ends everywhere she turned. She compared the dead ends to being at the bottom of a well. Using this image, the therapist designed an imagery exercise whereby Tania was instructed to imagine being at the bottom of a well and at the same time to pay attention to her feelings. She felt that she was not worthy to get out of the well and that there was no way to get out, but she wanted to find a way out. She was instructed to find a way out. In her image she saw herself putting her back against the wall of the well and using her hands and feet, she gradually pushed herself to the top. In being able to bring herself out of the well, she felt that she could do it and experienced a sense of relief. She added that she should not be afraid to become afraid, but spend more energy in doing what she wanted to do and confident that she could do it (89).

In a later session, Tania reported that the exercise in which she pushed herself out of the well changed her thinking about bringing about change. She realized that she was responsible for her change. The fact that she was able to push herself out of the well influenced her thinking in that she knew that she was capable for pulling herself out of a difficult situation (90).

Process in becoming assertive with others

During therapy, Tania acquired new ways to maintain her autonomy and "authority" when relating with others, which were different from the way she was when she was younger. As a teenager she was unwilling to listen to others and always wanted to have the last word. She felt powerless with others, and her way of taking power, which she called "false power," was to take control over a person, which she pushed to overkill as this was safe for her (265: 274). When she did not have the last word, she "sulked and became contrary" and acted out (265: 272). She disliked herself for wanting to have the last word and for acting out. During therapy, things changed. She did not have to have the last word and put up a false front (265: 292–302; 320). She tried to say what was on her mind and regarded others as equals. She no longer had a need to prove herself, and she felt comfortable to be herself and if others could accept her for being that way, that was fine, and if they couldn't, it was their problem. She was able to let herself "be seen and heard" (265: 334).

The following are examples of how Tania changed in the way she related to and became assertive with others, and in the way she brought about greater internal harmony between her sense of obligations and her core needs.

A first task for Tania to become assertive was for her to recognize when she complied with the wishes of others rather than to respond from what she felt was appropriate for her. As an example, Tania agreed to take on a community project only to realize that she accepted it for the wrong reasons, such as not being rejected by others or being displeasing. When she became aware of her motives, she informed those concerned and withdrew from the project (91). This behavior was markedly different from those of the past when she feared expressing her true interests. Now she became more forthright in expressing herself in the presence of others (122).

A second task in becoming assertive was Tania's determination to live more from her beliefs, thoughts, feelings, and needs and to break away from the deeply ingrained habit of complying with the wishes of others. She felt that she could not continue to blame others for what happened in her life as she could do something about it. She also had the sense that others were as insecure as she was and that they were also influenced by the external in the same way that she was. This helped her see herself as an equal to others (137).

A third task was to set limits to the demands of others without feeling guilty. She managed her guilt by putting things into perspective (150). Tania observed that in setting limits and asserting her thoughts, feelings, and needs, there was a willingness on the part of the other to engage in a give-and-take relationship (175).

Fourth, Tania became aware that she made assumptions regarding the motives of others, that she responded to others in terms of her feelings, and that she was not as empathic as she would like to have been. She became committed to become more empathic toward others and to form perceptions of others not based on her feelings but on facts (123).

A fifth task was for Tania to learn how to take care of herself while at the same time to take care of or be present to others. For example, Tana felt stretched by caring for a woman friend who was depressed, demanding, and complaining. Tania discovered that by setting limits to the time spent with her, she was taking care of both herself and of her friend (207). With regard to a visit from her family, Tania took the position that she would be herself, not put on a mask, and not have any expectations of them. She decided to be herself and be with them (221).

In summary, over the course of therapy, Tania tended to become more socially engaged with people, more compassionate toward and accepting of others, learned to set limits, was able to appreciate that a person's behaviors were influenced by past experiences, and understood herself better by understanding others (150; 177). She came to realize that it was better do what she "thought was correct" even if she was wrong rather than to be dependent on someone else (54: 233). She learned that rather than avoid situations, it was far better to be up-front and disclose her thoughts and feelings. In doing so, she felt more genuine and natural, this increased her self-confidence, and she felt like herself and was accepting of herself (243). In the past Tania was often puzzled by her friends telling her to "be yourself." It "dawned" on her now what "people talked about when they said things like be yourself' (230: 388). This was a transforming moment for her and a great relief as it took off the pressure she had felt.

Treatment of Obsessive Thoughts and Compulsive Behaviors

In having accepted her feelings, transformed her representations, reworked her psychic and self-structures, accepted her core needs, and developed more effective coping strategies and assertiveness skills, Tania was prepared to address and resolve her obsessive thoughts and compulsive behaviors and to bring them in line with reality.

Tania's obsessive thoughts entailed the fear of morally and psychologically harming and contaminating others, and her compulsive behaviors included hand-washing, checking behaviors, the picking up of broken glass, nails, and worms from the street, procrastination, and religious practices. The emergence of her obsessions and compulsions seemed to have followed a temporal sequence, which was as follows: first, fear of contaminating, then checking behavior and handwashing, and last, picking up glass and worms, and sorting garbage.

The primary technique used to resolve the compulsions was TDI (Meier & Boivin, 2011, 2022), in which Tania was asked to face her obsessions and compulsions and find a way let go of them. The use of imagery provided Tania an opportunity to develop the belief that she could, in imagery and eventually in reality, let go of her compulsions. The use of imagery also helped Tania have a better grasp of the dynamics (e.g., fears, unmet needs) underlying her obsessions and compulsions. At the termination of therapy, Tania had worked through all her obsessions and compulsions and continued to remain free from them 13 years after therapy terminated.

This section presents Tania's efforts and successes in freeing herself from her obsessive thoughts and compulsive behaviors. The client factors and therapeutic techniques that facilitated this process are briefly described.

Fear of morally hurting others

At the root of Tania's obsessive thoughts and compulsive behaviors was her fear of morally and psychologically harming the young and the vulnerable and of being punished for it. When Tania was ten years of age, she heard a clergyman say that to scandalize (i.e., morally hurt) a little child is a great crime in God's eyes and such a person would be better off having a millstone tied to his neck and being dropped into the sea (226: 211–223; 228: 52; 373). This horrified her and subsequently she became overly conscious about her own behaviors lest she morally hurt others. In addition to the message from the church, Tania's family ingrained in her to be a good example to others including her siblings, peers, and the elderly (226: 211–223). She regretted being taught this as it caused her to focus on the small things and give them too much importance and to make them out to be big issues (228: 47–54).

With messages such as these from church officials and her parents, Tania began to feel obligated not to harm others. To protect herself "from offending God" and to be punished by Him and to avoid being judged by people, she became overly conscientious not to morally or psychologically harm others. Her unreasonable sense of obligation not to harm, led to her many compulsions (228: 102–104). Tania realized that her obsessions and compulsions had a common theme in that the things she worried about were not the real issues (228: 102–104). Gradually, she realized that she was not responsible for protect others in this fashion and she was able to let go of the obsessive thought.

Fear of contaminating people

Tania's obsessions about contamination included people and religious objects (158: 242). Her fear of contaminating people was about passing on germs to them. For example, she feared that when she went to a lady's room, she might have left germs on the faucets and that the germs would be picked up by the next person using the faucet. She struggled against returning to wash the faucets. She said to herself, "Don't do this; please don't do this" (158: 261). After many such repetitions, she finally let go of the fear of contaminating others in this fashion.

Her concern about contamination included sacred objects such as the Good Book (i.e., Bible) (63: 164, 182). When handling the Good Book (Book), Tana had to wash her hands (63: 126) and be careful not to place the Book on something that was dirty and would soil it (158: 271–272, 282). To help her overcome her fear of contaminating the Book, the therapist engaged her in an imagery exercise wherein she was to imagine placing the Book on the arm of the chair as she attended to another activity such as watching television. Initially this was difficult for her as she feared that she had placed the dirty remote control for the television on the arm of the chair and this would contaminate the Book. After a short internal struggle, she experienced a change in her attitude and managed to place the Book on the arm of the chair. The therapist then suggested that she try to integrate the Book into her daily life rather than the reverse. Up until that moment, she had tried to be as perfect as the Book; she had tried to adapt herself to something outside of herself rather than to integrate the Book into her daily life. In the imagery exercise she was able to bring the Book into her daily life and to make it a part of her life. This was a profound experience that changed her attitude about the Book. She felt free and normal after the exercise (182). The thing that helped her most was the therapist suggesting that Tania bring the Book into her world rather than she entering the world of the Book (183). Many sessions later, Tania stated she no longer had a need to treat the Book in a special way (287) and was not compelled to wash her hands before touching it or to place it on a clean surface (316: 185).

Compulsive handwashing

Tania's compulsive handwashing began about five months before she sought therapy (10: 87–90) when she was a member of a charismatic group with some individuals seeing "evil here and evil there" (126: 156). It had its beginning also when she placed the Book on clean places as before that, she "didn't seem to worry about most things like that" (162: 68). Her handwashing decreased with an increase in checking behavior, but increased a hundredfold when her checking behavior diminished (63: 164).

To assess Tania's compulsion to wash her hands, the therapist designed a TDI. She was asked to describe situations where she felt compelled to wash her hands. After she named a few situations (e.g., before going to church), she was asked not to give in to her compulsion to wash her hands. She struggled intensely not to give in, her face turned red, she felt upset, and tears dropped from her eyes. She felt that in not washing her hands, she was not making herself good enough and living up to her unrealistic standards. To negate the difference between how she saw herself and who she wanted to be, she felt a need to cleanse herself, that is, wash her hands. She looked upon her compulsion to wash her hands with a sense of humor, saying that nothing was changed except that she "has cleaner hands and drier hands" (161: 219).

In a subsequent TDI exercise, Tania was asked, as she was about to go to church and partake of the Eucharist service, to think that her hands were clean enough even after touching various things such as doorknobs. As she struggled to achieve the task, she suddenly realized that she "equated dust or anything like that with evil" (162: 134) and that she was "trying to live without a body" (162: 149). The awareness that dust, dirt, and the body are not evil, was a great sense of relief. She added that all the self-talk that she had been doing did "not accomplish what the imagery exercise accomplished for her" (162), that is, dealing with her handwashing.

Tania became aware of what motivated her handwashing. When she felt compelled to wash her hands, she experienced an inner voice, that was connected to the past, as saying, "wash your hands right now" (225: 108). She pictured this voice as being that of her mother, who was fussy about cleanliness. The words that she heard were "you have to be perfect; you have to be good; you have to behave yourself" (225: 130). Tania had the sense that a person was watching her and accusing her of something about which Tania felt guilty (225: 144). In terms what she would like to say to the inner voice, she felt conflicted as one part was saying, "this is ridiculous," and the other part was saying, "but what if" it isn't perfect and you annoy and anger God (225: 204, 209).

Without it being a direct target of therapy, Tania's compulsion to wash her hands began to decrease in frequency during the second year in therapy (55: 187–192; 226: 162–166). By the fourth year in therapy, her compulsion to wash her hands greatly diminished and it was more like normal (223), and by the seventh year in therapy, compulsive handwashing was no longer a problem (247; 287; 373). She was helped to let go of compulsive handwashing by a change in attitude toward dirt. She told herself that if "God created everything, He's not going to be overly upset if I have dirt on my hands" (227: 73–76). She also began to think more rationally and reminded herself that "if God wanted to be one with us, and he did hang out with fisherman, then there had to be dust, dirt and fish" (247: 151–152). Humorously, she stated that she let "God take care of the dirt" (316: 164).

Removing worms from streets

Tania's preoccupation about her avoidance to hurt animals, particularly those not able to take care of themselves such as worms, began during the third year in therapy when she became involved with the pro-life moment (217: 230, 245; 226: 104–108; 245). She associated worms with the helpless unborn fetus (245). She assumed responsibility for assuring that worms did not get hurt. When she saw a worm on the sidewalk or on a pedestrian and bicycle path, she avoided stepping on it, or she would pick it up and put it on the grass (166: 29).

Tania realized that her concerns were irrational, but she had no power over her thoughts (246). Humorously she stated that "if they were a little brighter, they'd go in another direction than on the street" (166: 43). She was less concerned about preventing worms from being killed (166: 178) and "protecting them," but more concerned about not wanting "to see them get hurt and suffer" (166: 178; 227: 209; 247: 266–267; 277: 177), as she would then see this as being her fault. If the worm was dead, it did not bother her; but she would not want to kill a worm (217: 90–104; 226: 60–61).

To help Tania assume responsibility only for the worms that she could potentially hurt, the therapist designed a TDI. She was asked to let go of her responsibility toward worms that was not essential and to maintain a sense of responsibility that was important and describe what this experience was like (166: 240–255). She responded that the imagery exercise helped her think more clearly. When she gets obsessed "with what she thinks is her responsibility, she does not think clearly and finds it easier to do something about it no matter how ridiculous it seems" (166: 262–263). Tania became aware that her worry about the worms was connected "with my being very afraid that I'm going to get in trouble, that God is going to be very angry" (227: 50–51). Eventually she did not feel compelled to pick up worms (287) and stated that the worms "are on their own" (316: 129).

Becoming Autonomous and Assertive with Others

The therapy with Tania progressed through four overlapping foci. The first focus was on helping Tania pay attention to her subjective experiences and accept and validate them as genuine parts of herself. The second focus involved Tania transforming her representations, reworking her psychic structure, and accessing and accepting her core needs. The third focus helped Tania develop more effective coping strategies and assertive skills and ameliorate her obsessions and compulsions. In having become empowered and having worked through her obsessions and compulsions, Tania, in the fourth focus, turned her attention to her external lived world and strove to relate to people in an honest, genuine, authentic, and assertive manner (303).

This section presents Tania's struggles to become assertive with the therapist and with church officials. The technique that was used most frequently to develop assertive experiences and skills was TDI as it provided Tania the opportunity to experience herself in a new, different, and authentic way when relating to real people.

The client–therapist relationship

Beginning in the second year of therapy, Tania became more vocal about her feelings regarding the therapist and the therapy process, which differed drastically from the way she was at the beginning of therapy when she was reserved and withdrawn. Tania was brought up by teachers, church officials, and parents who gave her advice, and she expected the same from the therapist; she expected to be told how to deal with her obsessive thoughts and compulsive behaviors. She stated, "I would like for you to have all the answers and tell them to me" (54: 110–117) and again "Why don't you tell me what is wrong with me?" (63: 50). She felt that the therapist knew the answer but he "won't tell her" and that he was "keeping secrets from her" (63: 88–94). The therapist redirected her questions and statements back to her for her to consider and to explore. This angered her since the therapist in asking her to come up with answers to her questions, disarmed her. In reconsidering her request, she stated that "maybe I don't want you to tell me the answers because I feel better when I figure them out myself" (54: 115).

Tania expressed her doubt as to whether the therapist cared for her and yet was confronted by his caring behavior toward her. She assumed that the therapist expected her to change. The therapist shared with her that he expected her to be honest with herself and that she strive to achieve the goals that she had set out for herself.

Tania from time to time questioned the value of continuing with therapy and felt that she had to do it on her own. She felt that the therapist was trying to convince her that feelings matter, which she was not ready to accept. The therapist commented on his observation of the therapeutic relationship, which was that she had invited the therapist to understand and get to know her. That is, she pulled him toward her and then she pushed him away. She recognized this to be so and laughed about her behavior (71). Although there were times that Tania thought of terminating therapy, she accepted that in coming to therapy, she had a different experience than she had outside of therapy. She also felt that she as a person and what she thought and felt, mattered, and she was being listened to (79).

The clergy and the church

Toward the end of therapy and in 14 consecutive sessions (359–372), Tania expressed her feelings toward the clergy and church officials. Tania observed that the clergyman at the church she attended was very conservative, which reminded her of her childhood experiences. She felt curtailed, treated like a child who could not think for herself, and feared that she would slide into the old way of thinking and the old attitude from which she has progressively tried to free herself (277). When the clergyman was first assigned to the church that she attended, he unilaterally dissolved the church council, which angered Tania and other members of the council. As well, his teaching approach was that of hell, fire, and brimstone, which reminded her of her childhood (365). The clergyman tried to change her thinking, but she refused to give her "heart and soul" over to him (372b). Tania was one of very few who spoke up and stood up to him (355; 356; 371).

In her interactions with the clergyman, Tania became aware that she was settling some unfinished childhood experiences. She also became aware that in the past, she was like the clergyman who thought in black and white terms and was inflexible in her thinking and unwilling to compromise. She became aware that she was projecting her struggles onto the clergyman. Gradually she was able to soften her negative attitude toward him, made compromises, and accepted him for doing things his way (367; 369). When the clergyman left at the end of the year, Tania was happy, but also felt guilty thinking that she won her case against him. The victory was revenge for the things that had happened to her when she was young as the clergyman, like her parents, teachers, and church officials, dominated and controlled her and others (372).

Therapeutic Gains and Changes

This section presents Tania's determination to change her behaviors and to overcome her obsessions and compulsions. It also discusses her reported changes and transformations.

Determination to change her obsessions, compulsions, and behaviors

From the beginning of therapy, Tania intensely wished that she could free herself from her obsessions and compulsions and be able "to make [her] own decisions and judgements without having to depend on somebody else all the time" (9: 78–79). More specifically, she wanted to change her negative attitude, not let herself be influenced by the criticisms and comments of others, and stop making assumptions about the actions and behaviors of others (169).

However, she felt stuck in her old ways, felt hopeless, and thought that it was safer to "stay as you are" (3: 50, 62, 71). She struggled to keep herself motivated to work toward change as she did not "know how to change anything" (9: 53).

Tania was "very tempted to give up trying to change anything, but then [she would] always be curious and wonder, well maybe something would have happened" (9: 62–65). For her, it did not matter that she had a problem or where it came from; rather, what mattered was to get rid of it (4: 208–209). She thought that the only thing she could change was her attitude, but "that's hopeless too" (3: 204–205). Tania added that "it is not easy to change your attitude [i.e., perception] of something. I think that I would have to be brainwashed in the same way that I was brainwashed into the first attitude" (27: 177–184).

Although Tania was frustrated with her slow progress to change, she realized that for change to occur, she had to take responsibility and not blame others or circumstances. She also became aware that she relied on others, and not on herself, for the direction of change (52).

While she had the impression that nothing was happening, she suddenly perceived "results and changes" (55.27). It dawned on her that a human being is valued regardless of how they act; the act does not define the person (55: 38–43). With this major change in her attitude, persons became special to her (55: 82–83). Consequently, Tania saw herself as separate from what she did. In the past, she had viewed herself and others in terms of what they did or did not do (55: 87–94). In seeing herself more as a person rather than as her actions, helped Tania accept herself and others. She also felt that things did not have to be perfect and nor did she have to be controlled and become a robot. Her relationships changed as she felt less intimidated by people and more on the same level as they (55: 300–301).

Reported therapeutic changes and gains

About twice a year the therapist and Tania reviewed the progress of therapy and established mutually agreed-upon future goals. At the same time, Tania reported the therapeutic gains that took place both at the level of her "inner world" and at the level of her "outer world." The changes at the level of the inner world consisted of Tania accepting and validating her inner experiences, transforming her representations, reworking her psychic structure, accessing and accepting her core needs, and developing an attitude toward it being correct to be assertive. The changes at the level of the outer world comprised resolving her compulsions and relating assertively with others. The change process was not linear but cyclical, with relapses that at times discouraged Tania (57–59; 113). Tania reported that by being on the path of making her desired changes, she felt "mentally and physically" healthier than she had ever felt (225: 9–16).

Although Tania would spontaneously report perceived changes through the course of therapy, the major perceived changes were articulated during sessions 128–136, 152, 184, 255, and 344. Briefly, these changes, in the words of the client, are the following: developed a more positive sense of self; responded to her unmet core childhood and growth needs; let go of control; set limits to her availability and learned to compromise; became more assertive by overcoming her paralysis; shifted from feeling obligated to taking responsibility; felt better able to live in and enjoy the moment; became more open and forthright with others and accepting of herself; grew tolerant of the views of others and changed her black and white thinking; became empathic of others and began to see them as they were; became self-determined and self-directed: better able to regulate emotions; diminished compulsive behaviors; and developed a new perception of and relationship with God.

Interventions That Contributed to Transformations and Changes

During the last two therapy sessions, Tania spontaneously offered her perception of the therapeutic techniques and factors that contributed to her changed transformations and changes. These are briefly presented with excerpts from the therapy session.

Techniques and interventions

Tania found the use of questions helpful because they encouraged her to focus on her inner experience, especially her feelings. Being asked to use the pronoun, "I" instead of "You" helped her own her experiences. The Gestalt Two-Chair technique helped her express her feeling and see the perspective of others. TDI helped her get in touch with her experiences as it offered new opportunities to experience herself in a different way. She also found it helpful when the therapist asked her to stay with her feelings "a little while longer" as this developed the courage to be her own person (340; 341).

Relational and self factors

Tania mentioned three self and relational factors that contributed to overcoming her obsessions and compulsions. A first factor was Tania accepting that she had a problem that she needed to deal with. Being intellectually aware that she had a problem was not enough (276: 78–79). She had to reach the point where she had "to be able to accept it as a fact" (276: 89–91). Accepting that she had a problem "freed" her from "hammering herself over the head all the time" (276: 95–96).

A second major factor was Tania's shift in her thinking and attitude from living by rules and regulations to living more from relationships. In living from relationships, there was no fear, but there was love and trust that others would have her best interests at heart. Love and trust were two defining characteristics of her changed attitude. With this change came her ability to relate to and connect in a real way with real people. She added that "maybe now is the time that I strike out on my own, but I feel now I have (struck out on my own) and that I can cope" and that "I'm ready to graduate" (316: 286–287; 294). A major shift was seeing God not as someone out to get her, but as a person who wants to have a loving relationship and who she trusts has her best interest at heart (275).

A third factor was the realization that the therapist believed in her and that she could overcome her obsessions and compulsions. She stated, "I gathered from you, that you believed that I can beat this, that it can be done, that made a big difference" (276: 44–48). This belief was supported by the therapist asking her to perform a task using TDI. An added therapist quality was that she felt supported by him even when he "did not say anything [which] drove [her]crazy as she thought that he had all of the answers" (316: 251–252). With the therapist's support, "she did not feel so alone and even though she was all over the place," when she left the session, she "felt so much more centered and grounded" (316: 254–255). Prior to therapy, she "was going around carrying all these things inside of [her] head and living in a totally different world with all of this junk and nobody knew any of it" (316: 266–268). Another therapist quality was her feeling that he cared for her. However, she struggled with this for many years until a session before leaving for Christmas vacation. As she left the office, the therapist put his arm around her shoulder and in that moment, she felt he cared for her, which made a huge difference for her (340).

In overcoming her obsessions and compulsions, she was left with a vacuum and without direction as to where to turn as she entered new relational and self territories. Gradually she found her way and became involved with church functions taking on a leadership role, took up dancing, pursued her biking, and spent more time with her friends. As well, she began to think in terms of "relationships" more than in terms of "dos and don'ts [and she] felt less boxed in" (276: 66–67). Last, she differentiated between obligations and responsibilities, and felt free to commit herself to activities and to do the things that she wanted to do.

References

Bowlby, J. (1988). *A secure base: Parent-child attachment and healthy human development.* New York: Basic Books.

Gendlin, E.T. (1996). *Focusing-oriented psychotherapy: A manual of the experiential method.* New York: Guilford Press.

Ivey, A.E. (1983). *Intentional Interviewing and Counseling.* Monterey: Ca.: Brooks/Cole.

Klein, M. (1959). Our adult world and its roots in infancy. In M. Klein (Ed.), *Envy and gratitude and other works 1946–1963* (pp. 247–263). New York: Delacorte.

Mahler, M.S., Pine, F., & Bergman, A, (1975). *Psychological birth of the human infant.* New York: Basic Books.

Meier, A., & Boivin, M. (1984). *Phases of the counseling process: Operational criteria.* Unpublished manuscript, Ottawa, Ontario: St. Paul University.

Meier, A., & Boivin, M. (1987a). Self-discovery approach to counseling. *Pastoral Sciences, 6,* 145–168.

Meier, A., & Boivin, M. (1987b*). Manual of operational criteria, coding guidelines and training procedures for the use of the "counseling phases criteria".* Unpublished manuscript, Ottawa, Ontario: St. Paul University.

Meier, A., & Boivin, M. (1992). *A seven-phase model of the change process and its clinical application.* Paper presented at the 8th annual conference of the Society for the Exploration of Psychotherapy Integration, San Diego, California.

Meier, A., & Boivin, M. (1998). *Treatment changes to compulsive behaviors in obsessive compulsive disorders: A case study using theme-analysis.* Paper presented at the 29th annual meeting of the Society for Psychotherapy Research, Snowbird, Utah, June 24–28, 1998.

Meier, A., & Boivin, M. (2000). The achievement of greater selfhood: The application of theme-analysis to a case study. *Psychotherapy Research, 10*(1), 57–77.

Meier, A., & Boivin, M. (2011). *Counselling and therapy techniques: Theory and practice.* London, UK: Sage Publishers.

Meier, A., & Boivin, M. (2022). *Self-in-relationship psychotherapy: A complete guide to theory and practice.* London, UK: Routledge.

Perls, F. (1969). *Gestalt therapy verbatim.* Toronto: Bantam Books.

Part II

Couple and Family Therapy

Chapter 5

Self-in-Relationship Couple and Family Psychotherapy (SIRCFP)

This chapter presents the application of Self-in-Relationship Psychotherapy (SIRP) to couple and family therapy. The approach is called Self-in-Relationship Couple/Family Psychotherapy (SIRCFP).

The distinguishing characteristic of SIRCFP is that it gives primacy to core relational, self, and physical intimacy needs in transforming repetitive negative couple and/or family interactional patterns. Several couple and family therapists have paid attention to relational and self needs. Satir, Banmen, Gerber and Gomori (1991) consider the need for self-worth to be related to the satisfaction of the universal yearning and longing to "be loved, accepted, validated and confirmed" (p. 151). Hendrix (1996, 2008) and Shaddock (2000) theorized that the underlying motivation for all people is the desire for "reliable emotional connection" (p. xiii). Greenberg & Johnson (1988), Greenberg & Goldman (2008), Johnson (2004), and Gottman & Gottman (2008) include attachment needs in their practice of couple and family therapy. However, they do not directly work with attachment needs; rather, they work with the emotions associated with attachment injuries in the context of negative interactional patterns. In summary, the couple and family therapists who include the concept of needs in their theory and practice, limit themselves to the inclusion of self-worth and connection and/or attachment needs.

This chapter begins by presenting SIRCFP's assumptions and principles. This is followed by a presentation of its major constructs, therapy goals, therapy interventions and techniques, the change process, and the role of the therapist. It concludes by describing the practice of couple and family therapy.

Assumptions and Principles of SIRCFP

The assumptions and principles that guide the practice of SIRCFP are derived from the philosophical foundations presented in chapter 10 and from the authors' clinical practice. The following are SIRCFP's major assumptions and principles regarding the practice of couple and family therapy.

DOI: 10.4324/9781032655291-8

1. A family comprises a complex unit of distinctive and unique interactive relationships. Parents have a relationship with each other; they have, as a couple and as individuals, a relationship with each of their children; and each child has a unique relationship with his parents and with his sibling(s).

2. In healthy couple and family living, each person forms a relationship with the others and at the same time strives to be an autonomous and an independent person. A healthy couple and family foster connections and separations, emotional bonding and autonomy, and they strive to find a balance between them.

3. The glue that holds the couple and/or the family together is that each member experiences that their core relational, self, and physical intimacy needs are respected, honored, embraced, and are a significant part of the couple and family life. These fulfilled core needs form the energy for the life of the couple and family.

4. Couple and family problems often occur when an individual's core needs are not respected and do not become part of the couple and family life. A person's relational and self problems often manifest themselves in symptoms and behaviors such as anxiety, depression, anger, somatic complaints, antisocial behaviors, eating disorders, and addictions.

5. A person's inner world (i.e., internal working model) that is formed through his early negative relationships with significant others and through his experiences with the depriving and/or critical and demanding external world, are factors that contribute to individual, couple, and/or family negative interactional patterns.

6. Although the focus in couple and family therapy is on the interactional patterns, it is often necessary to focus on an individual's organization of his inner world, such as his psychic- and self-structures and determine how they contribute to the interactional patterns. Each person lives from two places. He lives from his own strivings and he lives from the expectations of the relationship with his partner and/or the members of the family.

7. The primary agent of change in transforming repetitive negative interactional patterns is the uncovering and naming of the unmet core relational, self, and/ or physical intimacy needs and to have them embraced by the couple and/or family and to orient their relationships accordingly.

8. SIRCFP focuses on the present, on the here-and-now, rather than on the here and there, or on the here and then. It assumes that what is carried over from the past is experienced in the present, and the concerns and worries of tomorrow are also experienced in the present.

9. Psychotherapy is assumed to be a fluid, dynamic, and recursive process. It unfolds in unique ways and finds its own path depending upon the direction given by the core needs of the participants. The therapist follows the leads of the members and helps them achieve their goals. Psychotherapy cannot be programmed, nor can it be designed to follow predetermined steps.

Major Constructs of SIRCFP

The defining characteristic of SIRCFP is placing unmet core relational, self, and physical intimacy needs at the center and at the heart of understanding and treating repetitive negative interactional patterns. The position is that individual, couple, and family problems surface when an individual's core relational, self, and physical intimacy needs are not sufficiently understood, accepted, and integrated into the significant relationships. The goal of therapy is to help individuals, couples, and families identify their unmet core needs, to link them to their struggles and problems, and to develop personal and relational patterns that validate, accept, and embrace their core needs.

This section presents the SIRP constructs that are pertinent to SIRCFP. These constructs are explained in greater detail in the first chapter. The major explanatory constructs are adopted from psychodynamic- and experiential-oriented theories and from developmental psychology. The names of the original constructs are maintained and where necessary, their meanings are slightly modified to accommodate the SIRCFP approach. This group of constructs provides the conceptual tools to explain the relational problems, perform an assessment, establish therapy goals, and plan and carry out treatment.

The constructs provide the focus for the analysis of the negative interactional patterns in couple and family therapy. Therapy is tailored according to and in keeping with the relational, self, and physical intimacy needs of the participants. The integration of the unmet core needs sets up a process that leads to changes in communication style, relational patterns, and coping strategies.

Core Relational, Self, and Physical Intimacy Needs

The core needs are grouped according to relational, self, and physical intimacy needs. The grouping is based partly on the writings of developmental psychologists and partly on the research and the theories of the present psychotherapists (Meier & Boivin, 2022). However, the authors arrived at the significance of human needs primarily from their clinical work with children, adolescents, and adults in the context of individual, couple, and family therapy.

In working with core needs, it is important to differentiate between needs that were not met (i.e., not satisfied) in childhood and needs that were met in childhood but are not met in adolescence and/or in adult relationships. A characteristic of an unmet childhood need is that it is unquenchable, whereas a characteristic of a need that was satisfied in childhood but was not met in adolescence and in adulthood, referred to as an unmet growth need, is that when it is responded to, the person feels satisfied and moves on with daily living.

Core relational needs

The core relational needs comprise the need for emotional bonding with a significant caregiver (safe-anchorage) and the need to become autonomous, that is, to psychologically separate from the caregiver and to individuate (Mahler, Pine & Bergman, 1975). These two relational needs are referred to as the "need for emotional bonding" and the "need for autonomy."

The "need for emotional bonding" refers to a need for an emotional and psychological closeness that is characterized by affection and trust between people. The term "emotional bonding" is used when referring to the infant/child–parent relationship and the term "emotional closeness" and/or "emotional connection," is used when referring to the post-infancy/child–parent relationship.

The "need for autonomy" implies psychological separateness and individuation. Psychological separateness refers to experiencing oneself as different and separate from the other. Individuation refers to being one's own person and living from one's preferences, values, and desires. To be autonomous means being the origin of one's own behaviors (Deci & Ryan, 2002), to develop one's own interests, values, and goals in life and have the freedom to make choices and decisions. To be autonomous also implies taking distance from a relationship to be present to oneself, to ruminate, reflect, and see life issues and challenges in a broader perspective. In terms of couple and family relationships, the need for autonomy is often expressed in terms of a member wanting the freedom to be his own person, to make decisions and choices, to have a voice in matters important to him, and to pursue his interests.

Core self needs

The core self needs include the "striving to be competent" and the "striving to be significant." The child needs the caregiver's admiration and affirmations to foster his sense of omnipotence, empowerment, and competency, and to experience that he is a good and lovable person for just being who he is. He also needs to be admired and affirmed for his movement out of the emotionally bonded relationship and toward autonomy. These self needs are referred to as the "need for competency" and the "need for significance" (Meier & Boivin, 2011, p. 155).

Whereas the relational needs are about being connected to others and being one's own person in the presence of others, the self needs are about the subjective experience that one has about oneself, that is, a sense of *being* competent and a sense of *being* significant. The "need for competency" refers to the striving to be effective in one's ongoing interactions with others (relational competency) and to experience opportunities to exercise and express one's capacities (self-competency in relation to oneself) (Deci & Ryan, 2002). The "need for significance" refers to the striving to be lovable, significant, worthwhile, and likable, and to being a good person and attractive in relation to others.

The development of the "self-needs" begins in early childhood with affirmations and validations from caregivers. With consistent positive validations, the child gradually develops a sense of competency and significance and requires less feedback from others regarding the two self needs. With the development of the self needs, a person is equipped to perform a realistic evaluation of self, becomes less dependent on the positive and negative judgments of others, and can maintain his sense of competency and significance despite negative responses from others.

Core physical intimacy needs

The core physical intimacy needs include the need for "sensual contact" and the "need for sexual intimacy." The "need for sensual contact" refers to the need for physical contact (e.g., hugs, cuddles) and/or physical presence (e.g., to be in the same physical space), but not with the intent of sexual intimacy. The need for sensual contact is associated with an infant's need for physical touch and emotional bonding.

Sensual contacts expand to include the urge for sexual intimacy when the infant/child begins to experience pleasure by physically touching erogenous parts of his body. These early pleasurable experiences gradually seek as their goal, in later years, pleasure in genital expression. The pleasurable experiences awaken the urge for physical contact with the intention of genital expression.

In summary, the relational, self, and physical intimacy needs play out together and impact each other. The way caregivers acknowledge and affirm them, and how they are realized and integrated affect all aspects of the personality. When these needs go unmet, problems are apt to occur. However, it is important to remember that unmet needs do not inevitably lead to personal and relational problems. One cannot make predictions about the outcome when needs go unmet, but one can possibly postdict, that is, trace a problem back to an unmet relational, self, and/or physical intimacy need.

Psychic Structure

Psychic structure is a combination of hereditary inheritance or biological factors, the acquired social heritage, that is, the internalization of society behaviors and values to live by, and a capacity to integrate these for the benefit of the person. It defines the dominant organization of an individual's mind, way of managing internal conflicts, and manner of establishing relationships.

According to Freud (1923), the psychic structure comprises three parts: the innate energy system (i.e., the id, which embraces the instincts), the acquired social heritage (i.e., the superego, which comprises acceptable behaviors and values by which to live), and the creative capacity to think, plan, and act (i.e., the ego). The ego ensures that both the instincts of the id and the demands and expectations of the superego work together for the benefit of the person. It is the encounter between an infant/child's innate instincts and the societal demands and expectations that leads to their encoding and to the development of internal structures (i.e., superego) that are an amalgam of an infant/child's instincts, the expectations of significant others, and the demands of reality. The id, ego, and superego together, as one unit, form a complex organizing principle that influences all human interactions.

It should be noted that Freud did not use the word "instincts" when speaking about the energy of persons. He used the term "instincts" with regard to animals and the German word *Triebe* when speaking about people. *Triebe* refers to an urge, drive, or wish, very similar to a need or desire (Bettelheim, 1983).

SIRCFP has adopted but modified Freud's (1923) tripartite organization of the psychic structure in the following ways. It has replaced the *instincts* of the id with the construct of core needs; the *life instinct* with the relational need for emotional bonding; the physical intimacy needs with sensual contact; and sexual intimacy and the *death instinct*, that is aggression, with the need for autonomy. SIRCFP does not consider aggression to be innate but an emotional reaction to interference in the pursuit of one's innate needs. The striving for autonomy, however, is innate; it is an innate need to move away from the emotional bond of the caregiver, to psychologically separate and to individuate and become autonomous. These core needs are assumed to be the prime motivators of much of human behavior and interaction.

The modification of the two instincts is consistent with Freud's (1938) reformulation of the instincts where he wrote, "The aim of the first of these basic instincts [Eros] is to establish ever greater unities and to preserve them thus–in short, to together; the aim of the second is, on the contrary, to undo connections (and so to destroy things)" (p. 148).

The SIRCFP approach embraces Freud's (1923) concept of the ego, which is innate and potentially present at birth, and is described as a "coherent organization of mental processes" (p. 17). The ego is an active agent and its functions, briefly, include perception, thinking, memory, planning, motility, and action. The ego can be thought of in terms of adaptive functions and defensive functions. An adaptive ego is flexible, resourceful, and resilient, and is capable of managing the challenges of daily living and the life problems that it faces in a creative, realistic, and rewarding manner. The ego in its defensive mode responds to intrapsychic conflicts and attempts to mediate between the core needs of the id, the prohibitions of the superego, and the demands of reality. In its defensive mode, it protects one from danger and threats to one's psychological well-being.

SIRCFP adopts Freud's concepts of superego, which comprises all of that which is socially inherited in terms of acceptable behaviors and conduct, and in terms of values and ideals to live by. Freud (1923) used the term "conscience" when referring to socially acceptable and unacceptable behaviors and the term "ego ideal" to refer to values and ideals to live by. The superego can be considered moderate, severe, or harsh in its function (Jacobson, 1964). A moderate superego integrates prohibitions without compromising a person's innate needs and preferences. A severe superego is demanding of self and of others, tends to be perfectionist, feels obligated (rather than responsible), and has a need to be in control. A harsh superego is punitive, guilt ridden, and may self-harm and entertain suicidal thoughts.

Self-Structure and Sense of Self

The self is thought to be potentially but not actively, present at birth. Human infants generally are born with a (nuclear) self already in place, that is, with a biologically determined psychological entity (Brinich & Shelley, 2002, p. 46). The baby's self is thought of as a "virtual self" (Kohut, 1977, p. 101) that begins as a bodily sense of self (Allport. 1967).

The baby's potential self interacts with the caregiver's sense of "what is self," and from this interaction emerges the infant/child's organization of a cohesive self that is cognitive and affective in nature and is stored as an internal representation of self (Kohut, 1971; Mahler et al., 1975; Winnicott, 1965; Stern, 1985). At the beginning of an infant's life, the ego is dominant, but with the development of a self, the "living self" becomes the "organizing center of the ego's activities" (Kohut, 1971, p. 120). An infant/child's first perception of self is dependent on how others see him, but as he matures, he forms his own sense of self based on his experiences.

Two of the components that the constitute the self are a sense of significance and a sense of competency, which are inferred from Kohut's (1977) study of narcissistically wounded clients. The sense of significance is made up of idealized images of self and world, and develops from the child's involvement with powerful others to whom the child can look up and with whom he can merge as an image of calmness, infallibility, and omnipotence (Kohut & Wolf, 1978). The sense of competency comprises the grandiose and exhibitionistic self-images that are the result of interchanges with (mirroring) caregivers who with joy and approval, confirm the child's innate vigor, greatness, perfection, and expanding states of mind (Kohut, 1977).

The sense of significance and the sense of competency, as presented by Kohut, are perceived as states. That is, the person experiences himself to be significant and to be competent. SIRCFP considers competency and significance to be core needs, which are included under the construct, the self. However, these two core self needs are not considered to be of the same order as the relational and physical intimacy needs, which are more inherently psychophysiologically rooted.

Communication Styles and Patterns

Communication refers to how people verbally and nonverbally "convey information, make meaning with one another, and respond – internally and externally" (Satir et al., 1991, p. 31). This includes the "words, tone, and quality of expression" (Luthman & Kirschenbaum, 1974, p. 59). An individual's pattern of communication can be influenced by the person communicated to (e.g., if that person is an angry or loving person) and by one's own internal dialogue.

Internal dialogue refers to the internal communication that a person carries on within himself, which Meichenbaum (1977) refers to as self-talk. The internal dialogue takes place between the three agents of the psychic structure, that is, between the inner child (i.e., id) and the ego, and between the superego and the ego. Each of the constituents of the psychic structure has its own unique voice. The id represents the voice of the child (e.g., is needy, angry), the superego the voice of the parent (e.g., demanding, authoritative), and the ego the voice of reason and adaptive capacities. An individual's psyche can be organized with a domineering superego that does not accept the needs/urges of the id, or with a dominant id that rebels against the demands of the superego. When the ego fails to harmonize the needs of the id and the demands of the superego, the individual's style of communication may at one time be skewed toward being demanding, critical, and controlling, and at another time toward being needy, whining, complaining, and angry.

The pattern of internal dialogue may be externalized in the communication with real people. Satir (1972) and Satir and associates (1991) refer to the externalization of the styles of communication in terms of survival stances that include placating (i.e., disregards one's own feelings of worth and hands them over to someone else), blaming (i.e., discounts others and counts only the self and context), being super-reasonable (e.g., focuses on facts, not feelings), and irrelevant (e.g., distracts from the real issue) (pp. 36–52). An individual's style of communication can reveal many aspects of his personality, including his psychic and self-structures, unmet needs, and coping strategies.

Relational Patterns and Projective Identifications

Relational patterns differ from projective identifications. The differences between these two types of relating are described.

Relational patterns

Relational patterns are repeated and consistent ways in which an individual inter-acts with and responds to the people (e.g., parents, partner, and friends) with whom he is in a relationship. These patterns depict how an individual relates with another without expecting a specific response. The individual might even be oblivious to how others might be responding to him. It can be said that a relational pattern is a one-direction relational pattern.

Relational patterns are learned at a very young age. The core relational, self, and physical intimacy needs propel the person to develop meaningful relations, and these needs together with the responses from others influence the quality and nature of the individual's manner of relating. In a "good enough" (Winnicott, 1965) home environment, the infant/child and adolescent acquire the skills to develop meaningful, satisfying, and intimate relationships. They learn to problem solve, negotiate differences between competing needs, make compromises, reconcile conflicts, repair relational injuries, and to be empathic toward others. When the infant/child is exposed to an environment that is not good enough, he might acquire relational patterns that are helpful at that age, but they become problematic in ado-lescence and adulthood.

The patterns of relating can be adaptive or maladaptive (Benjamin, 2006; Conroy & Pincus, 2006). Adaptive patterns are characterized by interpersonal friendliness, flexibility, moderate engagement with and differentiated from others. Maladaptive patterns contain hostility, controlling or submitting to others, and disconnection in normal settings. These patterns are learned through the processes of identification, recapitulation, and introjection (Benjamin, 2006). Identification refers to behaving like an important other person; recapitulation is behaving as if the other person is still present and in charge; and introjection refers to treating the self in the same way as an important other person did. These processes can lead to maladaptive relational patterns and to projective dentifications.

The more common relational patterns include the caregiver, the Alpha, the parent, the codependent, and the push-pull (Van Edwards, 2022). The caregiver relational pattern strives to fix, to take care of, or to improve others and the person that they are with. The Alpha person wants to be in charge, dictate the rules, and likes to be in relationships where he can be the chief decision-maker. A person may relate to the other as a parent and treat their partner as a child. In a codependent relationship, both persons give up a lot of their individuality; may become completely reliant on the other person for social, emotional, and psychological support; and may stop having their own friends or activities. In a push-pull relationship, one person might always be pushing for more intimacy and for more time together, and the other person might be pulling away and want more space for himself/herself. The more that the "pusher" wants time together, the more the "puller" moves away and declares that he needs more space and time for himself. These relational patterns are maladaptive when they become rigid, compulsive, intensive, and ineffective.

Projective identifications

Projective identifications differ from interpersonal patterns. Interpersonal patterns refer to a style of relating to others without expecting a specific type of response. In projective identifications, the individual expects a specific response from others to his projection. As a relational dynamic, "a projective identification combines a projection and identification in an interactional way" (Ogden, 1989, p. 25). For example, an individual in his relationship with his partner might project an image of himself as being an expert in parenting and expect his partner to identify with this projected image of himself and say, "yes, you are an expert and I am not."

Klein introduced the concept of projective identification to explain the conflicted interaction between the therapist and the child. In Klein's (1946, 1959) description of this concept, she states that the individual (i.e., the child) projects his aggressive instincts that he found unbearable, onto the other, and then assumes that the other person is aggressive and potentially a persecutor. By projecting his aggression onto the other, the individual gets rid of it; however, the individual remains connected (by virtue of his ego) relationally with the other. By assuming that the other is aggressive, the individual indirectly manages his own aggression (Ogden, 1989, p. 25; Segal, 2004, p. 37). Klein's notion of projective identification is a one-person projective identification since the individual who projects also identifies with that which is projected. The person to whom it is projected does not respond to the projection.

Cashdan (1988) viewed the concept of projective identification as a two-person process to include a relational stance, metacommunication, and an induction process. Projective identifications are perceived to be repetitive and compulsive interpersonal patterns.

Four types of projective identification, according to Cashdan (1988), are: (a) Dependency – the need to be taken care of, feeling helpless and dependent on the other; (b) Power – portraying oneself as being more competent than one's partner and wanting to be in charge; (c) Ingratiation – laying on guilt trips to get the needed response from the other; and (d) Sexuality – using one's sexuality (e.g., flirting, dress, teasing/seduction) to create sexual arousal in the other so as to get his/her attention. In projective identifications, an individual takes a specific stance (e.g., sense of helplessness), which induces from his partner a specific response (e.g., a caretaking response).

Projective identifications are often driven by unmet childhood needs. Individuals enter a relationship with the hope that their partners will respond to their unmet childhood needs. For example, one partner may want to be validated as being competent, and the other partner may want to be validated as being significant. The meeting of their mutual needs results in a two-person projective identification as each respond to the needs of the other. Although initially both respond to each other's needs, nevertheless, as the relationship shifts from the honeymoon stage, through power struggle and then to real love (Hendrix, 2008), one or both partners may no longer want to respond to their partner's unmet childhood needs, either because they are frustrated that their own unmet childhood needs are not being responded to or because they have outgrown the relationship. When this occurs, their relational pattern is no longer referred to as projective identification since one partner does not identify with the stance of the other, such as being helpless or being more competent than the partner.

The relational patterns and the projective identifications can provide useful information regarding the degree to which an individual's core relational, self, and physical intimacy needs are striving to be responded to, and how the individual copes with unmet core needs. In observing the pattern, the therapist can also determine whether the relational pattern is symptomatic of unmet childhood needs or unmet growth needs. One can also assess whether the relational pattern is an externalization of the individual's own internal struggle or whether it is related to the individual's current relationship.

Stress and Coping Strategies

An infant/child will experience that his significant caregivers will not always be attuned to his feelings and core needs. Prolonged stress in not having his core needs met, might lead to developmental injuries. To protect himself from the wounding at various developmental stages, the infant/child develop defensive and reactive patterns that are maintained throughout his adult life.

The experience of stress connotes three elements: a stressor; the effect of the stressor on a person, couple, and/or family (i.e., distress); and conscious and unconscious coping strategies to deal with the stressor and its effects. The stressors that a person, couple, and family might experience can be thought of in terms of external stressors and internal stressors. The external stressors can be multiple and include physical and mental illness, work-related stressors, a challenged member of the family, loss of occupation, poverty, marginalization, demanding persons, addictions, infidelity, and a death in the family, to name a few. Internal stressors might include self-depreciation, feelings of shame and guilt, the striving for perfectionism, feeling obligated and duty-bound, anger for failing to self-regulate and to control one's relationships and environment.

The stressors might affect the person psychologically and physically, and indirectly affect the couple and family relationships. Psychologically, the person might become anxious, depressed, and angry and externalize these feelings in acting-out behaviors, be it in the couple, family, school, workplace, or socially. Physically, the person might convert the strong negative feelings into bodily ailments. The individual's psychological and physical symptoms may have an enormous impact on couple and family living.

The individual's strategies to cope with the stressors can be considered in terms of unconscious and conscious mechanisms. The unconscious mechanisms can be grouped according to primary and secondary defense mechanisms. The primary unconscious defense mechanisms could include repression, dissociation, denial, and splitting. The secondary defense mechanisms include projection, rationalization, reaction formation, and undoing, to mention a few. These are well described in the literature (Sadock, Sadock & Ruiz, 2014). The conscious coping strategies include problem solving, negotiation, compromise, the healing of psychological injuries, and the repairing of broken relationships. Psychological injuries are healed and broken relationships are repaired particularly by the offender acknowledging and making apologies, and the offended accepting the apology and forgiving the offender (Meier, 2001). The capacities to acknowledge and apologize for causing hurt, and the capacity to forgive are essential for meaningful and satisfying couple and family relationships.

Therapy Goals

The goals for couple and family therapy are largely determined by the dynamics underlying the couple and family's presenting problems and by the theoretical orientation of the therapist. The problems that clients present to therapy are typically interactional and behavioral in nature, and may include problems regarding communication, relationships, emotional and sexual intimacy, and coping strategies. From the perspective of SIRCFP, the presenting problems lie deeper than the surface and are believed to be sourced by unseen underlying personal and relational dynamics. The goal of SIRCFP is to uncover the underlying dynamics of the presenting problems and to develop more effective communication, relational, intimacy, and coping capacities.

Therapy begins with the clients presenting their view of the presenting problem, describing how it has affected them, and by providing clinical material for the therapist to formulate a conceptualization and to plan treatment. Following this information, the therapist, guided by his theory, leads the clients toward their expressed goals. The therapist works primarily with the clients' subjective experiences rather than with the content and keeps therapy focused in the here and now and in process. According to SIRCFP, couple and family therapy encompasses the following goals:

1. The primary goal of couple and family therapy is for the participants to explore, uncover, and become aware of their mutual unmet core needs, and for the core needs of everyone to be embraced, honored, and integrated into their couple and/or family relationships.
2. Understand how the unmet core needs have formed the participants' perceptions of themselves and of their partner and/or of their family members, and how the perceptions and/or the projection of their perceptions influences their dysfunctional interactional patterns.
3. Increase participants' awareness and understanding of how a couple and/or a family's patterns of interaction influences their effectiveness in everyday living and how such patterns affect, and are affected by, the satisfaction of individuals and by their psychological health.
4. Increase and support the separation and individuation process of a couple and family members as they move toward differentiation and autonomy.
5. Develop and maintain healthy relational boundaries and a respect for privacy.
6. Develop coping skills that more effectively address differences of opinion, disagreements, and relational conflicts.
7. Develop relational skills such as empathy and the ability to problem solve, negotiate, compromise, and repair relational ruptures.
8. Support the desire of a partner and of a family member to participate in making decisions about matters that affect him or her.
9. Enhance positive views of self and raise self-esteem.
10. Encourage self-expression, self-actualization, and relational authenticity.
11. Empower each member to be autonomous, to respect the same need in others, and to develop and maintain meaningful relationships.
12. Modify roles, rules, and coalitions according to the needs of one's partner and/or of the family members.

Therapy Interventions and Techniques

SIRCFP fosters exploration, insight, and action. SIRCFP helps clients explore the underlying dynamics of their presenting problems. The goal of the exploration is to link current problems to predisposing factors, that is, to vulnerabilities, and to gain insight into the origin of one's problem. Insight is followed by integrating the insight in new behaviors and interactions. To carry out these tasks, SIRCFP employs interventions that are common to all therapies, adopts advanced interventions from selected theoretical orientations, and adapts them to its theoretical orientation.

In his work with couples and families, a SIRCFP-oriented therapist begins by creating a safe, protective, and caring environment so that the partners and the members of a family feel free to express their intimate thoughts, feelings, and needs. The therapist's goal is to establish a therapeutic relationship with each partner and with each member of the family. The therapeutic relationship becomes the vehicle through which healing takes place and more effective communication and relationship skills and coping strategies are developed. The interventions that the therapist uses to accomplish these goals and tasks include active listening, empathic responding, open-ended questions, paraphrases, and summaries of the therapy content (Ivey, Gluckstern, & Ivey, 2006).

The use of advanced techniques may also be required in couple and family therapy. There may be situations when partners of a couple and members of the family find it difficult to express their thoughts and their deeper lying feelings and needs. They may not know how to express them, or they may fear to express them because of the past negative responses to them from their partner or members of the family. In situations such as these, SIRCFP might design a technique or adapt a technique from selected psychotherapeutic approaches to help the individual access his thoughts, feelings, and needs and learn how to express them. The couple and family therapist might adopt techniques from Gestalt therapy (Perls, 1969), Imago therapy (Hendrix, 2008), behavioral therapy (Wolpe, 1990), humanistic experiential therapy (Greenberg & Johnson, 1988; Greenberg & Goldman, 2008; Johnson, 2004), and object relationship therapy (Scharff & Scharff, 2014). A SIRCFP therapist adapts these techniques for use within the context of SIRCFP constructs.

The interventions and techniques that a SIRCFP therapist uses, can be considered in terms of those that facilitate the dialogue between the partners and the members of a family, and those that create new possibilities for the development of more effective communication and relational skills and provide corrective emotional experiences. SIRCFP assumes that for transformations and changes to take place, something new must enter or be introduced into the dialogue to challenge deeply engrained perceptions, projections, and behaviors. The following are some of the interventions that facilitate the dialogue between partners and among members of a family, and some of the techniques that create new possibilities and provide corrective emotional experiences.

Interventions That Facilitate Dialogue

A SIRCFP therapist uses interventions that support open and honest communication, and encourages the couple or members of the family to work together to create meaningful bonds. The therapist does not focus on negative emotions and the history of their problems, but focuses on what will help the clients to work toward developing the types of relationships that they desire.

Active listening: This refers to attentively listening to the client, understanding, and responding to what he is saying; it entails remembering this information (Nichols, 2009). It includes being attentive, requesting clarification, being attuned to, and reflecting feelings and asking open-ended and probing questions. Active listening takes its lead from what the client is saying; it is non-directive.

Active listening implies listening to the words spoken and to the emotional tone with which they are spoken. Words may be spoken out of anger or may be spoken cautiously and out of fear. The client might speak about something that is serious in a light-hearted tone. At an appropriate moment, the therapist might share his observation with the client and explore the client's feeling and track it to its origin, which often is to an unmet need.

Introspective Empathic immersion: This entails immersing oneself introspectively and empathically into the client's internal struggles, understanding how the clients have structured their subjective experiences (i.e., psychic structure and self-structure), assessing how the structures inform their interactions, and deciding how to transform these psychic and self-structures. In introspective empathic immersion, the psychotherapist vicariously experiences the client's struggles and subjective experiences as if they are his own, sees the world through the client's eyes, and responds in an authentic, accurate, and fitting manner.

Empathy becomes relevant to a therapist–client interaction when it results in an action that follows directly from the therapist's experience-near observations. Kohut noted the link between empathy and action in the introspective empathic immersion concept. Kohut (1981) states that "introspection and empathy are informers of appropriate action" (p. 529). Empathic immersion is a slow, long-term, and plodding process by which the therapist "tastes to an attenuated degree the flavor of the client's experience while maintaining his or her objectivity" (The New York Institute for Psychoanalytic Self Psychology, 2022).

Reflective statements: Reflection in therapy is like holding up a mirror and repeating the client's words back to him exactly as he said them. Reflective statements are more encompassing than Rogerian (Rogers, 1961) empathic responses, which focus on feelings that are accurately communicated to the client. In using reflective statements, the therapist might reflect the whole sentence or a feeling, thought, or core need from what the client said. In using reflective statements, the therapist tries to match the tone and the feeling of the words spoken.

The therapist uses reflective statements to establish rapport and build a relationship with the client. He also uses it to help a client to feel understood, to encourage the client to be open and express himself, and to help the client become aware of his emotions and feelings. The client might also be asked to be reflective and to reflect on a statement made by a partner, a member of the family, or by the therapist.

Validation statements: This means accepting the clients for who they are, where they are with their emotions, and how they perceive themselves and others. It means to accept them for their feelings, values, and ideals (Osipow, Walsh & Tosi, 1984). To validate does not mean to approve or to agree with what is said, or try to change the person; rather, it means that the therapist understands where the clients are coming from and accepts them without judgment. It is another way to communicate to the clients that the therapist sees them, that the clients are important, and that the therapist and clients' relationships matter (Rathus & Miller, 2015).

Validation begins by showing an interest in the client and by being present. The therapist can show his validation by his body language, by maintaining eye contact, and by other nonverbal means of communication. Validations are important to develop meaningful connections, and consistent and purposeful validations help build relationships. The therapist also tries to help partners and family members validate each other, accept the other without judgement and with a desire to know more about where they are coming from.

Process questions: The term "process" refers to the flow of experience and how it may change as new material (e.g., feelings, thoughts, memories) emerges. With regard to therapy, process refers to accessing the client's internal experience and working with aspects of it. Process questions focus on the client and his internal experience. In the therapist's work with a client, the client may discuss something important to the therapist. The therapist permits him to tell the story and listens until the client invites him for help. After the initial sessions that are often focused on the externals such as work and relationships, the therapist asks process questions that focus on the client's internal experience. The therapist helps the client reflect on ideas or feelings that seem significant, works in the here and now (emotions being experienced in a moment), and focuses on themes, patterns, and affects such as being prone to feeling hurt, dismissed, and depressed. The therapist aligns himself with and validates the client's self-directed and forward-moving internal transformations and behavioral changes.

Open-ended questions: This type of question is phrased as a statement that requires more than a simple answer like yes or no; it requires a longer answer. Open-ended questions keep the conversation going and encourage the client to speak. The therapist uses open-ended questions to clarify his understanding of what the client is feeling or saying. The advantages of open-ended questions are that they allow for unlimited responses and offer a deeper understanding of the client's experiences. Examples of open-ended questions are: "How do you see the couple/family problem?" "What are you experiencing now?" "How do you feel about hearing what your partner/son/daughter stated?" and so on. Questions such as these do not have set answers, but ask the client to speak from his bodily felt experience.

Techniques That Create New Possibilities and Provide Corrective Experiences

There are numerous techniques available to create new possibilities, help alter dysfunctional interactional patterns, and provide corrective emotional experiences in couple and family therapy. Each therapeutic approach has developed techniques to achieve its therapeutic goals (Gurman, 2008). SIRCFP adopted several of these techniques and adapted them to achieve its primary goal, which is to help clients uncover their unmet core needs and orient their lives according to them.

I-You statement: Buber (2010) makes a distinction between a monologue and a dialogue. A dialogue is an I-You (*ich-du*) relationship. Both persons in the conversation experience the other as a person like themselves, and there is mutual respect and a genuine interest in the other's thoughts, feelings, and needs.

An I-You statement asks the individual (i.e., speaker) to begin his responses using "I" statements rather than to begin his responses with words such as "It" and "You." In using "It" statements, such as "it hurts when you scold me," one keeps a bit distant from one's feelings. In using "I" statements, the feeling is felt more intensely and one feels more vulnerable, which renders a dialogue more intimate. To begin a response with a "You" statement might be understood as making criticism, scolding, judging, or blaming. By asking partners of a couple and members of a family to begin responses with "I" statements, this provides a way to keep the therapy focused on the here and now. It also helps the couple and members of the family become aware of their feelings and needs to assert them.

Translating complaints into assertive statements: Continued complaining about marital dissatisfaction or family unhappiness does not help make things better. The therapist can ask a partner or family member to change a complaining, blaming, or absolute statement into an assertive statement. By making an assertive statement, the client makes a more effective and appropriate statement, a statement that he feared to make in the past. An assertive statement is focused and controlled. It minimizes an emotional reaction. The minimizing of an emotional reaction is referred to as reciprocal inhibition, meaning that anxiety and relaxation cannot coexist (Wolpe, 1990). This change in communication shifts the level of conversation from that which keeps them divided to that which brings them closer together and establishes greater emotional bonds. A positive response to an individual's assertion on the part of a partner or of a family member may provide a corrective emotional experience. The individual may develop the sense that he can engage in open and honest communication, and be heard and respected even if others may not agree with him. Examples of how a therapist may elicit assertive statements are the following: "How would you like it to be?" "What needs to happen for the couple/ family relationship to improve?" and "What is missing in your relationship?" The therapist pays particular attention to statements about the relational and self needs that might not be positively acknowledged and responded to.

Structured dialogue: To help a partner or member of a family improve their communication and relationship skills, the therapist may initiate a structured dialogue. A structured dialogue comprises three elements, namely, mirroring, empathizing, and validating statements (Hendrix, 2008). In mirroring, a partner or member of the family is asked to paraphrase what the other said in the same tone without altering the meaning in any way. In empathizing, a person, the receiver, is to imagine and describe the feelings of the other person, that is, to describe what the other said. A validating statement offers an understanding of where the other person is coming from. In performing these tasks, the individual experiences a new and more satisfying way of communicating.

Evocative questions: These types of questions are designed to elicit, from the client, a strong response, be it a feeling, thought, or need. Evocative questions are created to help a client look within and bring forth answers to what he is experiencing, how he would like his relationships to be, and/or how he would go about acquiring his desired behaviors. Rather than imposing his ideas about the client's behaviors, the therapist, by using evocative questions, draws out the client's own thoughts, ideas, and feelings about his behavior and how he might change it. When a client arrives at his own discoveries about his behaviors, change is more likely to occur and endure. The role of the therapist is to support the client in a nonjudgmental, accepting, and affirming way in his search for answers to his feelings, thoughts, needs, and behaviors.

Miller and Rollnick (2013) used evocative questions to motivate behavior change. They coined questions for four areas, desire, ability, reason, and need (i.e., urgency) to make changes. Two areas, specifically, desire and ability, are particularly relevant for a SIRCFP therapist. With regard to desire, the therapist can ask evocative questions such as: "How would you like things to be different in your family and/or couple relationship?" "How would you like to feel rather than to be depressed?" With regard to ability to make changes, the therapist might ask: "If you want your relationships to change, how might you do it?" and "What do you think that you might be able to change?" Evocative questions, as illustrated above, help the client draw on his inner wisdom for answers, and the answers may lead to being enabled and result in the pursuit of a life that he wants to live.

Confrontation: Ivey and Gluckstern (1984) define a confrontation as

> pointing out the discrepancies between or among attitudes, thoughts, and behaviors. In a confrontation, individuals are faced directly with the fact they may be saying something other than that which they mean, or are doing something other than that which they say. (p. 32)

Egan (1982) provides an experiential-oriented description of a confrontation. He states that a confrontation "is an invitation to examine some form of behavior that seems to be self-defeating or harmful to others and to change the behavior if it is found to be so" (p. 186). Through confrontation, clients develop alternate perspectives regarding their feelings, experiences, and behaviors.

Confrontation can be used to challenge discrepancies between what clients think or feel, and what they say, between what they say and what they do, between what they are and what they wish to be, and between their expressed values and their actual behavior. Confrontations can also be used to challenge client distortions of reality, such as viewing a parent that a client fears as being cold and aloof. By the same token, confrontations can be used to challenge defeating attitudes and beliefs

(Egan, 1982). Confrontations can also be used to challenge distorted messages such as a parent saying that their son went to a faraway university rather than admitting that he could not tolerate the tension at home and wanted to distance himself from the home as far as possible (Cormier, Nurius & Osborn, 2015).

It is for the therapist to recognize what is going on, or to infer what is going and to honestly and directly point this out to the clients (Brammer & MacDonald, 2002). Ivey (1983, 1986) states that it is equally as important to work toward resolving discrepancies, mixed messages, and conflicts. A SIRCFP therapist points out discrepancies and works with the client to resolve them. The focus is not on changing behavior but on experientially examining the behavior. For example, if a client is sitting with his arms crossed, the therapist will not ask, "How come you are crossing your arms?" This only creates defensiveness. Rather, the therapist will ask, "What are you experiencing now?" The focus is not on the behavior but on the feelings, thoughts, and motives (i.e., core needs) that prompted the behavior. Questions such as the latter deepen the experience and make for a more positive dialogue.

Connecting with a bodily felt feeling: For partners of a couple and members of a family who tend to be overly logical and practical and/or are anxious, it might be useful to ask them to put aside their thoughts and preoccupations and to focus on their bodily felt feelings (Gendlin, 1996). It is asking them to clear a space so that what is hidden and lies deeper can emerge. At the same time, they are invited to connect with their bodily felt feeling and to follow it to where it leads them. When the bodily felt feeling has taken them to a place that feels real and genuine, they are asked to describe where and how they feel it in their body. After they have described where and how they feel it in their body, the therapist links the bodily felt feeling to a psychological experience or state, and shares it with them. For example, if a client states that he feels a heavy weight on his shoulders, the therapist asks him if he experiences life to be like that. If the client acknowledges it to be so, the individual and the therapist explore the factors in his life that bring about this feeling of heaviness.

Emotional Heightening: Feelings are one path that leads clients to their unmet core needs. For this reason, it is important for clients to be able to access and at times to heighten their feelings. Therapists can help clients heighten their feelings in two distinct ways. One way is for the therapist to intentionally use language to increase the emotional intensity of their interventions and thereby change a client's emotional arousal. The therapist might use evocative language (as described above), images, and metaphors, which encourages clients to go deeper into a particular emotion or feeling and ultimately to the unmet core need that triggered the feeling (Meier & Boivin, 2011). In response to a client's statement, the therapist might say: "You feel trapped and can't break free." "Regardless how hard you try to do the right thing, it is never good enough." "You find when your dad is around, you are walking on eggshells." With regard to emotions, Greenberg (2010) differentiates between primary and secondary emotions. Secondary emotions such as anger are a reaction against a primary emotion such as hurt. SIRCFP views the pattern with regard to emotions as beginning with secondary emotions, which when explored, lead to primary emotions. The exploration of primary emotions then leads to the unmet core need.

A second method to increase clients' emotional arousal is to use a Gestalt technique called "exaggeration" (Korb, Gorrell & Van de Riet, 1989, p. 103). In using this technique, a client is asked to repeat a statement that he made with more emotional intensity. Feelings that have not been dealt with may surface more clearly when a client repeats a statement with more emotional intensity. The therapist and the client then explore the emotion and trace it to its roots, which often is to an unmet core need. This technique is particularly helpful for clients who are shy, withdrawn, verbally retentive, and manifest with a flat affect and tend to be cerebral. With regard to couple and family therapy, the heightening of the emotions encourages the couple and/or family members to confront difficult topics together, express vulnerable emotions, and express how they would like to live their relationships.

Role Reversal: Role reversal means taking on or playing the role of another with the goal of feeling what it is like to be the other person. The individual assuming the role of another, is invited to experience and articulate the attitude and emotions of the other and to show this by the way he speaks and by his posture. The individual tries to demonstrate the other person's emotions, thoughts, needs, and intrapersonal conflicts explicitly and deeply (Yablonsky, 1976). The acting out in role-reversal can happen in many ways depending on the needs of the individual.

The use of role-reversals can be particularly helpful for couples to acquire some understanding of their partner's emotions, longings, thoughts, and perceptions by playing the role of their partner. In couple therapy, for example, the partners swap their traditional roles and routines in their relationship. Role-reversal helps an individual observe himself or herself as if in a mirror. Yablonsky (1976) gives the example of a daughter, in playing her mother's role, was able to see the role of the daughter from the mother's perspective. He provides the daughter's description: "From the vantage point of my mother, I saw for the first time that she feels badly about her age and her looks and is putting me down because she has begun to compete with me" (p. 116).

The Change Process in Couple and Family Therapy

Satir and associates (1991) and Bader and Pearson (1988) present models of the change process that comprise stages that a couple and/or a family passes through during psychotherapy. Satir and associates postulate six stages, Status Quo, Entry of a New Element, Chaos, Integration, Practice, and New Status Quo (pp. 98–99).

Bader and Pearson view couple stages in terms of Mahler and associates' (1975) four developmental phases, symbiosis, differentiation, practicing, and rapprochement, and their various combinations and interactions.

Meier and Boivin (1998, 2000) and Meier, Boivin, and Meier (2006, 2008) present a process model of the change process, namely, a Seven-Phase Model of the Change Process (SPMCP), that describes the process of change in individual, couple, and family psychotherapy. The seven phases are: Problem definition; Exploratory; Awareness/insight; Commitment; Experimentation/action; Integration/consolidation; and Termination. According to the SPMCP, psychotherapy begins with a Definition of the Problem (Phase 1) from the perspective of the members of the couple and family. This is followed by the Exploration of the Problem (Phase 2) in terms of its beginning, precipitators, intensity, and the difficulties experienced in bringing about a resolution. This often leads to greater chaos and relational disorganization. The exploratory work, which brings to awareness that which lies beneath the presenting problem, is followed by a new Awareness/insight (Phase 3), which becomes the basis for a Commitment (Phase 4) to make changes in their relationships. The members then begin to try out (Phase 5) the new behaviors that emanate from their awareness and attempt to implement them in their relationships. The members retain that which works and they let go of that which does not work. This phase is followed by an Integration/consolidation (Phase 6) of the new behaviors that fit in with their personal life and with their relationships. Following this phase, the therapist and members discuss the Termination (Phase) of therapy.

In brief, the significant phases of change are exploration, awareness/insight, and practice/experimentation. During psychotherapy, the therapist carefully leads the couple and the family through these phases. However, with resourceful couples and families, therapy might be terminated with the awareness/insight phase. An individual's progress through the seven phases is driven by a striving to fulfill core relational, self, and/or physical intimacy needs.

The Role of the Therapist in Couple and Family Therapy

It is incumbent upon the therapist to provide the structure for the couple and family therapy sessions. He informs the participants of the rules of engagement, which are presented in the form of a contract, discussed and signed by all parties involved.

As a general SIRCFP principle, clients are given a significant voice in their own change process, and therapy is conducted within the context of the clients' own expectations regarding change (Duncan and Miller, 2000). Therapy takes its lead from the clients' subjective experiences and from their desire for self-expansion in the development of meaningful relationships. When the clients have determined the direction for change, the therapist uses his conceptual and technical skills to help them achieve the desired goals. In the process of providing couple and family therapy, the therapist becomes an engaged and active participant and assumes many tasks, some of which are the following.

First, through his caring, accepting, and respectful attitude, the therapist provides a safe place for the participants to share their intimate feelings, needs, and thoughts about their relationships with their partner or family members. The therapist assures that all participants have relatively equal talk time, are not talked over or interrupted, and do not have others speak for them or complete their statements.

Second, the therapist endeavors to *meet* the partners of a couple as unique persons, the couple as a unit, the members of the family as unique persons, and the family as a unit, before he endeavors to address the cluster of their problems in their entirety. The purpose is to keep the focus on the persons and not on the cluster of problems, and to contextualize their problems in the individuals' psychosocial histories and current lived experiences.

Third, the therapist uses his conceptual skills to understand each member's frame of reference and his/her perceived place within the couple or family relationship. The therapist views relationships both from an interpersonal and an intrapersonal perspective.

Fourth, the therapist encourages the members to speak directly to the appropriate person and not to direct their statements toward the therapist. When this happens, the therapist redirects the member toward the appropriate person and encourages a dialogue or interaction between the parties concerned.

Fifth, the therapist keeps an eye on the therapy process and determines whether it is ready to move forward and, if so, guides it in that direction. This implies that assessment conceptualization, and treatment are ongoing and adjusted accordingly.

Sixth, the therapist is vigilant regarding client negative transferences and helps the client analyze them and use the insight gained for personal and relational changes. These transferences can be directed toward the therapist, a partner, or a family member. The therapist informs the participants that angry outbursts and destructive comments and behaviors will not be tolerated, and he helps the individuals contain them (Scharff & Scharff, 2008). This is not to say that a participant cannot voice his anger; however, it needs to be contained.

Seventh, the therapist accesses his own feelings (i.e., countertransference) about the interactions between members in order to have not only an intellectual understanding of the interaction but also an intuitive understanding of the process. He might choose to share his countertransference in a safe and effective way to help the interactions move forward.

Eight, the therapist develops a sense of how the members, who might be from a different geographical setting (i.e., rural, urban) and culture, form and shape a couple or family relationship and uses this information to facilitate this process. The therapist works within the context of the clients' historical and cultural backgrounds.

Ninth, when necessary, the therapist arranges to see a subsystem of a family (e.g., one or two members) for individual therapy that is keyed to their relational issues. The therapist obtains permission from other members to proceed in such cases. As much as possible, the same therapist, if qualified, offers therapy to the various subsystems to assure continuity between the various modalities of therapy, such as family, dyadic, or individual. A therapist working in an institution might be limited as to the modalities of therapy that he is permitted to offer.

Couple and Family Therapy in Practice

SIRCFP includes individual assessment sessions as part of the couple and family therapy. These sessions typically take place prior to seeing the couple and the family.

There are therapists, however, who begin couple and family therapy by seeing the couple and family first, which is followed by individual sessions for each partner and/or each family member. Their rationale for beginning this way is for the couple and family to meet, as a unit, the therapist, and for the therapist to meet them as a unit rather than as individuals. Seeing them first as a couple and a family conveys the message that "the history and current functioning of the relationship" is the focus of the therapy sessions (Baucom, Epstein, LaTaillade, Kirby, 2008, p. 41). The initial couple and family sessions are followed by individual assessment sessions with each partner of a couple and with each member of the family.

SIRCFP takes a different approach. It begins by seeing each member of the couple and each member of the family for an individual session prior to seeing them as a couple and as a family. Early in his practice as a couple and family therapist, the author (A.M.) became aware that when the partners of the couple and members of a family were seen for an individual assessment session prior to meeting them as a couple or as a family, therapy became more quickly focused and the underlying issues became more apparent and were directly addressed. An understanding of each member's psychosocial history, how they internalized their experiences, and how these experiences together with their core self, relational, and physical intimacy needs influenced their interactions, was extremely helpful in addressing the real couple and family issues. Upon completion of the individual assessment sessions, the couple and family are seen together. The therapist provides an assessment of their relational and interactional struggles and collaboratively plans treatment.

Individual Assessment Sessions

What are the goals of including individual assessment sessions at the beginning of and, when appropriate, during couple and family therapy? How is the material from the individual sessions useful to form a psychosocial assessment and plan treatment? These questions are now addressed.

Goals for including individual assessment sessions

There are several goals in seeing each person individually prior to the actual commencement of couple or family therapy. First, it gives the individual and the therapist an opportunity to get to know each other, to develop a relationship, and to form a safe place for the individual to share his thoughts, feelings, and needs. The individual session provides the opportunity for the therapist to *meet the person of the client* before fully *meeting his symptoms*; symptoms are understood within the context of the client's culture, relationships, and life experiences.

Second, it provides the individual an opportunity to discuss the process of therapy and its expectations and approach.

Third, it gives the individual an opportunity to speak about things that he would not want to speak about in either couple or family therapy but that are important for the therapist to know because of their impact on therapy. For example, the individual might be having an affair, is dishonest about finances, or has a drug issue. All of these have an impact on his relationships and are issues in considering whether couple and/or family therapy is appropriate.

Fourth, the therapist, in the assessment session, obtains important background information about the individual, which might include family of origin experiences, previous and present relationships, schooling and work experiences, use of leisure time, traumas and abuses, and addictions, to mention a few. In obtaining this information, the therapist focuses particularly on relational and self issues and unmet core child and/or growth needs. This information can be useful in understanding the unique psychological formation of each individual and how this might play out in relationships. The information is also useful in making an assessment, in formulating a conceptualization of the individual's personal and relational struggles, and in beginning to visualize how the person's internal dynamics might play out in relationships and in therapy.

All information from individual sessions, be it prior to the commencement of or during the couple and family sessions, are kept confidential and not shared by the therapist in any of the couple and/or family sessions. It is left to the individual to share this information if he deems it important.

Secrets, such as infidelities, however, are treated differently. The person who revealed the secret in an individual session is informed that he/she must share the secret with his/her partner because if not shared, it places the therapist and the person with the secret in a "position of colluding with the involved partner and undermines the couple therapy goal of working of improving the relationship" (Baucom, et al., 2008, p. 41). It is only when the affair is known that the therapist can "work with the couple's expression of disappointment, envy, rage, love and sadness" (Scharff & Scharff, 2008, p. 189). If the partner concerned refuses to share the secret, he/she is asked to "find a way to terminate couple therapy" (Baucom et al., 2008, p. 41).

Psychosocial history, assessments, and conceptualizations

To obtain relevant information to perform an assessment and a conceptualization for everyone's concerns, SIRCFP uses the SIRP:Semi-Structured Assessment Interview (SIRP-SSAI; Appendix A). The major topics covered in the interview and the items keyed to each topic have been designed to provide information regarding the SIRP constructs that become part of the analysis in couple and family therapy. Of particular importance is for the therapist to obtain information about childhood history to determine whether there was emotional neglect or physical and sexual abuse that may have resulted in unmet core needs, behavioral problems, and relational difficulties.

In addition to gathering the psychosocial history, the therapist also assesses the individual's willingness and readiness to improve the couple and/or family relationships. With regard to couple therapy, the therapist may ask the following questions: (1) Do you want to be with your partner? (2) Do you still have "chemistry" for your partner? and (3) Are you romantically engaged and have regular sex? Based on the interview, the therapist also assesses the individual's capacity for empathy, that is, to attune to the needs and feelings of the partner and of the children and vice versa.

Following the interview, the therapist provides a written psychosocial history for everyone that includes information regarding the major topics of the SIRP: SSAI. The report is used to assess the SIRCFP constructs using the Self-in-Relationship Psychotherapy Assessment Form (SIRP–AF; Appendix B). The last step is to formulate a conceptualization regarding an individual's problems that includes the precipitating, the predisposing, the perpetuating, and the protective factors (See Meier & Boivin, 2022, chapter 5). These conceptualizations provide the therapist with important information as what to expect in the dynamic interactions between each member of the couple and of the family and regarding the dynamic of the unit.

In brief, for the individual sessions, the therapist: (1) asks each person to describe the relational problem from his perspective; (2) obtains a thorough psychosocial history; (3) prepares a report based on the information from the psychosocial history; (4) codes the clinical material using the SIRP Assessment Form; (5) formulates a conceptualization for an individual's presenting problems; (6) forms an impression as to how the psychosocial profile of those interviewed are complementary and how they may be a potential source of self and relational issues; and (7) assesses an individual's readiness for therapy.

Couple and Family Therapy Sessions – Assessments and Interventions

After completing the individual assessment sessions, the therapist arranges for a couple and/or family meeting. The therapist shares with the couple and the family his assessment of their relational problems and together they formulate a plan for treatment. This and subsequent meetings focus on the repetitive negative inter-actional patterns, that is, on the nature and quality of the interactions between and among the individuals, and on helping the individuals establish more satisfying and nurturing patterns.

There are many aspects of the interactional patterns to observe, analyze, and potentially to modify. The interactional patterns comprise the communication style, relational patterns, and coping (and self-protective) strategies. The interactional patterns are a function of (i.e., motivated by) an individual's psychic structure, self-structure, coping strategies, and unmet core needs. The observations regarding these components of the interactional patterns provide the primary data for forming the assessments and for determining the goals for couple and family therapy.

The principal goal of couple and family therapy, according to SIRCFP, is to uncover the unmet core needs of the individuals, to name them, and to work toward having them become a significant factor in the development of new, satisfying, and nurturing couple and family relationships. One usually does not arrive at the unmet core needs quickly or directly. Often one arrives at them through the analysis of the couple and/or the family's communication style, relational patterns, and coping (and self-protective) strategies and the individual's psychic- and self-structures. Thus, it is incumbent upon the therapist to analyze these dimensions and to bring to light the unmet core needs and design interventions that will achieve the desired couple and family goals. It is not sufficient to simply uncover the unmet core needs of the individual members; it also important to work toward implementing them in their relationships and in their individual lives.

The following are the major components of the interactional patterns that a ther-apist might pay attention to and analyze as the couple and family therapy unfolds. Not all of the components necessarily form a part of the analysis and of the therapy for each couple or family as each couple and family is unique. The therapist focuses on the pertinent components of the interactional pattern that require reshaping.

The following are six of the components that a therapist might pay attention to, analyze, and address. For each component, areas of exploration using open-ended question are suggested. These serve only as a guide as in the process of therapy, other more pertinent issues may emerge that require detailed exploration and analysis.

Analysis of the communication style

One of the first components of the interactional pattern of couples and families that therapists pay attention to is their style of communication. The therapist might observe in couple therapy that neither one nor the other listens to what is being said by their partner. They seem to have their own narrative and do not engage in the narrative of their partner. That is, they do not talk about the same issue. Second, a partner or member of a family might make assumptions about another person's behaviors or statements and treat the assumption as a fact and react emotionally or behave accordingly. Third, the therapist might observe in couple therapy that one partner tends to attack, blame, and criticize, while the other partner tends to defend and justify his/her actions and behaviors. They are engaged in what seems like a power struggle. Fourth, in listening to the couple's conversation, one might get the sense that one speaks to the other from a parental position, while the other speaks from a child's position. Fifth, the partner of a couple or members of a family may use distancing and separating language rather than endearing and bonding language. Similar styles of relating may also be observed among members in family therapy.

The therapist presents to the couple and family members his observations regarding their style of communicating, asks for their feedback, and then engages in a discussion as to how to improve their style of communicating. For example, the therapist might ask the individual to use "I" and "You" statements rather than to begin his statements with "You," which sound more like scolding and judging, whereas as the former sound more like assertive statements and seem to be without judgment. That is, the therapist can help them reframe judgments into assertiveness statements and to practice this in therapy.

Based on these preliminary observations, the therapist might begin to formulate a hypothesis as to which unmet core relational, self, and physical intimacy needs are propelling the couple or family's negative style of communication. The therapist may also begin to think in terms of other components of the interactional pattern, such as the psychic- and self-structures of each member and try to understand how these might be externalized and consequently affect the style of communicating.

Analysis of relational patterns

A second component of the interactional pattern that a therapist pays careful attention to is the relational pattern of the couple and of the members of the family. The therapist may observe that there is a lot of tension in a family where one member is domineering, another member is passive but present, another member is withdrawn and disinterested, and the fourth is resentful and angry. One might also observe that one of the parents is controlling and oppressive and wants things to go his/her way (e.g., projective identification), while the other parent is passive, needy, and quiet, and the children feel helpless, immobilized, and unprotected. The therapist might observe that there is not much love in the family and there is a lack of empathic capacity to attune to the feelings and needs of others. The couple can come across as being more like roommates than a couple, and the family might come across as being a group of individuals doing their own thing; they are not a family. The therapist may observe that the language spoken is more attuned to keeping distant from others and keeping others at a distance rather than encouraging closeness, intimacy, endearment, and collaboration.

The therapist may provide his impression of the relational dynamics of the couple and the family and explore with them what it is that is keeping them from being loving, caring, endearing, supportive, and empathic toward each other. The therapist might use the session to help one member or the other to reframe judgmental and angry statements into assertive statements that indicate what he/she wants from his/her partner or from other family members. For example, the therapist may help a teenager who is angry and withdrawn to express to his parents his need to have a say in matters that pertain to him rather than being told what to do and how to do it. The therapist might ask the parents to respond as to how they might feel about what they heard from their son.

The therapist could use the information from the analysis of the relational pattern to affirm or to revise his original hypothesis regarding which unmet core needs are impacting the couple and family relationships and to revise, if necessary, treatment goals. The therapist might also begin to formulate how the individual's psychic- and self-structures are being played out in the relationships and how to address them and transform them so that the individuals move toward having the nurturing and supportive relationships that they so desperately desire.

Analysis of the psychic structure

The impact that a person's psychic structure (i.e., inner world) has on the formation and maintenance of a relationship is more difficult to analyze. However, the therapist can pick up cues from the analysis of the individual's communication style, relational pattern, and coping strategies. Statements such as "when I do things for myself, I feel selfish and guilty" and "I should be helping out more with the chores but I don't feel like it" provide clues to a person's psychic structure. In both examples, the therapist observes that there is an inner struggle, with one part wanting to do things for himself and the other part demanding that he comply with the wishes of others. The therapist listens for such statements and determines whether the individual's internal struggle is externalized in his relationships and if so, the therapist makes a link between the two. It is possible that an individual who is demanding of himself, may also be demanding of others in terms of putting emphasis on duties, obligations, and being busy, and downplaying the need for pleasure, fun, and play. The function of psychic-structure may also be observed in statements such as "I have to do things in a specific sequence and if I don't, I fear that something bad will happen." The ritual might serve to protect the person from being scolded and reprimanded for making mistakes and causing harm to others.

The therapist and the individual together analyze and try to resolve the intra-psychic struggles within couple or family therapy as it is useful for the others to understand the individual's struggle and to be of help to him. The therapist reviews his assessment of the person's unmet core needs and makes adjustments if needed.

Intrapsychic work in couple and/or family therapy is frowned upon by most systems-oriented therapists. Napier and Whitaker (1978) state that working with couples and families begins with couple and family therapy, and when the family has resolved their major relationship conflicts, the conflicts that remain are then of an "intrapsychic nature, remnants of past experience that continue to trouble the person" (p. 275). They add that if a person wants to work on his personal difficulties, then there is reason to meet with him individually. SIRCFP takes a slightly different approach and incorporates intrapsychic work into couple and family therapy. This is particularly true if an individual's internal problems are standing in the way of couple and family therapy moving forward. SIRCFP questions whether couple and family problems can be said to be resolved when one or more members continue to have intrapsychic struggles. If the therapist arranges to see a member individually, he will ask permission from the client and from the other members.

Analysis of self-structure

The perception that an individual has of himself in relationship to others can play a significant role in the development, quality, and maintenance of intimate relationships. Both low self-esteem and feeling inadequate can lead to self-depreciation and self-criticism and possibly to depression and to other disorders. The therapist can obtain information about an individual's view about himself by listening to statements such as "I am stupid in not being able to ace the exam" or "I do not like myself for not being a good father and a good partner" or "I am just not good enough." In these statements the therapist understands that the client's unmet core needs are to be "significant" and "competent."

The therapist and client can work together on these needs in the context of the couple and family therapy. The therapist can help the client understand the origins of his unmet needs, such as an absent parent during childhood, and bullying at school, and share them with the others. Such sharing may motivate those present to show their empathy toward the client and provide meaningful support.

Analysis of the coping strategies

As the therapist observes how the couple and family communicate and relate with each other, he also pays attention to how they deal with relational conflicts and with differences of opinion, ideas, interests, and needs. Are such conflicts and differences addressed, dismissed, minimized, and/or catastrophized? For example, a teenager may want to have a voice in matters that concern his life such as the choice of friends, the type of athletic activity, the form of music, and the selection of education and career. The therapist assesses the extent to which the parents support the teenager in such choices or the extent to which the parents determine the teenager's choices. The therapist may also assess the couple and members of the family's capacity to negotiate, compromise, apologize for hurt caused, forgive the offender, and to repair ruptures in relationships.

To help the couple and members of the family develop more effective coping skills, the therapist could engage an individual, such as a teenager, with one of his parents in a discussion about a matter significant to him. The therapist can help the teenager and the parent listen to each other, stay on topic, and come to a decision. That is, rather than the two engaging in an argument, the therapist helps both be direct, thoughtful, focused, and assertive rather than being defensive and feeling judged.

Coping strategies can be used to deal with life's day-to-day situations and they can also be employed to protect oneself from psychological hurts. In the latter case, the therapist can ask himself what is the member protecting himself from? He can determine whether his impression is consistent with the hypothesis that he formulated based on the couple and family's communication and relational difficulties, or whether the hypothesis and the treatment goals need to be revised.

Analysis of the unmet core needs

An important aspect of SIRCFP is to help the individual uncover, accept, and integrate core relational, self, and physical intimacy needs and have them accepted and responded to by his partner or by his family members. The therapist reframes the client's experiences and then helps him identify, name, and express the unmet core needs. The process of identifying, naming, and working with the unmet needs begins at the commencement of therapy and is an integral part in the analysis of the communication style, relational patterns, and coping strategies. As the therapist and a partner or member of the family analyzes his communication style, relational patterns, and coping strategies, the therapist listens for and helps the participant identify, name, and express his unmet core needs. Two significant aspects in helping him express his needs are an analysis of the personal barriers that stand in the way of expressing them, and an analysis of the difficulty on part of his partner or his family members to accept his core needs (Meier & Boivin, 2022). The path to uncovering these needs may begin with feelings of anger, then move to hurt, and finally to the expression of unmet needs. Another path can begin with depression, move to anger, and then hurt and finally come to the unmet need.

Typically, one begins to work intensely and almost exclusively with unmet needs after a person has expressed and managed his/her negative feelings toward the other and the feelings have been acknowledged and validated. The work with needs is usually followed by an empathic shift toward their partner or member of the family. At this point, the partners and members of the family are more disposed to talk about their unmet needs in the couple and family relationships. It is anticipated that the recognition, acceptance, and validation of core needs moves progressively toward changes in communication style, relational pattern, coping strategies, and psychic and self-structures.

The observation that couples and members of a family engage in the expression of tender feelings and of their intimate needs following an empathic shift is consistent with the results from Meier and Boivin's (2006) research on the resolution of internal conflicts. In their study, they observed that following the expression of negative feelings and judgments, there was an empathic shift by one of the parts (e.g., Topdog, Underdog) in the conflict. This led to a discussion of their unmet needs and a willingness to collaborate in establishing a meaningful relationship.

This chapter presented the unique characteristics, principles, and assumptions of SIRCFP; its major theoretical constructs, therapy goals, and interventions; the phases of the change process in couple and family therapy; the role of the therapist; and the negative interactional patterns and their underlying dynamics that can be the focus of couple and family therapy. The following chapter applies SIRCFP to the therapy of a couple.

References

Allport, G.W. (1967). *Becoming: Basic considerations for a psychology of personality*. New Haven: Yale University Press.

Bader, E., & Pearson, P.T. (1988). *In quest of the mythical mate: A developmental approach to diagnosis and treatment in couple therapy*. New York: Brunner/Mazel.

Baucom, D.H., Epstein, N.B., LaTaillade, J.J., & Kirby, J.S. (2008). Cognitive-behavioral therapy. In A.S. Gurman (Ed.), *Clinical handbook of couple therapy*, 4th Edition (pp. 31–72). New York: Guilford Press.

Benjamin, L.S. (2006). *Interpersonal reconstructive therapy: Promoting change in nonresponders*. New York: Guilford Press.

Bettelheim, B. (1983). *Freud and man's soul: An important reinterpretation of Freudian theory*. Toronto: Random House.

Brammer, L., & MacDonald, G. (2002). *The helping relationship: Process and skills*, 8th Edition. London, UK: Pearson.

Brinich, P., & Shelley, C. (2002). *The Self and personality structure: Core concepts in therapy*. Buckingham, UK: Open University Press.

Buber, M. (2010). *I and thou*. New York: Charles Scribner's Sons.

Cashdan, S. (1988). *Object relations therapy: Using the relationship*. New York: W.W. Norton.

Conroy, D.E., & Pincus, A.L. (2006). A comparison of mean partialing and dual-hypothesis testing to evaluate stereotype effects when assessing profile similarity. *Journal of Personality Assessment, 86*(2), 142–149.

Cormier, S., Nurius, P., & Osborn, C. (2015). *Interviewing and change strategies for helpers*. Australia: Cengage Learning.

Deci, E.L., & Ryan, R.M. (2002). *Handbook of self-determination research*. Rochester, New York: University of Rochester Press.

Duncan, B.L., & Miller, S.D. (2000). The client's theory of change: Consulting the client in the integrative process. *Journal of Psychotherapy Integration, 10*(2), 169–187.

Egan, G. (1982). *The skilled helper: Model, skills, and methods for effective helping*. Monterey, CA: Brooks/Cole Publishing Company.

Freud, S. (1923). The Ego and the Id. *Standard Edition, 19*, 12–63.

Freud, S. (1938) An outline of psycho-analysis. *Standard Edition, 23*, 144–207.

Gendlin, E.T. (1996). *Focusing-oriented psychotherapy: A manual of the experiential method*. New York: Guilford Press.

Gottman J.M., & Gottman, J.S. (2008). Gottman method couple therapy. In A.S. Gurman (Ed.), *Clinical handbook of couple therapy*, 4th Edition (pp. 138–164). New York: Guilford Press.

Greenberg, L.S. (2010). Emotion-focused therapy: A clinical synthesis. *Focus, 8*, 32–42.

Greenberg, L.S., & Goldman, R.N (2008). *Emotion-focused couples therapy: The dynamics of emotion, love, and power*. Washington, D.C.: American Psychological Association.

Greenberg, L.S., & Johnson, S. (1988). *Emotionally focused therapy for couples*. New York: Guildford Press.

Gurman, A.S. (2008). *Clinical handbook of couple therapy*, 4th Edition. New York: The Guilford Press.

Hendrix, H. (1996). Foreword. In W. Luquet (Ed.), *Short-term couple therapy: The imago model in action* (pp. vii–x). New York: Routledge.

Hendrix, H. (2008). *Getting the love you want: A guide for couples*. New York: St. Martin's Press.

Ivey, A.E. (1986). *Developmental therapy: Theory in practice*. San Francisco: Jossey-Bass Publishers.

Ivey, A.E. (1983). *Intentional interviewing and counselling*. Monterey, California: Brooks/ Cole.

Ivey, A.E., & Gluckstern, N.B. (1984). *Basic influencing skills*, 2nd Edition. North Amherst, Massachusetts: Microtraining Associates.

Ivey, A.E., Gluckstern, N.B., & Ivey, M.B. (2006). *Basic attending skills*, 3rd Edition. North Amherst, Massachusetts: Microtraining Associates.

Jacobson, E. (1964). *The self and the object world*. New York: International Universities press.

Johnson, S.M (2004). *The practice of emotionally focused couple therapy: Creating connections*, 2nd Edition. New York: Brunner-Routledge.

Klein, M. (1946), Notes on some schizoid mechanisms. In M. Klein (Ed.), *Envy and gratitude and other works, 1946–1963* (pp. 1–24). New York: Delacorte Press/Seymour Lawrence.

Klein, M. (1959). Our adult world and its roots in infancy. In M. Klein (Ed.), *Envy and gratitude and other works 1946–1963 (Vol. 4)* (pp. 247–263). New York: Delacorte Press/ Seymour Lawrence.

Kohut, H. (1971). *The analysis of self*. New York: International Universities Press.

Kohut, H. (1977). *The restoration of the self*. New York: International Universities Press.

Kohut, H. (1981). On empathy. In P.H. Ornstein (Ed.), *The search for the self: Selected writings of Heinz Kohut: 1978–1981 (Vol. 4)* (pp. 525–535). New York: International Universities Press.

Kohut, H., & Wolfe, E.S. (1978). The disorders of the self and their treatment: An outline. *International Journal of Psycho-Analysis, 59*, 413–425.

Korb, M.P., Gorrell, J., & Van de Riet, V. (1989). *Gestalt therapy: Practice and theory*, 2nd Edition. Oxford, UK: Pergamon Press.

Luthman, S.G., & Kirschenbaum, M. (1974). *The dynamic family*. Palo Alto, CA: Science and Behavior books.

Mahler, M.S., Pine, F., & Bergman, A. (1975). *The psychological birth of the human infant*. New York: Basic Books.

Meichenbaum, D. (1977). *Cognitive-behavior modification: An integrative approach*. New York: Plenum.

Meier, A. (2001). Adult survivors of incest and capacity to forgive: An object relations perspective. In A. Meier & P. VanKatwyk (Eds.), *The challenge of forgiveness* (pp. 87–123). Saint Paul University, Ottawa, ON: Novalis.

Meier, A., & Boivin, M. (1998). *The seven-phase model of the change process: Theoretical foundation, definitions, coding guidelines, training procedures, and research data*, 5th Edition. Unpublished manuscript. Ottawa, Ontario: Saint Paul University.

Meier, A., & Boivin, M. (2000). The achievement of greater selfhood: The application of theme-analysis to a case study. *Psychotherapy Research, 10*(1), 60.

Meier, A., & Boivin, M. (2006). Intrapsychic conflicts, their formation, underlying dynamics and resolution: An object relations perspective. In A. Meier & M. Rovers (Eds.), *Through conflict to reconciliation* (pp. 295–328). Ottawa, Ontario: Novalis.

Meier, A., & Boivin, M. (2011). *Counselling and therapy techniques: Theory and practice.* London, England: Sage.

Meier, A., & Boivin, M. (2022). *Self-in-relationship psychotherapy: A complete clinical guide to theory and practice.* Oxford, UK: Routledge.

Meier, A., Boivin, M., & Meier, A. (2006). The treatment of depression: A case study using theme-analysis. *Counselling and Psychotherapy Research, 6*(2), 115–125.

Meier, A., Boivin, M., & Meier, M. (2008). Theme-Analysis: Procedures and application for psychotherapy research. *Qualitative Research in Psychology, 5*, 289–310.

Miller, R., & Rollnick, S. (2013). *Motivational interviewing: Helping people change*, 3rd Edition. New York: Guilford Press.

Napier, A., & Whitaker, C.A. (1978). *The family crucible.* London: Harper & Row.

Nichols, M.P. (2009). *The lost art of listening: How learning to listen can improve relationships.* New York: Guilford Press.

Ogden, T. (1989). *The primitive edge of experience.* Northvale, NJ: Jason Aronson.

Osipow, S.H., Walsh, W.B., & Tosi, J. (1984). *A survey of counseling methods.* Homewood, Illinois: The Dorsey Press.

Perls, F.S. (1969). *Gestalt therapy verbatim.* Toronto: Bantam Books.

Rathus, J.II., & Miller, A.L. (2015). *DBT skills manual for adolescents.* New York: Guilford Press.

Rogers, C.R. (1961). *On becoming a person.* Boston: Houghton Mifflin.

Sadock, B.J., Sadock, V.A., & Ruiz, P. (2014). *Kaplan and Sadock's synopsis of psychiatry Behavioral sciences clinical psychiatry*, 11th Edition. New York: Walter Kluwer.

Satir, V. (1972). *People making.* Palo Alto, CA: Science and Behavioral Books.

Satir, V., Banmen, J., Gerber, J., & Gomori, M. (1991). *The Satir model: Family therapy and beyond.* Palo Alto, CA: Science and Behavioral Books.

Scharff, D.E., & Scharff, J.S. (2014). An overview of psychodynamic couple therapy. In D.E. Scharff & J.S. Scharff (Eds.), *Psychoanalytic couple therapy: Foundations of theory and practice* (pp. 3–24). New York: Routledge.

Scharff, J.S., & Scharff, D.E. (2008). Object relations couple therapy. In A.S. Gurman (Ed.), *Clinical handbook of couple therapy*, 4th Edition (pp. 167–196). New York: Guilford Press.

Segal, J. (2004). *Melanie Klein*, 2nd Edition. London: Sage.

Shaddock, D. (2000). *Contexts and connections: An intersubjective systems approach to couple therapy.* New York: Basic Books.

Stern, D.S. (1985). *The interpersonal world of the infant: A view from psychoanalysis and developmental psychology.* New York: Basic Books.

The New York Institute for Psychoanalytic Self Psychology (2022). *Self psychology psychoanalysis: Empathy misinterpreted.* New York: Author.

Van Edwards, V. (2022). *The 5 relationship patterns: Which are you?* Retrieved from: www.scienceofpeople.com/relationship-patterns June, 2022.

Winnicott, D. (1965). *The family and individual development.* London: Tavistock Publishers.

Wolpe, J. (1990). *The practice of behavior therapy.* New York: Pergamon Press.

Yablonsky, L. (1976). *Psychodrama: Resolving emotional problems through role-playing.* New York: Basic Books.

Chapter 6

Case Illustration

Daniel and Sylvie

The application of Self-in-Relationship Couple and Family Psychotherapy (SIRCFP) to couple therapy is illustrated in the therapeutic work with Daniel and Sylvie, both in their late forties. They had been married for 21 years and had one teenage daughter. They requested therapy to help them to resolve their long-standing marital conflicts and abuses that spanned their entire 21 years together.

The application of SIRCFP in working with this couple begins by presenting the brief psychosocial histories for Daniel and Sylvie. This is followed by a description of the results from the application of the Self-in-Relationship Psychotherapy Assessment Form (SIRP-AF; Appendix B) to the psychosocial histories. Sylvie and Daniel's presenting problems are then conceptualized. The next part presents the goals of therapy, the therapy process, the orientation of the therapist, and the therapeutic relationship. The last part presents the treatment, which includes the analysis of the communication style, relational patterns, coping strategies, psychic- and self-structures, and the articulation of the unmet core needs.

Psychosocial Histories

Daniel's History

Daniel was brought up in a family where there was very little expression of affection and where discipline was adequate. His mother was the disciplinarian. He and his family did very few things together with the exception of going fishing. He thinks that he was brought up in a "good enough" but conservative home.

Daniel has a high school education and a three-year college diploma. He is president of his company, which provides both hardware and software computer services.

Daniel came across as being reserved and as having low energy. He did mention that he had not learned how to deal with his anger toward his wife and toward his employees. He tends to become helpless when confronted with conflict, opposition,

DOI: 10.4324/9781032655291-9

or anger. He avoids conflict and has not learned how to be helpful to resolve conflictual situations.

Regarding their marriage, and contrary to Sylvie's contention, Daniel stated that he does show his affection and love for her. In the face of Sylvie's criticisms of him, Daniel feels discouraged, and helpless. He also thinks that Sylvie finds him to be worthless and has placed him at the bottom of the totem pole. However, his view of himself is that he strives to be autonomous and feels that he is competent as a person and in his work.

Sylvie's History

Sylvie's upbringing was abusive and traumatic. Her father, an alcoholic, was a blue-collar worker and her mother was a stay-at-home mom. Both of her parents passed away about eight years prior to the beginning of couple therapy.

She mentioned that both her father and mother were physically abusive toward her, hit her, and used the strap until she was 17 years old. They were also mentally abusive by demeaning her, telling her that she was good for nothing, and calling her "stupid," which continued into her adult life. Her father, who at one time was caring and loving, and at other times abusive, also sexually abused Sylvie and her sister. The abuse began when Sylvie was ten years of age and continued until she was 13 years old. One of the instances of sexual abuse occurred when she was asleep, and when she woke up, he left her bedroom. She did not know whether the abuse was real or if it was a dream. She screamed to her mother for help, but when she arrived, the father was already in another room of the house. The sexual abuse stopped between the ages of 13 and 15, during the time that the father was in jail, but continued after his release until Sylvie was 16 years old. Rather than reporting the sexual abuse to her mother and risk splitting the family, she left home. The father sought counselling and promised not to abuse her again. She came home, only to have him resume the abuse. She then left home, was married, and had a transformative experience, and three years before he passed away, she forgave her father for his abusive behaviors.

Sylvie has grade 12 education and two years of university. Sylvie worked for six years in Daniel's company and then left the company because of the employees' complaints about Daniel, who was perceived not to affirm them nor to validate their work.

Regarding their marriage, Sylvie mentioned that it has had its ups and downs since the beginning. She reported that Daniel has been both physically and verbally abusive toward her. She was very bitter and angry toward Daniel for having deprived her of love, affection, and compliments. She blamed him for their marital problems. She mentioned that she had in the past burst out in anger and lost control of her anger and rage, and had been both verbally and physically abusive toward Daniel.

Results from the SIRP-AF

The results from the administration of the SIRP-AF to Daniel and Sylvie are summarized in Table 6.1. The results provide a glimpse into their inner worlds and how these might affect their potential communication and relational dynamics and patterns.

Daniel tends to relate to others as differentiated persons. He strives to be autonomous and competent. He has integrated social and cultural demands with his personal needs and reality, and tends to be genuine in his responses to others. He is predisposed to avoid conflict and stressors and to take a rational and matter-of-fact approach in solving such problems. Daniel appears to have the empathic capacity to understand the feelings and needs of others and to respond accordingly.

Regarding Sylvie, she tends to relate to others as being enmeshed, that is, as two undifferentiated persons. Her need to feel important and significant dominates her close relationships. She tends to be a pleaser and tries to draw people into caregiver positions to meet her expectations and demands. When they do not respond as expected, she feels rejected and unloved and acts out in anger and rage. Her relationships appear to be characterized by neediness, anger, rage, and lack of empathic understanding of others. Her sense of self is underdeveloped. She has not harmoniously integrated social and cultural expectations with her basic needs and with reality.

Conceptualizations

The conceptualizations for both Sylvie and Daniel are based on the psychosocial histories and on the results from the SIRP-AF. The conceptualization for each is presented and is followed by a comment regarding how their intrapsychic realities might interact in their intimate relationship.

Sylvie's presenting problems consisted of becoming angry and raging when slighted, unable to regulate her affect, feeling unloved, insignificant, and not complimented by Daniel. She fluctuated between being harsh and critical of him and being needy. In her relationship she tried to draw Daniel into being a caregiver (i.e., her projective identification), which he resisted. Her desires and her acting out behaviors were understandable given her history of emotional, physical, and sexual abuse and of feeling that she was "stupid" and would amount to nothing in life. As a young child she failed to develop an emotional bond with her "mother," a "bodily sense of self," and object constancy (i.e., internalization of positive qualities and behaviors of loving people). At the same time, she internalized the criticisms of her parents to form a harsh and critical superego. Sylvie was left with a *needy self,* *a harsh superego,* and an *ineffective ego* to reconcile her relational and self needs with her superego. She reenacted this relational and self-dynamics with Daniel in that she craved his love, attention, and affection, and became critical of him when he was not able to respond in the way she needed. Since she did not experience love

Table 6.1 Summary of results from the SIRP Assessment Forms

Construct	Daniel	Sylvie
1. Manner of relating to others: (PO = Part object [person relates to others as they are needed]; WO = Whole object [person relates to others according to needs of the other] (Score on a 5-point scale with PO = 1 and WO = 5)	3.5	1.5
2. Psychic Structure: (Au = Need to be autonomous; Eb = Need for emotional bonding; Superego (Acceptable behaviors) (1 = Weak striving; 5 = Strong striving)	Au = 3.5 ego = 3.5 superego = 3	Eb = 4 ego = 2 superego = 4
3. Self-Structure: (Comp = Need to be competent; Sign = Need to be significant) (Scored on a 5-point scale with 1 = Weak striving; 5 = Strong striving)	Comp = 3.5	Sign = 4
4. True Self (Living from): (Scored on a 5-point scale with minimally = 1; strongly = 5)	3.5	2
5. Coping Strategies	Defends Avoids	Blames Projects Devalues
6. Emotional Bond: (Secure; Striving; Avoiding; Disconnect)	Avoiding	Striving
7. Object Constancy; (On a 5-point scale with 1 = Not formed; 5 = Fully formed)	3.5	1.5
8. Characteristic Emotional State	Detached, reserved	Angry, Raging
9. Projective Identification: (Power; Dependency, Ingratiation; Sexuality, Rational)	Power	Dependent
10. Characteristic Developmental Phase: (Symbiosis; Differentiation; Practicing; Rapprochement; Integration/consolidation)	Integration/Consolidation	Different-iation
11. Characteristic Developmental Position: (On a 5-point scale with 1 = Paranoid Schizoid Position and 5 = Depressive Position)	3.5	2.0

as an infant and child, it was difficult for her to give love and to receive love, or to know when Daniel was not able to give more as he had no more to give.

Daniel's presenting problems included difficulty in managing Sylvie's emotional outbursts, graciously responding to Sylvie's affectional needs, openly facing and resolving conflicts rather than withdrawing from them, and accessing and expressing his own feelings and needs. When faced with conflicts, Daniel shut down and withdrew. Daniel resisted becoming Sylvie's caregiver as he cherished his sense of autonomy. Daniel's style of relating is comprehensible given that he was brought up in a home where there was very little expression of emotions and affection. He did not learn how to deal with conflicts; he was not encouraged to express his feelings; he suppressed them. He developed at a young age a sense of autonomy and competency that he was not willing to surrender. Daniel was left with *repressed needs and feelings*, a *moderate superego*, and a *super rational ego*. When he began a relationship with Sylvie, he reenacted a style of communicating and relating that he learned in childhood. This style comprised suppressing and regulating feelings, brushing aside conflicts, being rational, rigorously maintaining his sense of autonomy, and demonstrating an unwillingness to become Sylvie's caregiver.

In terms of their attractions, Sylvie saw in Daniel someone who was secure, strong, rational, and practical, whereas Daniel saw in Sylvie someone who was expressive, outgoing, passionate, and energetic. In their growth as a couple, one would expect that each would adopt and integrate some of the qualities of their partner. That is, Daniel would accept and integrate some of Sylvie's qualities and Sylvie would accept and integrate some of Daniel's qualities. Failing to accomplish this, and with the intense need on the part of Sylvie for love and affection and to feel significant, it is possible that Daniel would feel that he could not give enough to satisfy her and might feel inadequate as a husband, and that Sylvie, on her part, would feel deprived. This combination, it is anticipated, could lead to marital discord and potential emotional and psychological abuse. This dynamic would affect their manner of communication and the formation of their relational patterns.

Treatment: Goals, Process, Orientation, Interventions, and Therapeutic Relationship

The goals of treatment, the therapy process, therapist orientation and interventions, and the therapeutic relationship are briefly presented. In a letter from Sylvie one year after the termination of therapy (see excerpt from letter at end of chapter), she mentioned that they overcame many of the obstacles in their relationship and they were enjoying the relationship that they never dreamed to have.

Goals of Treatment

The short-term goal was to help the couple develop a more harmonious and satisfying relationship by improving their communication, relational, and coping skills. The long-term goal was for the couple to become aware of their unmet core self, relational, and physical intimacy needs and how these were impacting their relationship. The goal for Daniel was to become aware of the roots of his difficulties to express his core self and relational needs, and for Sylvie the goal was to help her to bring her core self and relational needs in line with realistic expectations. An overarching goal was to help the couple become aware of their core needs, accept them as part of being human, learn to freely express them and to respect the same in his/her partner, and to organize their personal lives and their couple relationship accordingly.

The Therapy Process

Daniel and Sylvie requested therapy to help them resolve their long-standing marital conflicts and abuses that spanned their entire 21 years together. Prior to the commencement of couple therapy, Daniel and Sylvie were seen individually for one assessment session. Following the individual assessment sessions, they were seen for 15 couple sessions. They terminated couple therapy after the fifteenth session. However, they returned six months later and continued for another 10 couple sessions. The purpose of the individual sessions was to obtain their psychosocial history and to assess how they internalized the events of their history to shape their inner worlds and form their relational expectations. Such information is helpful to understand their internal dynamics and how it would contribute to the relational dynamics. In the early therapy sessions, the couple was engaged in blaming and defensive dialogues and not talking about the issues that mattered. As therapy progressed, they became more congenial and open to considering the psychological place from which their partner came.

The treatment, in broad strokes, proceeded according to the following sequence: (a) description of the problems; (b) analysis of the communication style; (c) analysis of the relational pattern; (d) uncovering of the internal factors (e.g., psychic structure; self-structure) that might act as barriers to the development of healthier relational patterns; and (e) identifying of their unmet core needs and integrating them in their relational patterns.

Therapist Orientation

The therapist (A.M.), male, Canadian, was a doctoral-level trained and experienced developmental, psychodynamic, and humanistic-oriented individual and couple/family psychotherapist who worked full-time in a university graduate counseling and psychotherapy program and had a part-time private practice. The therapist's training in couple/family therapy was according to the Virginia Satir (Satir, 1972; Satir, Banmen, Gerber & Gomori 1991) and Luthman and Kirschenbaum (1974) models. Both models apply an experiential, psychodynamic, and relational approach in their theory and practice. The therapist had the great pleasure to meet Dr. Satir in person and to attend a weekend workshop on couple and family therapy.

Therapist Interventions

Interventions to facilitate fruitful dialogue

To facilitate a fruitful dialogue between Daniel and Sylvie, the therapist used reflective and validation statements and process and open-ended questions. Reflective statements were used in two different ways. In one way, the therapist reflected to the clients the feeling and need aspects of their statements. In a second way, the therapist asked either Daniel or Sylvie to repeat correctly what his/her partner said. The purpose was for the client to develop listening and observational skills.

Validation statements were used to let the clients know that the therapist understood where they were coming from and that he accepted them without judgment. To validate did not mean to approve or to agree with what the clients said or to try to change them. The therapist also tried to have the partners validate each other and to know more about where they were coming from.

In using process questions, the therapist followed the flow of clients' internal experiences and made changes as new material such as feelings, needs, and thoughts emerged in the session. The therapist helped the clients reflect on and process their thoughts, feelings, and unmet needs that seemed significant. The therapist worked with them in the here and now and focused on themes, patterns, and affects, such as being prone to feeling hurt, often feeling dismissed, and feeling depressed.

The therapist used open-ended questions to clarify his understanding of what the client was feeling or saying and to keep up the conversation. Open-ended questions required more than a simple answer such as yes or no.

Interventions to create new possibilities and provide corrective experiences

To create new possibilities, to alter dysfunctional interactional patterns, and to provide corrective experiences, the therapist used several available techniques. The techniques used include making I-You statements, translating complaints into assertive statements, engaging in confrontation, connecting with a bodily-felt feeling, and using emotional heightening.

The therapist encouraged the couple to use I-You statements (Buber, 2010), that is, to begin with an "I" statement rather than with a "You" or "It" statement. To begin with a "You" statement can sound like a scolding, blaming, or making a judgment, and to begin with an "It" statement is to keep distance from one's feelings. The use of I-You statements helped both Daniel and Sylvie experience the other as a person like himself/herself and respect the other and have a genuine interest in the other's feelings, needs, and thoughts.

A second technique used was asking the couple to translate complaints into assertive statements. In asking the couple to make assertive statements, it minimized an emotional reaction and rather than keeping them apart and at a distance, it brought them closer together and created a greater emotional bond. Translating complaints into assertive statements also demanded that they explore their feelings, thoughts, and needs.

Confrontation (Ivey & Gluckstern, 1984) was a third technique that the therapist used. He used this technique to point out between what a client thought or felt and what he said, between what he said and what he did, between what he is and what he wants to be, and between expressed values and his actual behavior. The focus was not on changing behavior but on experientially examining the behavior.

As a fourth technique, the therapist asked a client, such as Daniel, who was logical and cerebral, to put aside his thoughts and preoccupations and focus on his bodily felt feelings (Gendlin, 1996). This technique was used to help Daniel access deeper feelings and needs, which became material for the couple therapy sessions.

Emotional heightening (Korb, Gorrell & Van de Riet, 1989) was a fifth technique used in his therapy with Daniel and Sylvie, and particularly with Daniel, who tended to be soft spoken, retentive, and cerebral. Daniel was asked to repeat a statement that he made with more feeling and intensity. That which was expressed was then explored and traced to its roots, which often was to an unmet core need.

In brief, the therapist worked in the "here and now" as opposed to the "there and then" (Joyce & Sills, 2007, pp. 27), was actively engaged in therapeutic dialogue, and constantly checked back with the clients to assess what they were experiencing and processing, particularly when they demonstrated changes in behavior, tone of voice, and mood. The goal of therapy was to engage the clients in experiential learning and self-understanding, in order to better understand themselves and the nature of their relational difficulties, become skilled and empowered, take ownership of their own life, and become an agent of their own person within the context of their intimate and significant relationships.

Therapeutic Relationship

At the beginning of couple therapy, Daniel and Sylvie were in constant conflict. Sylvie was critical of Daniel, who either defended himself or became quiet. She tried to draw him into her thinking patterns and into her way of relating. He vehemently resisted. The therapist would ask them to stop with their dysfunctional way of communicating and relating, check out their assumptions, and use "I" and "You" statements rather than "You" or "It" statements. He also assigned exercises for them to do between sessions. Despite their conflicted relationship, they did collaborate and carried out communication exercises between sessions. They tended to be collaborative, responsive to the therapist's interventions, and had a strong motivation to improve their relationship. As therapy progressed, they became more reflective and attended to their subjective experience, and particularly their assumptions and projections and how they contributed to the marital discord. In the process, they accepted more responsibility to bring about the changes that they desired. Toward the end of therapy, they became more focused, reflective, poised, hopeful, and upbeat with themselves and with their relationship.

Treatment Aspects

Therapy with Sylvie and Daniel addressed the major overlapping components of the interactional patterns, which included: (a) analysis of the communication style; (b) analysis of the relational pattern; (c) the uncovering of the internal factors (e.g., psychic structure; self-structure) that might act as barriers to the development of healthier relational patterns; and (d) identification of the unmet core needs and integration of them into their relational patterns. As the therapist and Daniel and Sylvie addressed and worked through each of these components, the psychotherapist paid particular attention to the unmet core childhood and/or growth needs that were the source of the presenting problems. The therapist helped the couple identify their unmet core needs, name them, and make them become part of their personal lives and their couple relationship.

Analysis of Communication Style

In the analysis of Sylvie and Daniel's communication style, the therapist observed that their communication was marked by two characteristics, namely, an attack–defense behavior and a tendency to make assumptions and treat them as facts. The therapist pointed these out to the couple and helped them develop more effective communication skills. The focus was on *how* and *what* (e.g., feelings, core needs) to communicate and not on the *objective content* (e.g., work setting) of their communication.

Attack–defend pattern

In terms of their communication, it was observed that Sylvie tended to be bitter and angry toward Daniel; she was critical of him for not having been affectionate and loving toward her. Sylvie tended to use superlatives such as "never" and "always" to describe Daniel's lack of showing affection. She said that "he never looks at me," "he never holds my hand," and he "never hugs and kisses me." Daniel, on his part, would become defensive and justify his past behaviors, or he would withdraw, which only angered Sylvie more.

Daniel tended to use the words "it," "we," and "you" rather than "I." He found it difficult to find words to express his feelings and needs in the relationship. Sylvie also experienced difficulty coming up with words to express her feelings and needs. The therapist tried to help the couple improve their communication skills. During the couple's arguments in therapy, the therapist would intervene, stop the couple after they made an attacking or defensive statement, and help them improve upon it by asking them to say it in such a way that it more positively reflected their feelings, thoughts, and needs. The therapist asked them to practice speaking this way between the therapy sessions. They were asked to set aside 30 minutes two or three times per week to share with each other their positive feelings and needs with the hope that this would help them change their typical blaming-defensive and critical way of communicating. In follow-up sessions, both mentioned that for them to talk in an assertive way and to share their feelings and needs rather than to blame and defend, was difficult and would take some work.

Unchecked assumptions

A second characteristic of Sylvie and Daniel's communication pattern was that both made assumptions about the meaning of a statement made by their partner and treated their assumption as a fact, which led to repeated arguments. They did not check out their assumptions. Sylvie often began a conversation with Daniel, assuming what he meant by a certain statement. Following her interpretation (which was not what he meant) and with Daniel being defensive, she often lost it and raged toward him. She gradually became aware that what he meant was not what she thought it meant.

Sylvie stated that in not being able to communicate with each other, she did not understand Daniel nor what he was thinking or feeling. Consequently, she interpreted or inferred what he might be feeling with reference to his nonverbal behaviors. But this confused her since his words said one thing and his actions said something different. All of this led to her not being able to accept thoughtful gestures and affection from Daniel.

To help the couple with their discussions, the therapist suggested that both begin their discussion by putting their assumptions on hold, listen to the other and ask for clarification, and then focus on the topic or issue at hand and not bring in hurt feelings and issues of the past. In this way both would prevent the arousal of anger. As well, when Sylvie became angry, Daniel was to strive not to let her anger disable him, but move toward her in an understanding way. In the past when Sylvie became angry toward him, he withdrew, which only added to Sylvie's anger and rage. The therapist asked them to practice to withholding their interpretations and assumptions and to ask questions about what the other was thinking and feeling. This was intended as a way for the couple to check their assumptions and not jump to conclusions, which often brought forth automatic negative responses and behaviors.

Toward the end of therapy, Sylvie and Daniel acquired more efficient communication skills. This was illustrated in Sylvie discussing Daniel's business company with him. She felt that Daniel did not share enough about the company. This caused her to make assumptions about the company and finances. Daniel was reluctant to talk about the finances as he felt that it would anger Sylvie even more. The therapist encouraged the two to talk about it in therapy with the therapist guiding the discussion. Following this discussion, Sylvie heard Daniel say things that were reassuring.

Analysis of Relational Patterns

The main feature of Sylvie and Daniel's relational dynamics and pattern was Sylvie unconsciously trying to draw Daniel into forming a type of relationship where she was the "good" person and Daniel was the "bad" person (like her father). Consequently, she tried to draw Daniel into one of two positions (referred to as projective identifications). There were times when Sylvie tried to draw Daniel into playing the role of a father figure, to take care of her and say nice things such as "My sweet little girl." There were other times when she looked upon him as a child, was critical of him, and found him to be irresponsible and not caring. Daniel, on his part, felt pressured to be drawn into one of the two roles, but he resisted and tried to maintain the role of the adult and to relate to Sylvie as a lover, sweetheart, and friend.

Daniel's resistance to be drawn into Sylvie's projective identifications, enraged her as she felt unloved and insignificant to him. She lashed out, became critical of him, and called him a liar and described him as being cold, cruel, and as treating her like dirt. There were times when her rage resulted in physical altercations. This occurred particularly when Sylvie had expectations of Daniel with which he did not agree or became silent, and Sylvie interpreted his silence as a rejection of her. When Sylvie raged and demeaned him, Daniel found it difficult to remain in his role as an adult; he felt trapped and cornered as regardless to what he said or did, she did not accept it but continued to demean him.

Sylvie described Daniel as a person who was not capable of expressing his affection for her. She interpreted Daniel's difficulty to express his affection as the way her family responded to each other. She dismissed Daniel's affectionate gestures. When he expressed his affection for Sylvie by giving her a kiss before going to work, for example, she retorted by saying that his "behaviors are phony." Daniel found himself coming and going when he expressed his affection toward Sylvie as on the one hand, she begged for it, and on the other hand, when he was affectionate toward her, she pushed him away by being very critical of him.

She also accused him of never complimenting her. When Daniel expressed his love for her during one of the therapy sessions, she could not accept that he loved her. Daniel stated that it was difficult for him to compliment Sylvie. He gave the example of finding it difficult to compliment her for a good meal when he liked only the chicken but not the way the vegetables were cooked. Because he was not able to validate her for both, he felt he could not compliment her. Also, he feared that if he complimented her on a good meal, she would think that the compliment was about the meal and not an expression of his love for her. Daniel, on his part, when Sylvie did not accept his love and compliments and became frustrated and angry, shut down emotionally, withdrew, and became angry toward her. Sylvie, in turn would become angry hearing this, and they would find themselves in an escalating argument. Daniel felt that in her eyes, he was at the bottom of the totem pole.

The goal of therapy was to help them understand the underlying dynamics of their relational pattern and their feelings and expectations of their partner, learn to listen to each other, develop empathic capacity to tune into and respond to the feelings and needs of the other, become more spontaneous in their relationship, and be available to relate to the other at one time in a supportive and caring way, and at another time as relying on receiving the same from their partner. These goals remained the focus for the 25 therapy sessions. With these goals in mind, the therapist discussed with them a new way of relating, which included speaking to each other using "I" and "You" statements and expressing their feelings, thoughts, and needs in the here and now rather than letting them build up. This was difficult for them, but they managed to speak to each other about their experiences in the here and now using "I" and "You" statements. However, they continued to add words or phrases that aroused anger or defensiveness in the other. Nevertheless, both felt more hopeful and optimistic as they felt that something very different and positive had emerged. The therapist also suggested that for the time being, rather than focusing on the past hurts and disappointments, they focus on doing things that were pleasurable. At this suggestion, Sylvie's mood changed and she showed interest in Daniel.

The exploratory work that was carried on in therapy, led Sylvie to question whether her anger and rage toward Daniel came from the bad times in their relationship or whether they came from her relationship with her abusive father. In reading a self-help book, she saw a link between her unresolved feelings toward her father and her behavior toward Daniel. Thus, she became aware that some of her bitter feelings came from the relationship and some came from her being mentally, physically, and sexually abused by her father. Sylvie often got down on herself and repeated to herself statements that she heard when she was young such as "you are stupid" and you are "good for nothing." When she got down on herself, she became enraged toward Daniel (i.e., projected the feelings that she could not repress or tolerate). With this insight, Sylvie began to make changes in her relationship with Daniel, and Daniel on his part began to relate to her in a non-defensive way. This pattern of relating was new to both. She was able to speak to Daniel about conflictual issues with humor and detachment.

Sylvie was also helped by reading a book written by a pastor-psychologist who discussed relationships in terms of a blessing and a curse. The pastor-psychologist believed that in relationships, a person either blesses the other or curses the other and that the blessing or curse that is given is returned to the sender. This thought had a profound effect on Sylvie and helped her change the way she spoke to Daniel. She tried to give blessings, and the blessings given were returned to her.

Analysis of Psychic Structure

With the development of more effective communication and relational skills, Sylvie and Daniel began to focus more on themselves to better understand what it was that they brought to their relationship. Sylvie became aware, as mentioned earlier, that she brought into the relationship a lot of childhood baggage stemming from the abusive relationships with her parents. In some respects, she became (through internalization) her critical, demanding, and demeaning parents, first toward herself and second toward Daniel. She had fleeting thoughts where she heard herself repeat things that she, as a child, heard from her parents, such as "you are stupid" and you will "amount to nothing." Her "inner child" responded to these judgments in hurt, anger, and rage. In her relationship with Daniel, Sylvie played out these two roles. She could be critical, demanding, and demeaning, particularly when he did not respond positively to her need for compliments and expressions of affection. At other times she was needy and wanted him to compliment her and say things such as "my sweet little girl," but she rejected his compliments and expressions of affection stating that they were "phony." That is, she fluctuated between being the "internal critical parent" and being the "neglected and needy child," or in Freudian terms, between the superego and the id. Daniel on his part, tried to walk a middle road, that is, not be drawn in by her "internal parent" nor by her "inner child." He tried to be the adult for her. In Freudian terms, Daniel represented Sylvie's ego and tried to bring reason and reality to her personal struggles and to their relationship.

During therapy, the couple, particularly Sylvie, reworked and transformed their psychic structure. As mentioned earlier, Sylvie was profoundly affected by her insight that the "blessings" and "curses" that she gave to others were reciprocated. This insight led to a significant change regarding her "internal critical parent" in that it became more moderate in its demands, judgments, and sense of duty. The consequence was that Daniel too made changes in his psychic structure as he became keen to listen to Sylvie's needs and to respond to them without withdrawing and becoming angry.

Analysis of Self-Structure

Issues regarding self-worth, self-esteem, significance, and competency were present from the beginning of therapy; however, these were only indirectly addressed as part of improving communication and relational skills. The latter skills were thought to be foundational to support working through self issues and maintaining the improvements.

Throughout the therapy sessions, Daniel maintained his sense of autonomy and competency both in terms of relationships and his business practices. Sylvie constantly criticized him for not having the capacity to be compassionate and affectionate, and she often acted out in rage toward him. He did not let her criticisms nor her raging outbursts undermine his view of himself; he remained steadfast in his belief about himself. Sylvie on her part, often felt insignificant, worthless, and unlovable and was not ready to address these. Daniel, however, did not agree with Sylvie's perception of herself. He remained steady and persistent in his wish for her to accept his compliments and expressions of affection.

With the working through and transformation of her psychic structure, particularly her "internal critical parent," Sylvie began to perceive herself as significant to Daniel and to accept his compliments and expressions of affection. With her transformed view of herself, Sylvie became more accepting of Daniel as a person with his unique characteristics. As well, the communication and relational advances became more solidified.

Analysis of Coping Strategies

An important part of therapy with Sylvie and Daniel was to help them not only understand the roots of their communication and relational problems, but also develop more effective coping skills to address relational and personal problems when they emerged. The assessment of their coping strategies included an analysis of both their skills and capabilities to deal with issues external to themselves and issues internal to themselves.

During the analysis of their communication styles and relational dynamics and patterns, the couple became aware of the improvements that were needed and they worked toward implementing them. For example, they improved their capacities to listen, to withhold assumptions, and to ask for clarifications, and they changed their attack and defensive way of communicating to being more direct, nonjudgmental, and assertive.

However, the development of the capacities to deal with the external issues depended in part on Daniel and Sylvie's individual psychological work. Daniel, on his part, explored his tendency to be avoidant, to have difficulty in facing conflicts, to sweep relational issues under the rug, and to form emotional connections. Sylvie explored her tendency to make assumptions, to have strong emotional outbursts and rages toward Daniel, and her strong desire to be validated for being a worthwhile person. She also investigated her tendency to fluctuate between being critical and demanding on one hand, and being needy and dependent on the other. She linked these and other internal struggles to her emotional and physical abuse on the part of her parents and her sexual abuse on the part of her father. The insights that both Sylvie and Daniel gained from their personal work, which took place during couple therapy, added greatly to the development of their communication and relational skills.

Exploration and Integration of Core Needs

The exploration and integration of Sylvie and Daniel's mutual core relational, self, and physical intimacy needs was an integral and essential aspect of their therapy. This topic was in the forefront from the beginning of the therapy. It came up in the analysis of communication where Sylvie wanted Daniel to express his love and affection for her and to show that she was significant to him. It came up in the analysis of their relational dynamics and pattern where Sylvie, in her neediness, tried to draw Daniel into a caregiver role, which he resisted to maintain his need to be autonomous.

Addressing and trying to implement their individual core needs was not possible in the early sessions of couple therapy because of the negative feelings that characterized their relationship. The negative feelings toward each other inhibited the expression of tender feelings, a phenomenon referred to as reciprocal inhibition (Wolpe, 1990). The goal was not simply for them to practice expressing tender feelings and showing them behaviorally. Before this could occur, both Sylvie and

Daniel had to do personal work on themselves. Daniel worked on his tendency to avoid conflict and take distance when he felt hurt. Sylvie worked on trying to curb her tendency to emotionally act out and rage when Daniel did not respond to her in the way she wanted. Before both were able to express their personal and intimate needs, they succeeded in transforming their inner worlds, that is, their psychic structures and self-structures. In doing so, they became kinder toward themselves and consequently kinder toward their partner.

Toward the last therapy sessions, both had worked out their angry feelings toward each other and became more understanding of and empathic toward their partner. At the same time, both were more able to become tender toward the other and express their affection and to provide meaningful compliments. When Sylvie was asked by the therapist what she wanted in her relationship, she stated that she wants better times, to have fun and be playful. Daniel echoed her sentiment. The couple would not have been able to express these needs at the beginning of therapy. The core needs for Sylvie were for significance and emotional connection, and the core needs for Daniel were for autonomy and emotional connection. To help the couple identify their core needs and to express them, and to accept and respond positively to their partner's core needs guided couple therapy from beginning to termination.

As Sylvie and Daniel approached the termination of therapy, they were able to solve many of their marital conflicts and became more compassionate and affectionate partners. They developed more effective communication and relationship skills, which they were determined to continue to practice to improve the quality of their relationship. They became more responsive to the relational, self, and physical intimacy needs of their partner.

Evaluation of Couple Therapy

There were no outcome measures administered at the beginning nor at the termination of therapy. However, one year after the termination of therapy, the therapist received an unsolicited letter from Sylvie, who described the improvements in their couple relationship. These are excerpts from her letter.

"Since we left counselling, we have been enjoying a relationship that had completely eluded us in the past [...] Your patient input and guidance is a major factor for this change in us."

"You had inspired me to do a lot of reality checks and that was something that I took time to do. I began to realize that I could be way off base in my conclusions and it helped me to stop acting on what I perceived and to put to rest the anger and hurt that maybe only I brought to myself."

"I realized the way I reacted to Daniel and circumstances was MY perception of things not necessarily the truth. When I allowed these things deep into my spirit, I was able to stop allowing resentment and anger take over my life."

"As Daniel observed the changes that began in me, he began to react to me in a nondefensive and caring way [...] which was new to both of us."

"I never thought I would be 'comfortable' nor feel as though I belong in this relationship but now, I know it would have been disastrous had I left it, at least to me."

In summary, this chapter presented couple and family therapy according to SIRCFP. The unit of analysis was the couple's interactional pattern, which comprised communication style, relational patterns, coping strategies, and psychic- and self-structures. These dimensions were viewed considering unmet core needs, which when identified, accepted, and embraced led to improved communication skills and relational patterns.

References

Buber, M. (2010). *I and thou*. New York: Charles Scribner's Sons.

Gendlin, E.T. (1996). *Focusing-oriented psychotherapy: A manual of the experiential method*. New York: Guilford Press.

Ivey, A.E., & Gluckstern, N.B. (1984). *Basic influencing skills* 2nd Edition. North Amherst, Massachusetts: Microtraining Associates.

Joyce, P., & Sills, C. (2007). *Skills in Gestalt counselling and psychotherapy*. New York: Sage.

Korb, M.P., Gorrell, J., & Van de Riet, V. (1989). *Gestalt therapy: Practice and theory*, 2nd Edition. Oxford, UK: Pergamon Press.

Luthman, S.G., & Kirschenbaum, M. (1974). *The dynamic family*. Palo Alto, CA: Science and Behavior Books.

Satir, V. (1972). *People making*. Palo Alto, CA: Science and Behavioral Books.

Satir, V., Banmen, J., Gerber, J., & Gomori, M. (1991). *The Satir model: Family therapy and beyond*. Palo Alto, CA: Science and Behavioral Books.

Wolpe, J. (1990). *The practice of behavior therapy*. Oxford, UK: Pergamon Press.

Part III

Parent–Child Therapy

Chapter 7

Self-in-Relationship Child Psychotherapy

The beginning of child psychotherapy can be traced back to the practices and writings by Sigmund Freud, Hermine Hug-Hellmuth, Melanie Klein, and Anna Freud. These innovators used play in their therapy with children. Sigmund Freud (1909) was the first to use play in therapy to try to uncover his client's (Hans) unconscious fears and concerns. Hermine Hug-Hellmuth (1921) began using play as part of her treatment of children in 1920, and ten years later, Melanie Klein and Anna Freud formulated their theories and practices of psychoanalytic play therapy (Gil, 2014).

Klein believed that one can work with children's horrifying and unrealistic nature of their fantasies in the same way that one works with dreams and free associations. She hypothesized that a child projects his relational and internal struggles onto real persons and onto external objects. Anna Freud believed that one cannot work with the unconscious of the child. She emphasized the development of coping strategies and skills and used play to develop a relationship with her child clients (Lindon, 1972). Certain significant changes in the aim and methods of psychotherapeutic work with children were made with the application Rank's relationship therapy (1945). He was concerned with problems as they existed in the immediate present, regardless of their history. His theory was applied to child therapy by Allen, Taft, and Axline. Allen (1942) and Taft (1933) viewed the therapeutic relationship as being curative in its own right. They stressed the need for helping the child define himself in relation to the therapist. The therapy hour was conceived as a concentrated growth experience (Dorfman, 1951). Axline (1947), another pioneer in the use of play in therapy, emphasized the "power of the therapeutic relationship in conjunction with the child's natural growth process" as fundamental in helping the child individuate and develop self-esteem (cited by Webb, 1991, p. 26).

The early play therapists found play therapy to be a useful approach with children because children have not yet developed the abstract reasoning capacity and the verbal skills needed to adequately articulate their feelings, thoughts, needs, and behaviors (Hall, Kaduson & Schaefer, 2002). The belief is that through play, "the child will reveal meaningful information regarding his emotional problems and behaviors" (Johnson, Rasbury & Siegel, 1997). Hall and associates (2002)

DOI: 10.4324/9781032655291-11

concluded that "for children, toys are their words, and play is their conversation" (p. 515).

This chapter presents the application of Self-in-Relationship Psychotherapy (SIRP) in working with children and their parents. SIRP was originally designed as a therapy for adults (Meier & Boivin, 2022); however, it has been extended to working with children by the inclusion of play therapy techniques such as puppet play, drawing, storytelling, the turtle technique, and more than 50 other techniques (Hall et al., 2002; Schaefer & Cangelosi, 2016; Selva, 2020). The SIRP approach, when applied to child psychotherapy, is referred to as Self-in-Relationship Child Psychotherapy (SIRCP).

This chapter begins with a presentation of the core constructs of SIRP that are relevant to working with children and their parents. This is followed by a presentation of the definition of play therapy and its change mechanisms, therapeutic power, techniques, problems treated, and its effectiveness. It then proceeds to outline some therapeutic aspects such as the inclusion of parents in child therapy and the tasks, interventions, and qualities of the therapist.

Self-in-Relationship Psychotherapy's Core Constructs

In applying constructs from SIRP to working with children, it is helpful to keep in mind the process of psychologically separating and individuating (Mahler, Pine & Bergman, 1975). To psychologically separate means establishing that which is "me" from that which is "not me," and to individuate refers to forming one's own thoughts, preferences, values, choices, and goals and asserting them. The child's myriad of psychological and relational developments can be thought of as beginning in the separation and individuation process of the first three to four years of life. The separation and individuation process, which begins with the phase of symbiosis, has been conceptualized in terms of subphases, with developmental tasks associated with each subphase. It is within this process that the child develops representations of other, self, and the world; incorporates acceptable social behaviors and values; begins to develop his identity; and learns how to live out his core needs within a social context (Mahler et al., 1975; Stern, 1985). The separation and individuation processes are the concepts that bring a coherent unity to SIRP's constructs and interventions.

The SIRCP constructs that are relevant in working with children are briefly described and illustrated. At the heart of the SIRCP approach is the concept of core needs, which gives direction to a child's growth and development. The SIRCP constructs maintain their essential meaning but are worded in a way to reflect the life experience of the child. The reader can find a detailed description of the SIRP constructs and their operational definitions in the first chapter and in Meier and Boivin (2022).

The infant/child's initial relationship with others will be referred to as being with the mother. Mother can mean the birth mother or an adult, female or male, other than the birth mother.

Core Relational, Self, and Physical Intimacy Needs

The core needs have been organized according to three groups, namely relational, self, and physical intimacy needs. The relational needs comprise the need to emotionally bond with a significant other and the need to be autonomous. The self needs include the needs to feel competent and to feel significant. The physical intimacy needs comprise the need for sensual contact and the need for sexual intimacy (Meier & Boivin, 2022; Appendices B and C).

How does a child exhibit the strivings for these core needs? The child indicates its need for emotional bonding by shadowing the mother, by seeking for the mother when she is absent, and by wanting to have friends to play with. The child manifests its need to feel significant by seeking validation in pleasing the mother and in being a good child. The child manifests its budding need to feel competent, for example, by its first attempts to feed himself. He shows his growing need to be autonomous through his temper tantrums, which indicate that he is developing a mind of his own. He shows his need for sensual contact by the pleasure he shows in skin-to-skin touch as experienced in bathing, breastfeeding, in hugs, and in kisses.

Internal Representations of Other and Self

The degree to which the child's core needs are responded to by significant others will affect the child's perceptions of others, self, and the world. Based on these experiences with real people, the child forms cognitive and affective representations of others and self. When the experiences are pleasant, the child develops positive representations of others and the person is perceived as being "good," and when the experiences are unpleasant, the child forms negative representations of others and the person is perceived to be "bad" (Winnicott, 1962, p. 57).

Concomitant with the development of "good" and "bad" representations of others, the child also forms positive and negative representations of himself. When others respond positively to his core needs, the child perceives himself to be a "good" person, and when the other responds negatively to his core needs, the child feels "bad," thinking that it is his "badness" that kept the other from providing pleasant experiences and responding to his core needs. The good and bad representations of other and self form the child's subjective and imagined world; they represent the child's picture of the real world.

Psychic Organization

For the newborn to begin to live in a social world is a new experience that he must learn how to achieve. In his interactions with others and in the formation of representations of others and self, the child gradually learns what is expected of him regarding social behaviors and the values and ideals to live by. The child learns, through the processes of identification and internalization, how to live in the social world. The child becomes a social person by identifying with the behaviors, qualities, values, and functions of his caregivers and by internalizing and owning them.

The child's internalized socially acceptable behaviors and values become like an "internal working model" (Bowlby, 1988), that is, a template, that monitors and guides interactions with others and the world. The internalizations become like a "structure" or an "organization" within the person, which have come to be called, in psychodynamic terms, the superego (Freud, 1923). With the development of the superego, the child experiences being pulled by two forces, the demands of the superego and the strivings of his core needs. The Freudian concept of the id has been replaced by the concept of core needs (See Chapter 1). At the earliest age, the child is pulled by one or the other of the two forces, but with the maturation of perceptual and cognitive abilities and with the help of the parents, the child slowly learns, with as little conflict as possible, how to integrate his core needs and the social demands. The maturation of the perceptual and cognitive abilities ushers in a third force, namely, the ego, which has as its goal to negotiate the core needs of the child with the social demands and with reality. In the process, the child develops a psychic organization that comprises the superego, core needs, and the ego that function in harmony in the best interests of the child.

Self-Structure

The child begins to develop a sense of self from the experiences that he has in his interactions with and responses from his parents, siblings, and others, and from the experience in applying his cognitive and motoric skills in manipulating objects, The development of a sense of self begins by being unconditionally loved and by being admired for any advance in cognitive and motoric abilities. The received love and admiration feed the child's sense of omnipotence and nurture two of his core needs, namely, the needs for significance and competency. With the maturation of the child's perceptual and cognitive apparatuses and with the development of motoric skills, the child begins to explore the not-mother reality. His ability to manipulate objects and the admiration of his parents in seeing him do so, add to his sense of being significant (i.e., loved) and to his sense of being competent. The child begins to develop a sense of being significant and a sense of being competent by the parents being attuned to his feelings and needs and by validating him. As the child grows up, he uses the validations received from his parents as a basis to validate himself as a significant and competent person.

The child develops a self-structure that comprises two core needs, namely, the core needs to be significant and to be competent (Kohut, 1977). When one or the other of these two core needs is not adequately responded to by the parents, the child becomes vulnerable and may develop emotional and behavioral problems. The child might feel not loved, flawed, and incompetent when compared to his peers.

Coping Strategies and Emotional and Behavioral Problems

The infant/child inevitably experiences displeasure and frustration because the parents cannot consistently anticipate his biopsychosocial needs, or the child might experience emotional neglect, psychological, physical, and sexual abuse, and/or trauma. The way the child copes with this displeasures, frustration, trauma, and abuse is manifested by his behaviors. These behaviors can be thought of as acting in (internalizing) and acting out (externalizing) behaviors (Gil, 1991). Both types of behaviors may lead to emotional and behavioral problems.

Children who exhibit internalized behavior tend to be isolated, withdrawn, and not to interact with others but to try to deal with the emotional neglect and abuse on their own. They may show signs of depression, be anxious, be overcompliant, and lack spontaneity and playfulness. They may self-harm, disssociate, develop phobias, and demonstrate regressive behavior. These behaviors might be motivated by fear, guilt, and/or the need to please. Children who manifest externalized behavior direct their emotions outward toward others. Such children are aggressive, hostile, oppositional, and destructive. They can be violent and provocative and elicit abuse (Gil, 1991).

A SIRCP-oriented child therapist strives to understand the conditions that trigger internalizing and externalizing behaviors. The conditions are often assessed in terms of the child's relationships with significant others and cultural expectations. Conditions that lead to these behaviors may include emotional neglect, feeling that he does not belong, and psychological, physical, and sexual abuse. Another factor may be birth order, that is, being the eldest, youngest, or middle child. Identifying and addressing these conditions becomes an important aspect of therapy.

The SIRCP-oriented therapist looks beyond the behaviors and ascertains which of the child's core needs are not adequately responded to by the parents and by others. The therapist shares her assessment with the parents and helps them understand the child's needs and feelings, and develop parenting skills by giving a voice to the child to express his feelings and needs. The therapist uses this information to guide her therapy with the child and to remediate his behaviors by learning how to assert his feelings and needs and how to express them in a constructive way.

The therapist also tries to ascertain the mechanism that leads to the internalizing and externalizing behaviors. For a withdrawn child, it might be repression of his feelings and needs. With regard to an acting-out child, the mechanism might be displacement (i.e., a child who is angry at the father might express it toward his sibling or to a toy). For a child who can be loving at one moment and hostile another moment, the defense mechanism may be splitting, which means negating either the good or the bad qualities of a person and seeing them as being all good or all bad. In the case of a child who is excessively compliant and pleasing, the defense mechanism might be reaction-formation, which means that a child displays a behavior and emotion that is opposite to how he feels. Thus, an angry child might exhibit being kind, loving, and caring.

Characteristic Feeling State

A troubled child typically displays a characteristic feeling. Some children might be angry, hostile, oppositional, and destructive, whereas other children might be anxious, depressed, or sad. These feeling states are the child's way of saying that his core needs are not being met. The SIRCP psychotherapist pays attention to these feeling states and does not try to change them, but uses them to lead the child to the unmet core needs. This can be facilitated through play therapy and with the selection of toys that allow the child to project his unique feelings onto the toy. It is assumed that when the child begins to live from his needs with the help of the therapist and his parents, the characteristic feeling state diminishes and a more positive feeling state emerges.

Relational Pattern

There is a wide range of relational patterns that children may develop when they experience emotional neglect or are demeaned and oppressed by their parents and significant others. These relational patterns may include: approach and pursuit, with the child constantly clamoring the parent for love and affection; avoidance, with the child resisting emotional and physical intimacy; oppositional, in angrily resisting requests, advice, and direction from a parent; withdrawal. in being shy and noncommunicative; and well-behaved, in complying with the wishes of the parents and adults to avoid conflicts and reprimands.

The therapist's first task is not to change the child's relational pattern but to identify the child's unmet core relational and/or self needs that are driving the behaviors. When these have been identified, the therapist shares this with the parents, and then the therapist, parents, and child begin to work together to develop a parent–child climate where the child's needs and feelings are heard, understood, and adequately responded to. In her therapy with the child, the therapist organizes play activities that help the child express his feelings, needs, and thoughts. The therapist may set up activities through which the child vicariously fulfills his needs (e.g., by hugging and speaking to a stuffed teddy bear or doll, by caring for an ailing character). The therapist respects the child's relational pattern and yet at the same time tries to draw the child into relating in a more open, direct, and friendly manner.

Object Constancy and Self Constancy

A great achievement for the child is the development of object constancy and self constancy. Object constancy refers to the "maintenance of the representation of the absent love object" (i.e., mother) and implies "the unifying of the 'good' and 'bad' object into one whole representation." The establishment of affective object constancy "depends upon the gradual internalization of a constant, positively cathected inner image of the mother" (Mahler et al., 1975, pp. 109–110).

Object constancy differs from object permanence. Object permanence refers to the understanding that objects continue to exist even when they cannot be seen or heard. For example, a ball rolling under furniture still exists in the mind of the child, who will search for it. In object constancy, the child is in continual contact with the mother, and these contacts often take place under conditions of high arousal such as excitement, gratification, longing, and frustration. (Mahler et al., 1975, p. 111). The child develops the capacity to use the idea of mother to delay gratification, to comfort self, and to control inner moods through anticipation of future satisfaction (Edward, Ruskin & Turrini, 1981, p. 12).

Object constancy also implies the internalization of the mother's capacities to deal with frustration and anxiety and how to self-comfort. The child internalizes these functions, which become its internal capacities used to deal with separation and anxiety and to self-soothe and self-comfort. The attainment of affective object constancy permits the child to substitute for the mother, during her physical absence "a reliable internal image that remains relatively stable irrespective of the state of instinctual need or of inner discomfort" (Mahler et al., 1975, p. 110). This allows the child to function separately despite moderate degrees of tension and discomfort.

Self constancy is described as a stable individuality that comprises the attainment of two levels of the sense of identity, namely an awareness of being a separate and individual identity, and an awareness of gender identity (Mahler et al., 1975). A child who possesses self constancy, can say that I am the same me and the same member of the family whether it's when I am alone or when I am with others agreeing, opposing, or showing off my skills and bringing delight in a tempered calming-down. The continuity in time is paralleled by a continuity in space: my body–my mind–my name is all self-contained (the self as place) (Lichenberg, 1975).

Transitional Objects

Some children arrive for therapy carrying with them their favorite stuffed teddy bear, doll, and/or a small figurine in their pocket. It is essential for the psychotherapist to explore and understand the significance of the toy for the child. For some children, the toy may be a way for the child to bridge the known with the unknown, and the subjective with the new and objective reality. For other children, it might be a way to connect with the therapist in sharing something personal of themselves. In the former case, the toy can be thought of as a transitional object.

What then is a transitional object? How is it helpful to an infant or a child? To respond to these questions, it is necessary to realize that a child lives in two realms of experience; the one realm is subjective, psychical, located inside the self and manifesting itself mostly in dreams; the other is objective, environmental, and located outside of the self (Winnicott, 1971b). Between these two realms of experience there is an intermediate area of experience to which both the child's inner reality and the external reality contribute (Winnicott, 1951). In this realm, the subjective and the objective are fused. The child bridges the subjective and the objective by engaging in behaviors such as babbling and mannerisms like going over a song. These behaviors are referred to "transitional phenomena." The child might also latch on to a stuffed animal, a blanket, or a doll. These objects are referred to as "transitional objects" (Winnicott, 1971b, pp. 2–3). The word "transition" refers to two different modes of organizing experience, two different patterns of positioning for self in relation to others (Mitchell & Black, 1996, p. 128).

The transitional object is the child's first not-me possession. It is neither a subjective object nor merely an external object. It is something inanimate onto which the child projects his feelings as if the object were alive. It is a valued object (e.g., soft blanket) that the child uses during separation from the other and often uses in times of distress and in going to sleep. Symbolically, the transitional object stands for the breast or the object of the first relationship. It antedates reality testing (Winnicott, 1951, p. 236).

The intermediate realm is essential as creative living and health depend on its establishment (Winnicott, 1971b). In this realm, the child learns to renounce the tendency to hallucinatory wish-fulfillment in favor of adaptation to the environment. The child accomplishes this in the intermediate realm where he passes from omnipotent control (phantasy) to control by physical manipulation (i.e., reality testing). The child needs the illusion to create the situation, which is partly subjective and partly objective. Thus, a soft blanket is a real objectively perceived thing that acts like the comforting breast under the child's control (Winnicott, 1971a).

Winnicott (1971b) associated the intermediate realm of experience and transitional phenomena with the capacity to play. He stated that "playing is an experience, always a creative experience in the space-time continuum, a basic form of living" (p. 67). C. Winnicott (1989) added that play is the capacity to operate in the "limitless intermediate area where external and internal reality are compounded in the experience of living" (p. 3).

Play Therapy

This section begins with the definition of play therapy, its change mechanisms, and its therapeutic power. It concludes by presenting play therapy techniques, problems treated, and the effectiveness of play therapy. For the more practical aspects of play therapy such as setting up a play therapy room with regard to its physical space, appropriate furniture, and essential play items, authors such as Webb (1991), Lubimiv (1994), and Gil (2021) provide detailed and helpful suggestions.

Definition

Play therapy has been defined in various ways depending upon the play therapist's theoretical orientation and experience in their use to treat children's emotional and behavior problems. It has been defined as a "method of psychotherapy with children that utilizes both play and verbal communication to understand and help the child" (Webb, 1994, p. 3), a "powerful means of joining with the innate, creative, non-verbal capacities of children in order to engage and work therapeutically with them" (Short, 2015, p. 1), and

> a dynamic interpersonal relationship between a child [...] and a therapist [...] who provides selected play materials and facilitates the development of a safe relationship for the child [...] to fully express and explore self (feelings, thoughts, experiences, and behaviors) through play, the child's natural medium of communication for optimal growth and development. (Landreth, 2012, p. 11).

Bettelheim (1987) commented that

> the child's play is motivated by inner processes, desires, problems, and anxieties [...] play is the royal road to the child's conscious and unconscious inner world; if we want to understand her inner world and help her with it, we must learn to walk this road. (p. 35)

The Association for Play Therapy (APT; 2001) defines play therapy as "the systematic use of a theoretical model to establish an interpersonal process wherein trained play therapists use the therapeutic powers of play to help clients prevent or resolve psychological difficulties and achieve optimal growth and development" (p. 20) and as "a way of being with the child that honors their unique developmental level and looks for ways of helping in the language of the child–play" (Cited by Selva, 2020, p. 1).

In summary, for SIRCP, play therapy is a form of psychotherapy used with children to help them express and to project, in a protected and structured environment, their feelings, needs, fantasies, thoughts, and problems using play material. This takes place under the guidance of a therapist, who observes the behavior, affect, and conversation of the child to gain insight into his thoughts, feelings, and fantasies. The therapist helps the child understand and work through conflicts as they arise by identifying the unmet core needs. He helps the child live from core needs in his relationships with parents and peers.

Change Mechanisms and the Therapeutic Powers of Play

With regard to play being a mechanism for personal healing from injuries and for change, Nickerson (1973)

> views play activities as the main therapeutic approach for children because it is a natural medium for self-expression, facilitates a child's communication, allows for a cathartic release of feelings, can be renewing and constructive, and allows the adult a window to observe the child's world. Nickerson points out that the child feels at home in a play setting, readily relates to toys, and will play out concerns with them. (Cited by Gil, 1991, p. 27)

However, play by itself will usually not go beyond play. Chethik (1989) states that "play in itself will not ordinarily produce changes [...] the therapist's interventions and utilization of the play are critical" (p. 49). Gil (1991) adds that the therapist must serve as a participant–observer rather than a playmate. That is, play in therapy must be facilitated by an involved therapist in a meaningful way.

Schaefer and Drewes (2014) identified 20 therapeutic powers of play that they perceived to affect four different levels of development. The levels of development and how they are affected are: (a) facilitates communication (e.g., self-expression; access to the unconscious); (b) fosters emotional wellness (e.g., catharsis; abreaction; positive emotions; stress management); (c) enhances social relationships (e.g., empathy; social competence; therapeutic relationship; attachment); and (d) increases personal strengths (e.g., resiliency; creative problem solving; self-regulation; self-esteem). These four domains have been depicted in graphic form by Peabody and Schaefer (2016).

Kool and Lawver (2010), citing O'Connor (2002), state that the processes that accounts for lasting change in play therapy occurs at the cognitive, affective, and interpersonal domains. The change that takes place at the cognitive domain includes schema transformation, symbolic exchange, insight, and skill development. The changes that occur at the affective domain include abreaction, emotional experiencing, affective education, and emotional regulation. At the interpersonal domain, the changes include support and validation, corrective relationship, and supportive scaffolding.

Play Therapy Techniques

A host of play therapy techniques have been designed over the past three decades. Schaefer (2016) and Schaefer and Cangelosi (2016) presented 58 play therapy techniques and for each they explained its therapeutic rationale, therapeutic power, and empirical findings. Many of the techniques were designed with a specific goal in mind; however, they can also be used for other therapeutic goals.

In a recent publication, Kaduson, Congelosi and Schaefer (2019) recommended that specific techniques be keyed to the treatment of specific psychological disorders and adversities. That is, they are for prescriptive treatment, which implies that the techniques have inherent healing qualities. A SIRCP-oriented child psychotherapist believes that play therapy techniques have healing qualities when used intentionally by the therapist.

The play therapy techniques commonly used by a Self-in-Relationship Child psychotherapist include material that fosters symbolic play like puppet play, dollhouse play, sand play, storytelling, drawings, and plasticine. The techniques that the therapist selects are in part determined by the goal of a particular therapy session. In the techniques selected, the therapist allows the child to engage with them and to express his feelings, thoughts, and needs. The therapist may intervene to offer the child a new experience and to accelerate the progress.

Puppet play is a very flexible technique that can be used in many ways. The therapist might use a turtle puppet to re-enact a child's shyness and tendency to go into his shell. The therapist, in the voice of the puppet, might say that he is shy and he wishes to have a friend, and ask the child if he wants to be the puppet's friend. The child can relate to the shyness of the puppet and its need to have a friend. With the invitation from the puppet, the child might open up emotionally and become friends to the turtle puppet. The therapist can follow up by asking how the child feels in becoming a friend to the turtle puppet.

In dollhouse play, the child may be asked to select figurines and furniture from a collection of objects and construct his family, or the child may spontaneously set up the doll house. Following the construction, the child may be asked to describe who are the characters and what is going on. The story could reveal the child's frustrations, fears, his perceived place in the family and relationships, and what he desires to have from members of the family.

Sand play therapy involves the use of a sandbox, toy figurines, and sometimes water to create a miniature world that reflects the child's innermost thoughts, feelings, fears, struggles, and dreams. Following the construction, the child may be asked to tell a story, which might reveal his inner longings (Langham, 2020).

Problems Treated by Play Therapy

Play therapy has been applied to a wide range of children's emotional and behavioral problems. Gil (1991, 2017) has written at great length how to apply play therapy to children who are victims of emotional, physical, and sexual abuse, trauma, and of emotional neglect. Webb (1991, 2007, 2017) indicated how play therapy can be used to treat children and adolescents in crisis. Play therapy has also been used to treat autism, anxiety, attention deficit hyperactivity disorder (Selva, 2020), and selective mutism (Wonders, 2020).

From the perspective of SIRCP, it is essential that the psychotherapist be trained in child and pre-teen psychology. In order to have a deeper understanding of the child's inner world, struggles, and recovery, the training could be complemented by the reading of classical case studies such as *Dibs in Search of Self* (Axline, 1969), *Son Rise* (Kaufman, 1995), *The Boy Who Couldn't Stop Washing* (Rapaport, 1991), and *Dissociative Children* (Shirar, 1996), and more.

Effectiveness of Play Therapy

Several meta-analytic studies investigated the effectiveness of play therapy (PT), filial therapy (FT), and combined PT and FT for the treatment of the emotional and behavioral problems of children. Filial therapy is described as a "therapeutic intervention that can help children by teaching parents (and other paraprofessionals such as teachers) basic child-centered play therapy principles and methods to use with their children" (Bratton, Ray, Rhine & Jones, 2005b, p. 1). The treatment groups were compared to the nontreatment groups for effectiveness of treatment.

Effectiveness was calculated in terms of standard deviation units and the size of the standard deviation unit was interpreted using Cohen's $\underline{d}$ (Cohen, 1988).

The results from these studies indicate that PT, FT, and combined PT/FT were effective treatments for emotional and behavioral problems of children (Leblanc & Ritchie 2001, Bratton et al., 2005a, 2005b). In addition, it was observed that play therapy was more effective when parents were included in the treatment as compared to a professional working alone with a child. Play therapy was found to be effective for children of all ages and for both genders, and that it increases in effectiveness up to 35–40 sessions. Based on the research results, the authors cautiously suggested that a humanistic/nondirective approach when compared to a behavioral/directive approach appears to be more effective.

The research results are consistent with the observations of the SIRCP approach, which observed that child therapy is more effective when parents are included in treatment. It also observed that therapy is more effective when the therapist gives the child the freedom to explore his space, to express himself, and take the lead with minimal direction from the therapist.

Therapeutic Aspects

An SIRCP therapist utilizes both play therapy and verbal therapy in treating children. In the treatment, the psychotherapist is guided by developmental, psychodynamic, and humanistic principles of play therapy and includes parents in the treatment of the child. The manner of including parents in the treatment of the child and the qualities of the therapist are the topics of this section.

The Inclusion of Parents in the Child's Psychotherapy

The parents are included in the treatment of the child because they are the most important persons in the child's life. The way they are included may vary depending on the age and the needs of the child. For example, the child may want the parent to be present at the beginning of the therapy and later express his autonomy to be alone with the therapist and ask the parents to remain in the waiting room. The treatment of the child begins by meeting the parents as a couple, or individually when their schedules do not permit it.

When the therapist observes that the couple is conflicted regarding parenting, she suggests that each parent be seen for an individual session to better understand their position and their relationship and its impact on the child. If, on the other hand, the therapist observes that the parents are struggling with personal issues that interfere with their parenting, she might recommend that they seek the help of a professional to deal with their personal and/or couple issues.

The meeting of the parents as a couple or individually has several goals. One goal is to obtain information about their concerns regarding the emotional and behavioral difficulties and/or problems of their child. The parents may be asked to provide information regarding: the child's age at the onset and extent of the problems; how the problems relate to social interactions, school work, and extracurricular activities; the child's birth and nursing experiences; the separation experiences when being babysat or going to daycare; illnesses or traumas; any sources of stress; and custody arrangements. The therapist may ask how they have tried to respond to the child's problems and whether they have sought help from other professionals and if so, how it has been helpful.

A second goal is to discuss the practicalities of the therapy for the child. This includes the frequency and length of the sessions, how feedback will be given to the parents, and the fees per session. The psychotherapist describes her approach in treating children, and the parents are invited to ask questions about the approach. With their informed consent, the parents are then asked to sign forms that give the therapist permission to proceed with therapy and, when applicable, to take photographs of the child's productions. The parents are invited to provide the therapist with significant information between sessions concerning the child.

A third goal, if the parents are seen together, is to observe how they interact with each other, to assess their degree of agreement in parenting with regard to playtime, nursing, feeding, bedtime, and discipline. It is also an opportunity to assess how having a child has affected their couple relationship and whether they themselves have personal or relational issues with which they are struggling and that might affect their parenting.

A fourth goal is to discuss with the parents how they might participate in the treatment of their child. Their participation may take one of two forms. One form is, at times, for one or both to be present and to observe and to model at home how the therapist might help a child who is shy, angry, socially withdrawn, and the like. A second form, most often used, is for the parent to be invited to participate in an activity with the child, which can serve several purposes including practice. One purpose is for the therapist to assess the nature of the parent and child communication and interaction, the extent to which the parent can attune himself/herself to the needs and feelings of the child and be supportive, the child's ease in being close to the parent, and the child's capacity to ask for help or closeness. A second purpose is to actively facilitate the communication between child and parent and to improve their emotional closeness.

A fifth goal is to provide periodic feedback to the parent(s) based on the therapist's observations and to discuss possible changes that the parent might make in the way that they parent the child. The feedback takes place privately with parents as a couple or individually, that is, without the child being present. It is crucial to obtain the collaboration of the parent(s), to engage them and give them support and guidance. If the therapist observes that the parents are struggling with personal issues that interfere with their parenting, she might recommend that they seek the help of a professional to deal with the personal and/or couple issues. The therapist might help the parents see the link between the way they were raised and their way of parenting.

Therapist's Tasks, Interventions, and Qualities

The therapist's tasks and personal and relational qualities tend to meld into each other. That is to say, the way the therapist performs the tasks will be greatly influenced by her personal and relational capacities to understand the child's inner world and to attune to his needs and feelings.

Therapist's tasks

One of the therapist's tasks is to formulate as accurately as possible an assessment and a conceptualization of the child's presenting problem, to articulate the goals, and to design appropriate treatment. To perform these tasks, the therapist obtains relevant information from the parents and professionals, if involved. The therapist pays attention to the parent–child interactions and includes her observations with regard to how the child relates to her and how the child uses and relates to the play material. From these observations, the therapist begins to formulate a conceptualization regarding the underlying dynamics that influence the child's behaviors. This understanding is used to organize activities that lead to the healing of self and relational injuries.

A second task is for the therapist to choose play material that takes into consideration the child's age and presenting problem. The younger the child, the less developed are his verbal capacities and language skills; his natural and main activity is play. An older child, because of the increase in his capacities and language skills, may prefer play material that is more cognitively challenging. The therapist also chooses play material that has the potential for the child to express and release his unique feelings and to be creative. Play material can be thought of in terms of three categories: real-life toys (e.g., dollhouse, toy kitchen), which can serve as icebreakers for shy and timid children; aggressive toys (e.g., guns, ropes, mean looking figurines) that facilitate the release of anger and hostility through destruction; and creative toys (e.g., puppets, crayons) that provide the possibility for a wide range of expressive emotions that foster creativity (Kool & Lawver 2010). Whenever an object is unavailable for the child's story, it can often be created.

A third task is to assure that the office (i.e., play space) is comfortable and safe, and that the material provided is safe and safely used. It is important that all furnishings are safely secured and no potentially harmful objects are present. As for the toys, they are to be of the type that they will not cause harm to the child either in terms of their toxicity or of their structure (i.e., sharp and cutting edges). It is also important to provide consistency and predictability by always having the same material available to the child as over time they may become attached to a specific toy. Knowing that the toy will be there, at the same place, at the next session helps the child separate from it and leave it behind.

A fourth task is to be present to the child and to control the environment. To prevent disturbances during the session, a "do not disturb" sign is placed on the door and all communication devices are muted. Children respond very positively to feeling special and important during this hour.

A fifth task is for the therapist to set limits to the child's requests and behaviors in the office. The child is informed that it is not acceptable to breaks things or to hurt each other if more than one child is present. In setting limits, the therapist delivers them in a developmentally appropriate language with as much specificity as possible to the child. (Kool & Lawver, 2010).

Regarding a child's production during the therapy session, if a child would like to take the drawing home, the therapist can offer to make a copy of the original, which is kept in the child's file. However, if a drawing is made for a parent, the therapist allows the child to take the original home with him in order to foster a rapprochement. A child is not permitted to take a toy home and is reassured he will find it at its place next session.

Therapist's interventions and qualities

To work with young children requires special observational and attentive skills, specific interventions, and personal, relational, and attitudinal qualities. The therapist's qualities and interventions that characterize a SIRCP therapist are briefly presented.

First, the therapist must develop a warm and friendly relationship with the child in order to establish rapport as soon as possible (Axline, 1947, p. 75). The therapist accomplishes this primarily by being attuned to the needs and feelings of the child and by responding to them in an empathic way. The therapist is non-judgmental, allows self-expression, and establishes rules to create emotional and physical safety (VanFleet et al., 2010, p. 22). During an activity, the child notices that the therapist is paying attention and shows an interest in what he is doing. He may check in a subtle or obvious way. The undivided attention provided is like a holding environment.

Second, the therapist accepts the child exactly as he is, that is, regarding his initiatives and behaviors. The therapist refrains from making judgments and from giving direction to his activities when it is not asked for. The therapist gives the child free rein to pursue his activities.

Third, the therapist establishes an environment and an attitude of permissiveness so that the child feels free to play with the toys and to completely express his feelings. The therapist establishes permissiveness by using an accepting tone, maintaining a genuine interest in the child's play, and by behaving in a nonjudgmental and nondirective manner. Permissiveness means giving the child permission, within defined rules, to express whatever he is thinking and feeling while in the playroom (VanFleet et al., 2010, p. 25).

Fourth, the therapist pays attention to the feelings and needs that the child is expressing and reflects these back to him in a manner in which he can gain insight into his behavior. The therapist uses "empathic listening" that focuses on the child's feeling words, which helps establish acceptance, permissiveness, and a secure relationship with the child (VanFleet et al., 1977, p. 26). The therapist, however, may at times have to go beyond just listening and reflecting back feelings and needs. The therapist must know what it is to be the child. That is, she must enter the inner world of the child and experience what this is like (Axline, 1950). This entails "empathic-introspective immersion" into the child's inner world and feeding this back to the child (Kohut, 1977 p. 306).

Fifth, the therapist believes that every child has the innate potential to solve his problems through play if given an appropriate play therapy atmosphere. However, there are situations where the child's play may not move him toward solving his problems, and the therapist then intervenes to move the healing process forward. Accordingly, the therapist might create a situation that will facilitate the child in effectively dealing with an issue. For example, a child might construct his family in the playhouse and place himself distant from the other members of the family. The therapist might instruct him to move himself closer to the rest of the family and ask him how he feels about that. The healing process, in essence, comprises both "nurturing" and "nudging" (Mahler et al., 1975) as "play in itself will not ordinarily produce changes [...] the therapist's interventions and utilization of the play are critical" (Chethik, 1989, p. 49). Gil (1991) adds that the therapist "must serve as a participant-observer, rather than a playmate" (p. 28).

Sixth, the child is given the freedom to act and converse in any manner with the therapist. However, the therapist might, at times, suggest a specific action or behavior to broaden the assessment and guide treatment. During therapy, the child, for example, is given the freedom to choose figures to play with in the sand, or to use to construct a family in the playhouse, or be given the freedom to choose a stuffed animal with which to play. As the child is engaged in play, the therapist observes how he interacts with his constructions and with the inanimate objects. The therapist might ask the child to tell a story about his constructions and what is happening to gain an understanding of the child's internal working model.

Seventh, the therapist does not attempt to hurry the therapy; therapy is a gradual process. In play, the child learns about himself and how to be and relate in the world. This is a slow process and "cannot be hurried as the child needs time, space and acceptance to complete this process in a healthy fashion" (VanKleet et al., 2010, p. 37). The therapist, however, may have a general idea as to what the child needs to accomplish in therapy and gently guide the process, but the therapist allows the child to gradually arrive at this according to his pace.

Eighth, the therapist establishes those limitations in play therapy that anchor the session to the world of reality and make the child aware of his responsibilities in the relationship. In the establishment of limits, the child knows that the therapist will maintain an atmosphere of safety in the room, particularly when the child feels that he is not able to control his own emotions. Through the establishment of reasonable limits to his behavior and expression of his emotions, the child learns self-control and the appropriate expression of feelings. He learns to be responsible for his own behavior and expression of emotions (VanKleet et al., 2010, pp. 38–39).

In summary, it is essential that the play therapist be attuned to the feelings and needs of the child, follow the child's lead, use any material available, make it a play activity, balance play with nudging and nurturing, and "prioritize relationship when working with children and their families" (Gil, 2017, p. xii). But above all, the therapist must be "playful and inventive" (Lubimiv, 1994, p. 96).

References

Allen, F.H. (1942). *Psychotherapy with children*. New York: W.W. Norton.

Association for Play Therapy (2001). Play therapy. *Clovis CAL Association for Play Therapy News Letter, 20*.

Axline, V. (1947) *Play therapy*. Boston: Houghton-Mifflin.

Axline, V. (1950). Entering the child's world via play experiences. *Progressive Education, 27*, 68–75.

Axline, V. (1969). *Dibs: In search of self*. New York: Ballantine.

Bettelheim, B. (1987). *The importance of play*. Atlantic Monthly, March, 35–46.

Bowlby, J. (1988). *A secure base: Parent-child attachment and healthy human development*. New York: Basic Books.

Bratton, S.C., Ray, D., Rhine, T., & Jones, L. (2005a). The efficacy of play therapy with children: A meta-analytic review of treatment outcomes. *Professional Psychology: Research and Practice, 36*(4), 376–390.

Bratton, S.C., Ray, D., Rhine, T., & Jones, L. (2005b). *The efficacy of play therapy and filial therapy with children: Summary of the meta-analytic findings*. Retrieved from: https://cdn.ymaws.com/www.a4pt.org/resource/resmgr/publications/Meta-Analytic_Literature_Rev.pdf

Chethik, M. (1989). *Techniques of child therapy: Psychodynamic strategies*. New York: Guilford Press.

Cohen, J. (1988). *Statistical power analysis for the behavioral sciences*, 2nd Edition. Hillsdale, NJ: Erlbaum.

Dorfman, E. (1951). Play therapy. In C.R. Rogers, *Client-centered therapy: Its current practice, implications and theory* (pp. 235-277). Boston: Houghton Mifflin.

Edward, J., Ruskin, N., & Turrini, P. (1981). *Separation-Individuation: Theory and application*. New York: Gardner Press.

Freud, S. (1909). *The analysis of a phobia in a five-year-old boy*. London: Hogarth Press.

Freud, S. (1923). The Ego and the Id. *Standard Edition, 19*, 12–63.

Gil, E. (1991). *The healing power of play: Working with abused children*. New York: Guilford Press.

Gil, E. (2014). *Play in family therapy*, 2nd Edition. New York: Guilford Press.

Gil, E. (2017). *Posttraumatic play in children. What clinicians need to know*. New York: The Guilford Press.

Gil, E. (2021). *Cultural issues in play therapy*, 2nd Edition. New York: The Guilford Press.

Hall, T.M., Kaduson, H.G., & Schaefer, C.E. (2002). Fifteen effective play therapy techniques. *Professional Psychology: Research and Practice, 33*(6), 515–522.

Hug-Hellmuth, H. (1921). *A Young Girl's Diary*. New York: Thomas Seltzer.

Johnson, J.H., Rasbury, W.C., & Siegel, L.J. (1997). *Approaches to child treatment: Introduction to theory, research, and practice*, 2nd Edition. Boston, MA: Allyn and Bacon.

Kaduson, H.G., Cangelosi, D., & Schaefer, C.E. (2019). Basic principles and core practices of prescriptive play therapy. In H.G. Kaduson, D. Cangelosi, & C.E. Schaefer (Eds.), *Prescriptive play therapy: Tailoring interventions for specific childhood problems* (pp. 3-13). New York: Guilford Press.

Kaufman, B.N. (1995). *Son rise: The miracle continues*. Canada: H.J. Kramer

Kohut, H. (1977). *The restoration of the self*. New York: International Universities Press.

Kool, R., & Lawver, T. (2010). Play therapy: Considerations and applications for the practitioner. *Psychiatry (Edgmont)*, *7*(10), 19–24 (Published online, October, 2010).

Landreth, G.L. (2012). *Play therapy: The art of the relationship*, 2nd Edition. New York: Brunner-Routledge.

Langham, R. (2020). *The parent's guide to play therapy for children*. Retrieved from: https://parentingpod.com/play-therapy/

LeBlanc, M., & Ritchie, M. (2001). A meta-analysis of play therapy outcomes. *Counseling Psychology Quarterly*, *14*, 149–163.

Lichenberg, J. (1975). The development of a sense of self. *Journal of American Psychoanalytic Association*, *23*, 453.

Lindon, J.A. (1972). Melanie Klein's theory and technique: Her life and work. In P.I. Giovacchini (Ed.), *Tactics and techniques in psychoanalytic therapy* (pp. 33–61). New York: Science House Incorporated.

Lubimiv, G.P. (1994). *Wings for our children: Essentials of becoming a play therapist*. Burnstown, Ontario: The General Store Publishing House.

Mahler, M.S., Pine, F., & Bergman, A. (1975). *The psychological birth of the human infant*. New York: Basic Books.

Meier, A, & Boivin, M. (2022). *Self-in-relationship psychotherapy: A complete clinical guide to theory and practice*. Oxford UK: Routledge.

Mitchell, S.A., & Black, M.J. (1996). *Freud and beyond: A history of modern psychoanalytic thought*. New York: Basic Books.

Nickerson, E.T. (1973). Psychology of play and play therapy in classroom activities. *Educating Children*, Spring, 1–6.

O'Connor, K. (2002). The value and use of interpretation in play therapy. *Professional Psychology: Research and Practice*, (6), 523–528.

Peabody, M.A., & Schaefer, C. (2016). *The therapeutic powers of play: The heart and soul of play therapy*. Retrieved from: https://cdn.ymaws.com/www.a4pt.org/resource/ resmgr/ magazine articles/2019-20/Peabody_&_Schaefer.pdf

Rank, O. (1945), *Will therapy and truth and reality*. New York: Knopf.

Rapaport, J.L. (1991). *The boy who couldn't stop washing: The experience and treatment of obsessive-compulsive disorder*. New York: New American Library.

Schaefer, C.E. (2016). Short-term play therapy for children: Third edition. In C.E. Schaefer & H.D. Cangelosi (Eds.), *Essential play therapy techniques: Time-tested approaches*. New York: Guilford Press.

Schaefer, C.E., & Cangelosi, H.D. (2016). *Essential play therapy techniques: Time-tested approaches*. New York: Guilford Press.

Schaefer, C.E., & Drewes, A.A. (Eds.). (2014). *The therapeutic power of play: 20 core agents of change*, 2nd Edition. Hoboken, NJ: Wiley.

Selva, J. (2020). *50 play therapy techniques, toys and certification opportunities*. Retrieved from: https://positivepsychology.com/play-therapy

Shirar, L. (1996). *Dissociative children: Bridging the inner and outer worlds*. New York: W.W. Norton & Company.

Short, J. (2015). Play therapy: Working creatively with children. *InPsych, 37*(3).

Stern, D.N. (1985). *The interpersonal world of the infant*. New York: Basic Books.

Taft, J. (1933), *The dynamics of therapy in a controlled relationship*. New York: Macmillan.

VanFleet, R. Sywulak, A.E., & Sniscak, C.C. (1977). History, theory, principles, and variations of child-centered play therapy. In R. VanFleet, A.E. Sywulak & C.C. Sniscak (Eds.), *Child-centered play therapy* (pp. 20–42). New York: Guilford Press.

Webb, N.B. (Ed.) (1991). *Play therapy with children in crisis: A casebook for practitioners*. New York: Guilford Press.

Webb, N.B. (1994). *Techniques of play therapy: A clinical demonstration*. New York: Guilford Press.

Webb, N.B. (Ed.) (2007). *Play therapy with children in crisis, Third edition: Individual, family and group treatment*. New York: Guilford Press.

Webb, N.B. (Ed.) (2017). *Play therapy with children and adolescents in crisis*, 4th Edition. New York: Guilford Press.

Winnicott, C. (1989). D.W.W.: A reflection. In C. Winnicott, R. Shepherd, & M. Davis, (Eds.) (1989). *D.W. Winnicott: Psycho-analytic explorations* (pp. 1–18). Cambridge, MA.: Harvard University Press.

Winnicott, D. (1951). Transitional objects and transitional phenomena. In D. Winnicott (Ed.), *Through paediatrics to psychoanalysis* (pp. 229–242). New York: Basic Books.

Winnicott, D. (1962). Ego integration in child development. In D. Winnicott (Ed.) (1965), *The maturational processes and the facilitating environment* (pp. 56–63). New York: International Universities Press.

Winnicott, D. (1971a). *Therapeutic consultations in child psychiatry*. New York: Basic Books.

Winnicott, D. (1971b). *Playing and reality*. New York: Basic Books.

Wonders, L.L. (2020). Play therapy for children with selective mutism. In H.G. Kaduson, D. Cangelosi & C.E. Schaefer (Eds.), *Prescriptive play therapy: Tailoring interventions for specific childhood problems* (pp. 92–104). New York: The Guilford Press.

Chapter 8

Case Illustrations

André and Louis

This chapter presents the application of Self-in-Relationship Child Psychotherapy (SIRCP) to the treatment of two young boys. The first case is that of André, struggling with separation anxiety. The second case is that of Louis, wrestling with the aftereffects of parental alienation.

The Case of André – Resolving a Separation Anxiety Disorder

André, an 11-year-old boy, suffered from intense anxiety when his mother was absent from home and/or when he was at school. His greatest fear was to lose his mother and be permanently separated from her. No amount of reassurance on the part of the parents alleviated the anxiety, and for this reason they sought therapy for their son.

The presentation of André begins by differentiating between separation anxiety and Separation Anxiety Disorder (SAD). This is followed by a description of the presenting problem, background information, a conceptualization of the problem, and treatment goals and procedures.

Separation Anxiety and Separation Anxiety Disorder

Separation anxiety and SAD differ in several ways. Separation anxiety is part of the normal developmental process. The infant typically begins life being physically and emotionally bonded with her mother. With the maturation of cognitive and motoric skills, the infant gradually begins to take distance from her. When he begins to realize that he is separated from his mother, he begins to experience separation anxiety. This occurs around the eighth month and is reexperienced in a more intense way between the ages of three and four.

SAD, on the other hand, is a psychological condition in which an individual has an excessive level of anxiety when away from people to whom he has a strong emotional attachment, such as parents and caregivers. The anxiety can be overwhelming even when it involves brief separations such as going to school, remaining at

DOI: 10.4324/9781032655291-12

home while parents are away, and going to sleep. The child fears that his parents may die because of a car accident or illness. Those suffering from excessive levels of anxiety often go to extremes to avoid being away from their caregivers, protest leaving a parent, refuse to play with friends, or complain of physical illnesses. The key element is the child's excessive anxiety interferes with normal functioning at school, at home, and with their social life.

André met the criteria for SAD as presented in the *Diagnostic and Statistical Manual of Mental Disorders* (DSM–5) (American Psychiatric Association; APA, 2013). He experienced excessive stress in being away from home, feared losing his mother, and felt stressed in going to school. His anxiety, which persisted for over a year, impaired his relational, academic, and social functioning.

Presenting Problem and Background Information

The parents sought therapy for André because he began to exhibit intense anxiety over a year earlier when his mother, who was on a one-year sick leave from work, returned to work, which entailed traveling by car to meet her clients. When his mother, a salesperson for cosmetic products, left home for appointments, he became highly anxious. When he was at the babysitter or at school, he needed to call his mother every ten minutes to know where she was. When he did not accompany his parents, he feared that they might have an accident and get killed. He also became highly anxious when they arrived late to pick him up after school and feared they might not be at home when he arrived from school. He also feared to play outdoors with his friends for fear of losing his mother.

At times André became extremely anxious and too ill to go to school. At school, he trembled, cried a lot, was inconsolable, and complained of headaches and had trouble breathing. He had difficulty concentrating on his schoolwork.

Since the age of six months, his parents had had conflicts over finances. When André was five years of age, his father lost his job and started his own landscaping business, and his mother, after her workday, helped him with his business. The father was absent a lot because of his work. The mother was highly demanding of André, impatient in helping him with his homework, and not as emotionally available as André needed. Because of the parents' conflicts over finances, André feared that his parents would separate. His parents reassured him that they would stay together. The parents tried to help André feel more secure by traveling less and by working from their home offices. They also allowed him to sleep in their bedroom.

André was babysat at a private home from the age of six months to three years, attended a well-structured daycare from three to five years, and went to a school daycare for one year. Finding the school daycare too repressive, he was cared for at a private home from the ages of six to nine years. André made and maintained friends easily.

Assessment and Conceptualization

Many factors contributed to André's SAD. These included: the mother's changing moods, demands, impatience, and anger; tension and conflicts in the home caused by financial problems; the loss of playtime with his parents; the loss of friends because of a family move; illness of mother; and the parents having jobs that involved traveling.

The factor that precipitated André's SAD, however, was his mother's return to work. Prior to her illness and return to work, he managed his anxieties even though he had only tenuously completed the tasks of the separation and individuation process. The tasks that were not completed included forming a secure emotional bond with the physical mother and with the internalized mother (i.e., object constancy), psychologically separating from the mother, and maintaining emotional connection with her whether she was present or absent.

Treatment

The goal of treatment was to help André develop a secure emotional bond with his mother by helping him psychologically separate from her at his pace and form object constancy. It was assumed that by achieving psychological separation, establishing an emotional bond with his mother, and by developing object constancy, André would better manage his anxiety when she was absent.

Achieve psychological separation from mother

The goal was to help André to have a life separate from his mother and yet feel emotionally connected to her and to whom he could return when anxious. The main technique used to achieve this goal was a narrative using animal puppets. The therapist (M.B.) designed two exercises to facilitate psychological separation from his mother.

In the first exercise, the therapist created a story using two characters that embodied André's struggle to psychologically separate. The two characters were Mother Koala (MK) and Child Koala (CK). The two characters were joined to each other by a string of elastics and both characters, as suggested by André, had a paper heart taped to them representing their love for each other (Scene 1).

In the first step of this exercise, the therapist modeled how a scared CK experiments with moving away from his mother. The CK is attracted to leaving his mother and playing outside with friends, but is afraid to go without MK. He does not know if he can trust that MK will be at home when he returns. MK encourages and reassures him that she will stay at home and that he may come back whenever he chooses to, and she would like him to tell her what he did outside. Eventually, in the story, the CK was able to take distance from MK without feeling overly anxious and was able to enjoy playtime with his friends outdoors. He was able to trust his mother because she stayed inside the home, welcomed him when he came in, and showed interest in what he did.

In the second step of this exercise, André manipulated the CK. He experimented and practiced taking distance from MK with back-and-forth movements. He ended his story with the CK being able to successfully go out and play; however, he was not able to be away for long as he needed to be emotionally refueled.

In a second exercise, two new characters, Mother Kangaroo, and her child, were used to consolidate the experience of taking distance from the mother. Ribbons of different lengths were used to symbolize the various distances between Mother and child, depending if the child was at school, at the sitter, or with friends. The Mother and the child practiced separation (Scenes 2 to 4). The purpose was that after a period of practice, the child would be better able to tolerate being away from his mother for longer and longer periods of time knowing that the mother was available if needed. By experimenting with different distances from his mother, André was better able to tolerate his separation from his mother and know that she would be available if needed.

Image 8.1 André.

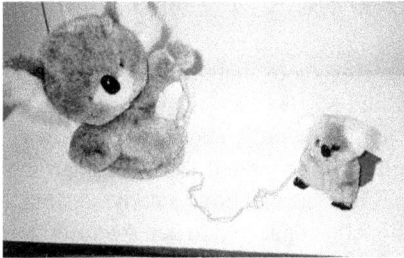

Scene 1. Practice with Koalas and elastic bands leaving mother to play with friends and coming back to her.

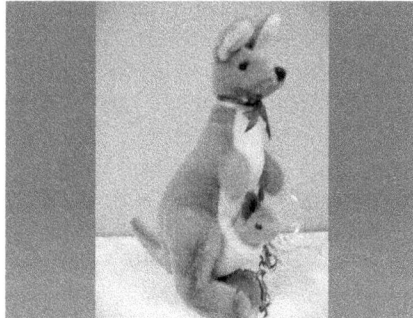

Scene 2. Child Kangaroo getting ready to leave Mother's pouch for different distances – outdoors, babysitter, school.

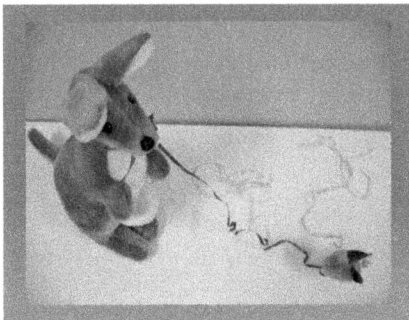

Scene 3: Child Kangaroo practices leaving Mother for farther destinations such as school.

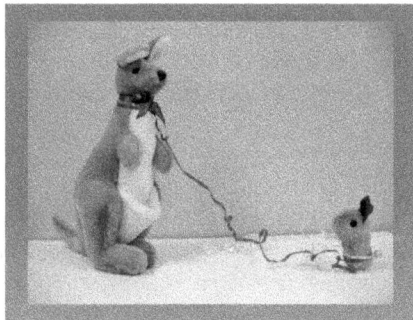

Scene 4: Child Kangaroo feels more secure leaving Mother for school.

Develop object constancy relative to his mother

The second goal of therapy was to help André establish object constancy by evoking images of his mother and thereby remain emotionally connected with her even in her absence without feeling abandoned whenever he did not see her. The therapeutic work focused on the two situations that caused him the greatest anxiety: when he was left with his sitter and when his mother left the office to drive by car to meet clients. Two techniques were used to address this goal.

The main technique was visualization. The first step was for the mother to describe to André the itinerary to her workplace. André was asked to visualize step by step (e.g., street name, bridges crossed) the itinerary that his mother took after leaving him with the sitter and arriving at her place of work. André was then asked, for the second time, to close his eyes and imagine the itinerary as the mother described it. The mother then left the office, and the therapist asked André to repeat the exercise to her. He succeeded in repeating it. After that he, on his own, diligently repeated the exercise daily when he was at the sitter. In grounding his perception of where his mother was, he was able to remain in contact with her.

The second technique used narratives with puppets of mother and child. In the first narrative, the Mother Koala (MK) and Child Koala (CK) puppets were joined by an elastic band (Scene 1). This represented the child's capacity to evoke an image of his mother and feel secure while he was separated from her. Because of his mental representation of the mother, André could be physically separated from his mother and he would still feel emotionally connected to her. According to André, the elastic band representing the bond between them was unbreakable. In the second narrative, the CK experimented with leaving the mother while they were connected by ribbons. André liked the Kangaroos' trick, as he called it, because it helped him conjure up a mental picture of his mother.

Engaging the Mother and the School in the Treatment

In order to help André achieve psychological separation and acquire object constancy, the therapist worked with both his mother and the school. It was the therapist's practice to include those who were involved in the child's life.

Work with the mother

In her meeting with the mother, the therapist pointed out the healthy emotional bond that was developing between her and André. The mother spoke about how she had changed her parenting of André. She was trying to back off from her expectations and demands of André and at the same time to be emotionally available and let him grow at his pace. She was also becoming more patient regarding his homework. In sessions with the mother and André, both expressed how they were understanding each other better and were doing things that promoted closeness and pleasure in being together. The therapist, in her individual session with the mother, recommended these types of interactions.

Work with the school

The therapist, André, and the school personnel worked together to create conditions of security and ways to diminish André's level of stress and anxiety within the limits of school rules and the availability of teachers. A major focus was to set up conditions whereby André would feel emotionally connected to his mother. A schedule, with the participation of André, was set up whereby he was able to contact his mother by phone. The schedule of contacts was made along natural breaks in the school day, and when the periods were too long for him, adjustments were made. All his teachers were informed of this and accepted to participate. Predictability and consistency were emphasized. The result was that the frequency of contacts diminished gradually and André, on his own, decided to skip some scheduled contacts.

Treatment Outcome and Follow-Up

André began to improve as soon as his mother understood her role in his insecurities, began to change her attitude and expectations toward him, and learned to respond to his need to connect with her. The schedule of contacts with the mother that was arranged with the school brought relief and security to André. This resulted in a gradual decrease of the number of phone contacts.

Upon completion of the exercises in therapy, André decided on his own to skip telephone contacts with mother and was able for the first time in six months to accept his mother's work outside of the home. The first signs of improvements were: he was able sleep in his own bed and to shower by himself; somatized less; played outside with his friends for 20 minutes; went to school with less stress and reluctance; and his school marks improved dramatically. He went to bed on his own and slept well, and he had no more physical complaints.

The successful resolution of André's separation anxiety was the establishment of a secure emotional bond with his mother, which led to the development of object constancy and the completing of psychological separation. Object constancy served as a home base from which he could find strength to deal with separation anxiety. He became confident that the mother's love would continue even in her absence and that the mother would be physically present when needed.

At a ten-month follow up, the mother reported that André's earlier problems for which he sought treatment, had disappeared. He became more secure and autonomous, he socialized with friends, was able to return home from school without a parent being present, was able to stay at a relative's home, and he no longer feared that his mother would die in a car accident. When André was a young adult, the therapist heard that André was doing very well in his studies and in sports. He was seen as a well-functioning young adult.

The Case of Louis – Resolving a Parental Loyalty Conflict

Louis, a nine-year-old boy, was referred for therapy because of his emotional struggles and physiological ailments, which were brought on, in part, by the mother alienating him from his father. Louis was troubled, anxious, somatized, was often sick, and was failing his year of school because of his numerous missed school days. He was very sensitive and introverted, with a tendency to dramatize situations such as conflicts with peers. He was referred for a medical examination to his family physician, who concluded that there were no physiological causes for his physical complaints and therefore he referred him for a psychological assessment and treatment.

In addition to dealing with the effects of parental alienation, Louis was also processing a profound loss of the recent death of his maternal grandmother who, with the grandfather, lived with Louis and his mother. Louis was very attached to his grandmother and described her as his friend and confidante. Louis did not have the same attachment to his maternal grandfather, who supported his mother's alienating behaviors.

The presentation of Louis begins with the concepts of parental alienation and parental alienation syndrome. This is followed by background information, a conceptualization of Louis's presenting problems, and the goals and approach of therapy. The last part presents Louis's resolution of an internal loyalty conflict.

Parental Alienation and Parental Alienation Syndrome

Parental alienation differs from parental alienation syndrome. Parental alienation involves "behaviors that a parent does to hurt or damage a relationship between a child and the other parent" (Farzad, 2019) and to the "psychological manipulation of a child, by saying and doing things that lead the child to look unfavorably on one parent or the other" (Champlin, Oldham, & Salvatoriello, 2017). Behaviors that are alienating include bad-mouthing the other partner in front of the child to gain his loyalty, preventing the child from spending time with the other parent, and undermining the authority of the other parent (Farzad, 2019).

The term "parental alienation syndrome" (PAS) is used to refer to the negative effects that parental alienation has on children. The negative effects include showing extreme but unwarranted fear and disrespect or hostility toward a parent (Gardner, 2001).

PAS has not been accepted as a diagnostic category (Wood, 1994; Hoult, 2006) as it is not listed as a medical or psychiatric syndrome in any medical, psychiatric, and psychological classification systems (Caplan, 2004; Dallam, 1999). The DSM-V (American Psychiatric Association, 2013) includes diagnostic categories that reflect the impact of parental behavior upon children, in particular Parent-Child Relational Problem (PCRP; V61.20) and Child Affected by Parental Relationship Distress (CAPRD; V61.29). These diagnoses relate to the mental health of the diagnosed individual rather than describe a disorder of the relationship between different people.

Although PAS is not included as a diagnostic category, there are negative effects associated with parental alienation. The DSM-5 defines CAPRD as a child whose parents are experiencing intimate partner distress, violence, acrimonious divorce, unfair disparagement of one partner by another, or parental alienation. Bernet, Wamboldt and Narrow (2016) proposed an expanded explanation clarifying that children may develop behavioral, cognitive, affective, and physical symptoms when they experience varying degrees of parental relationship distress. Parental alienation can cause a lifetime of psychological harm to a child and affect the child's future relationships as he grows older and well into adulthood (Farzad, 2019).

Louis's reported psychological and physical symptoms appear to be related, at least in great part, to parental alienation on behalf of his mother. His symptoms meet the broadened definition of CAPRD.

Background Information

Louis's parents separated when he was two years of age. The mother was given sole custody and his father had access once every second weekend. The mother had an enmeshed relationship with Louis and made it difficult for him to have a good relationship with his father. She made negative, hostile, and demeaning state-ments regarding Louis's father. These statements influenced Louis's perception of his father as he feared being with his father and engaging in activities with him. To please his mother, Louis began to falsely accuse his father of physically hurting him when Louis was deliberately hurting himself.

The parents went to court many times to settle issues, but the parental alienation on the part of the mother continued. When Louis was six years of age, it was determined by court that the mother was alienating her son from his father. The parents were informed how their conflict impacted on the development of their son and they had to agree on measures, such as never to criticize and talk negatively about their former partner in the presence of their son and not to use their son to resolve their marital conflicts. At the time of the referral, the conflict between the parents was less hostile.

When Louis was referred by the Youth Protection Services for therapy at the age of nine, he continued to experience an internal conflict of loyalty toward his parents. He felt that he did not have his mother's permission to love his father and to say to his father that he loved him. He did not talk about his feelings for fear of betraying one or the other parent. His mother was domineering, smothering, and overprotective, and he felt responsible for her happiness. The father observed that his son did not allow himself to have fun and to be happy when visiting him.

The long-lasting conflict between the parents deeply affected Louis. He was pulled in two directions without the capacity to make a choice. He was preoccupied with making mistakes and found ways to avoid being criticized. He had low self-esteem and self-confidence. He looked depressed and tired. He tended to lose his voice and have a nosebleed whenever he was afraid and stressed out.

Conceptualization

Louis's presenting problems included being anxious, somatizing, missing a significant number of days of school because of illness, and being torn in his love for his parents. For most of his life he had lived in a state of internal and external conflict, and in an environment where the mother in particular expressed hatred and hostility toward his father.

He craved to have a loving relationship with his father and form a secure emotional bond with him, but the mother's negativity stood in the way. Louis felt obligated to adhere to the demands of his mother and felt guilty (i.e., critical superego) when he did not comply.

Because of the state of conflict and negativity in the parents' relationship, and particularly because of his mother's negative, hostile, and demeaning attitude toward Louis's father, Louis's psychological, relational, and social development were skewed toward being critical of others and toward himself. He identified with his mother and internalized her critical attitude to form an internal critic (i.e., critical superego) by which he repressed his feelings of love (i.e., need for emotional bonding), particularly for his father. He had two competing internal forces, that of love and that of aggressivity.

He projected his love and aggressivity outward to form benevolent figures and malevolent figures. He populated his mind with benevolent figures (i.e., representations) such as his grandmother, grandfather, and his mother, and with a malevolent figure such as the father. Both destructive and constructive forces reigned within him. He split his world into good and bad people and his self into good and bad parts that corresponded to the projected good and bad people.

The defenses that he developed, such as splitting and suppression, were not capable to manage his angry and aggressive feelings, which leaked out in self-harm and somatizing. Louis struggled with unresolved emotions and thoughts from the past, which predisposed him to anxiety, somatic problems, and internal conflicts.

Goals of Therapy

The goals of therapy were twofold. The first goal was to help Louis grieve the death of his maternal grandmother. The second goal was to help Louis process and work through the effects of parental alienation. This entailed extricating himself from the parental conflict; resolving the internal loyalty conflict; feeling free to love both mother and father and be happy in their homes; connecting to and expressing his feelings, thoughts, and relational needs; differentiating from his mother; developing a sense of self; becoming autonomous and individuated; and developing more effective and adaptive ways to cope with stresses, anxieties, and relational and internal conflicts. In brief, the goal was to help him complete the developmental tasks of the separation and individuation process and to deal with the task of being loyal toward both parents.

Therapy Approach

The therapist was constantly mindful of the special observational and attentive skills, the unique interventions, and the personal and relational qualities that are essential when providing therapy to children. These unique skills, interventions, and qualities comprise an understanding of the conditions that trigger the presenting problems and the child's core needs that are not adequately responded to. The therapist searched for the underlying dynamics of the presenting problems. In addition to these skills, the therapist provided a warm, friendly, accepting, and permissive relationship so that Louis felt free to play with toys and to openly express his feelings and needs to the therapist and/or to project them using play material.

The therapist's approach in working with Louis combined verbal therapy with play therapy. In verbal exchanges, he opened up spontaneously and freely on the different areas of his life that upset him or excited him. Through play therapy, Louis projected his conflicts, feelings, and needs onto the chosen figures. After he built scenes consisting of persons and objects, the therapist asked him to tell her what was going on. Through the storytelling and the nudging of the therapist, Louis explored ways to deal with the difficulties in his life, and eventually found a resolution to the problem and experienced a transformation of his inner world that led to resolution of the internal loyalty conflict.

Resolution of the Aftereffects of Parental Alienation

In the first four sessions, Louis addressed his grief over the death of his grandmother, his sadness over his grandfather's illness, and his tendency to lose his voice whenever he was afraid. Using the sand tray, he projected scenes of danger, destruction, unpredictability, the incapacity of the mother and rescuers to help him, fear of his father, the need for saving the situation, and transforming it by moving away with the father and assuring safety and surveillance.

Louis arrived at the fifth session in a good mood because his mother was happy that he was enjoying his visits with his father, and she wanted him to let her know when he wanted to visit him. He also reported that his school marks were beginning to improve. He mentioned to the therapist that he had a story in mind that bothered him at school. Louis wanted to enact the story using the playhouse. He enacted the story across sessions 5, 6, and 7. For this chapter, the settings from sessions 5 and 7 are presented as they are a good illustration of the various aspects of his inner world that he projected onto characters.

The characters for the various settings included two merchants, parents, maternal grandparents, three children (a one-year-old and three-month-old girls; a ten-year-old boy), and a five-year-old cousin. The last setting, that is, session 7, also included a dog and Santa Claus with two reindeer and elves. Following each of the enactments, the therapist asked Louis to describe what was happening and she, with his permission, took photos of the settings.

Fifth Session – Family in Conflict

Setting 1: Chaotic home, violence, and destruction

This setting comprises malevolent and benevolent characters. The malevolent characters are two merchants and a cousin. The benevolent characters comprise the parents, the children, the grandparents and the ten-year-old boy.

The setting begins with the family asleep and while they are asleep, two merchants invade the unlocked house (Scene 5). One merchant scares the cousin and the other scares the children, who are in the washroom, and screams at them to return the money. He also scares the ten-year-old boy (in yellow top), who, when frightened, loses his balance, and falls out of the open window. In the morning, after the merchants leaves, the cousin plays with the decorations in the washroom and almost destroys the whole washroom. He throws the bath out the window. He tries to jump down with a parachute, falls from the top of the house (Scene 6). The bathwater runs into the living room.

In the morning after the merchants have left, the ten-year-old boy, who wanted to take his bath, saw the damage that the merchants did to the washroom. His science books are soaked with water. He shouts to his parents to get up to see the damage. The cousin returns to cause even more damage. He throws the bookshelf with its contents onto the floor, and overturns the parents' furniture on them and boy (Scene 7). The boy is so angry that he throws his sisters into the swimming pool, who die because they cannot swim, and he then trashes the kitchen, living room, and the school bus (Scene 8). The boy pitches his father into the swimming pool. The mother grabs the boy by the arm and throws him outside, and as he is on his way out, he trips over a science book and falls into the swimming pool. He then rescues his father, mother, little sisters, and his wet and damaged science books from the pool.

In the middle of the chaos, the grandparents arrive and inquire as to what was happening. They scold the cousin for the chaos that he created. The little boy is sad that he lost his science books, which his grandmother retrieves from the water. The grandfather offers to repair the damage done to the house, which he repairs. The cousin tries parachuting, loses his pants, and everyone except him found this funny. He cries, fixes his pants, and leaves to live in another house. The merchants do not return because everyone is there. The grandmother asks the children to hurry to finish with their baths and to clean up. The grandmother sets up a game of choo choo train using chairs. The grandfather takes his bath and he and the grandmother go to bed. Nobody wants to have dinner; everyone goes to bed. The boy sleeps with his grandparents (Scene 9).

Setting 2: Benevolent characters

The second setting comprised only benevolent characters, that is, the ten-year-old boy, his sister, his parents, and his grandparents. It is a sunny morning. In this setting the ten-year-old boy becomes interested in biology. He has a healthy breakfast and goes to school by bus. He comes home for lunch prepared by his grandfather. He does his homework at lunchtime. He brings home all his books in biology, sciences, and animals. His sister, in her excitement to help him, causes the books to fall on the floor, then she jumps into the pool without anyone knowing. The grandfather checks on her and he also falls headfirst into the pool (Scene 10). The grandmother goes upstairs and finds the science books on the floor (Scene 11). The father gets up and washes himself. The mother wakes up but does not know what is going on and goes to the roof to check and she gets stuck there. She calls her son, who did not know where the mother was. The father did not know either where she was. The boy is angry as he noticed another mess in his room. The boy then grabs his homework in biology, rushes to the bus, and goes to school.

Seventh Session – Resolution of Family Conflict

The seventh session comprised setting 3, which took place on Christmas Eve. Present in this setting are: the ten-year-old-boy, the parents, the grandparents, two girls, a cousin, two tigers, a dog, Santa, reindeer, elves, and the two merchants who became benevolent, and a jail in the background (Scene 12). This session is characterized by aggressivity, which eventually turns into joyful family life; it represents a resolution of family conflicts.

This setting begins with the family preparing for Christmas. The father runs his bath water and goes away. The mother puts the turkey in the oven, washes her hands, decorates the Christmas tree, gets herself ready for Christmas, and then watches a movie to relax. The girls wake up screaming and then come down and wash their hands. The youngest girl falls in the water and then gets out by herself. She and her sister then join her mother to watch a movie. Suddenly, a dog named Pretzel enters the house, jumps on the mother and father's decorations, tears up the father's police uniform, jumps in the bath with the father, then leaps through the window, and causes an avalanche of snow, and has not been seen since.

The ten-year-old boy goes to the pet shop to buy two tigers. The tigers scare and attack the mother and the girls, and then strike the boy. They turn the kitchen and entrance upside down, jump on the cousin, bite his two arms, and maul his leg so that he cannot walk. The cousin is sad and calls for his mother. The second tiger does the same to his second leg and calls him a spin top toy because he cannot walk (Scene 13). The first tiger than attacks the father in the bathtub; he falls down the stairs, and is knocked over but he is not dead.

The second tiger attacks in turn the grandmother and the grandfather. Both fall out of an open window (Scene 14). The grandmother is saved, and the grandfather goes to the top of the house and screams, "Hey Tiger." The tiger attacks the grandfather again and makes him fall, but the grandfather tricks the tiger by showing him a piece of steak to make him fall from the top of the house.

Image 8.2 Louis 01.

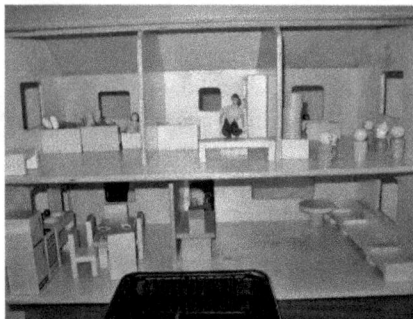

Scene 5. Family is asleep, merchants enter front door, create havoc in house.

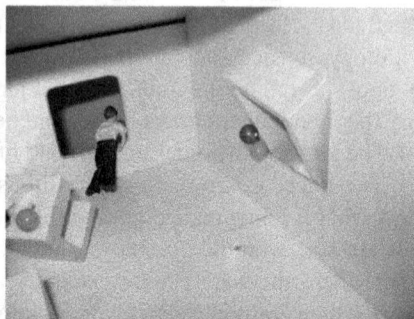

Scene 6. Cousin destroys washroom, falls out of window.

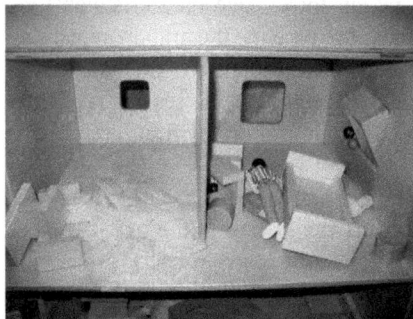

Scene 7. Boy asks parents to see the damage, and cousin pursues havoc and attacks parents and boy.

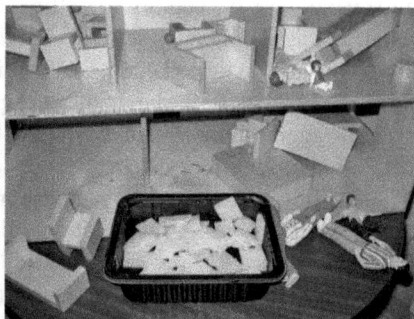

Scene 8. Boy is angry and attacks family members, the sisters die, and the books are soaked.

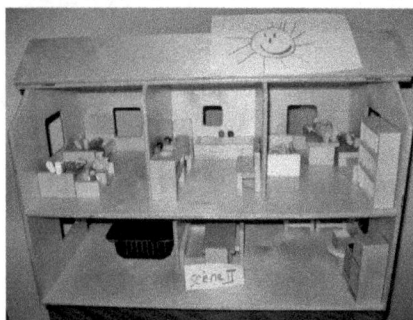

Scene 9. Early sunny morning. House back in order, family sleeping, boy sleeps with grandparents.

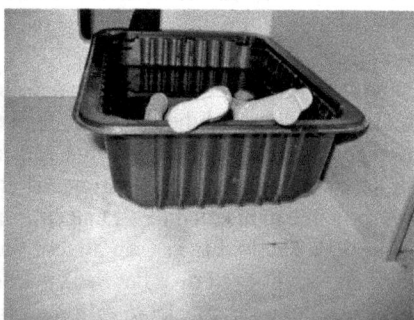

Scene 10. Grandfather falls into pool as he tries to rescue the boy's sister.

Image 8.3 Louis 02.

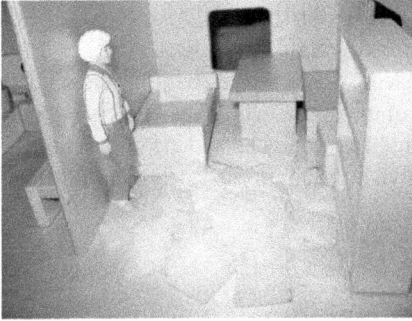

Scene 11. Grandmother sees books on the boy's bedroom floor.

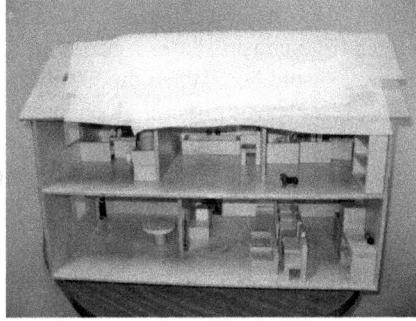

Scene 12. Christmas Eve and the family prepares for Christmas.

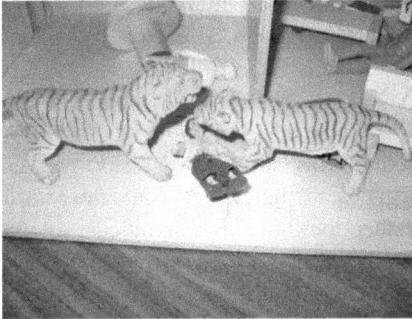

Scene 13. Cousin comes back and is attacked by tigers bought by the boy.

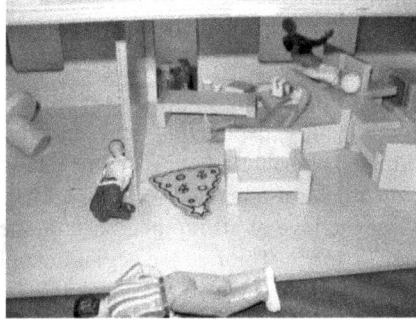

Scene 14. Grandparents are afraid of the menacing tiger, fall out of the windows, and are saved.

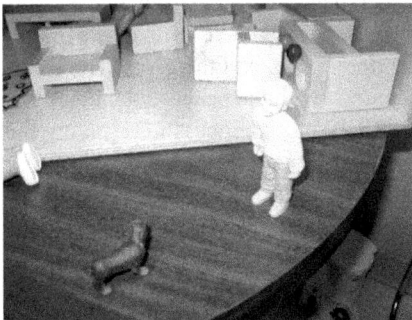

Scene 15. After the dog knocks down the tigers, the boy speaks to the dog and they put everything back in order for Christmas Eve.

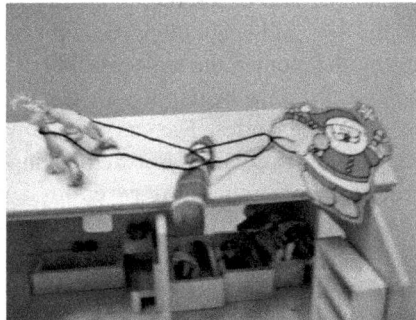

Scene 16. Santa arrives with reindeer and elves and leaves gifts for all including the dog.

Out of nowhere the dog returns and attacks and knocks down the tigers. The boy speaks to the dog and they together put everything back in order as it was Christmas Eve and they prepare a big gift (Scene 15). It is Christmas night; everyone goes to sleep. The cousin shares a bedroom with his grandparents. Pretzel sleeps with the ten-year-old boy. When the family is asleep, Santa arrives with his sleigh and reindeer, and leaves gifts for all on the roof of the house, which the elves bring into the house (Scene 16). On Christmas morning, everyone opens their gifts. There is also a gift for the dog. The two merchants visit the family to wish them a Merry Christmas.

Analysis and Discussion

The stories that Louis created in the two therapy sessions were complex. They consisted of many separate parts that comprised malevolent figures and benevolent figures and their relationships. The benevolent and malevolent figures represented parts of himself that were in conflict. The stories can be interpreted differently depending on the theory that is applied to their explanation. The explanation that follows is according to SIRCP.

There are several aspects of the stories that are notable. First, the mother in real life was angry, demanding, and critical of his father, and yet in the stories she is portrayed as being a caring and devoted mother. This can be interpreted as Louis idealizing his mother and splitting off her negative attributes as he could not afford to lose the love of his mother. Second, the father does not play a significant role in Louis's stories. Third, at the beginning of his story (first setting), the merchants and the cousin were malevolent characters, and at the end of the story (third setting), they became benevolent characters. Louis managed to transform the internal bad objects into good objects.

More generally, Louis's stories can be considered as externalizations (i.e., projections) of his internal struggles and conflicts. The stories begin with destructiveness, anger, and chaos represented by the merchants, the cousin, and the tigers and the dog, and end with peace and calm represented by the efforts of the grandmother, the mother, the ten-year-old boy, the dog, Santa, and the elves. The chaos and hostility at the beginning of the stories contrast with the peace and harmony at the end of the stories. The stories, in a way, represent his process in resolving the internal loyalty conflict. In externalizing his inner thoughts and feelings, in story form, Louis was able to draw on his inner resources (symbolized by his grandfather, grandmother, and the dog), to transform his aggressive urges into assertiveness, and his negative feelings (symbolized by the merchants, the cousin, and tigers) into more positive feelings and gradually resolve his conflicts and anxieties and to form a family with healthy relationships.

The dog was helpful to bring about harmony in the family. The dog, it appears, represents his split sense of self (i.e., the angry self and the caring self) and his inner resources (i.e., ego) that reversed the splitting and saw all characters and self in a realistic and positive way. This represents a transformation of his psychic- and self-structures that impacted the resolution of the internal loyalty conflict and brought about a sense of comfort in his relationships with his parents.

The energy that drove the resolution of his internal loyalty conflict, was Louis's desire to have the autonomy and freedom to choose to have an emotional relationship with his father. By the externalization of the benevolent and malevolent characters, and by the introduction of a third force (i.e., the transformed dog), Louis was able to resolve his conflict and was free to have a relationship with both his father and his mother. In SIRCP terms, Louis was able to reconcile superego demands with his core strivings to have a meaningful relationship with his father and mother by drawing on his inner ego resources.

By the termination of therapy, Louis was living full-time with his father with bi-monthly visits to his mother. He was enjoying a stable and conflict-free life in a caring and supportive family.

References

American Psychiatric Association (2013). *Diagnostic and Statistical Manual of Mental Disorders* (*DSM–5*). Washington, D.C.: Author.

Bernet, W., Wamboldt, M.Z., & Narrow, W.E. (2016). Child affected by parental relationship distress. *American Academy of Child and Adolescent Psychiatry, 55*(7), 571–579. Washington, D.C.

Caplan, P.J. (2004). What is it that's being called Parental Alienation Syndrome. In P.J. Caplan & L. Cosgrove (Eds.), *Bias in psychiatric diagnosis* (pp. 62). Washington, D.C.: Rowman & Littlefield.

Champlin, K., Oldham, C., & Salvatoriello, P. (Legal Team) (2017). *Parental alienation.* Retrieved from https://legaldictionary.net/parental-alienation/, September, 2019.

Dallam, S.J. (1999). The Parental Alienation Syndrome: Is it scientific? In E. St. Charles & L. Crook (Eds.), *Expose: The failure of family courts to protect children from abuse in custody disputes.* Sudbury/Manitoulin, Canada: Our Children Charitable Foundation.

Farzad, B.R. (2019). *What is parental alienation? What can you do about it?* Retrieved from https://farzadlaw.com/divorce-and-child-custody/what-is-parental-alienation/

Gardner, R.A. (2001). Parental Alienation Syndrome (PAS): Sixteen years later. *Academy Forum, 45*(1), 10–12. Retrieved March 31, 2009.

Hoult, J.A. (2006). The evidentiary admissibility of Parental Alienation Syndrome: Science, law, and policy. *Children's Legal Rights Journal, 26*(1), 1–61.

Wood, C.L. (1994). The parental alienation syndrome: A dangerous aura of reliability. *Loyola of Los Angeles Law Review, 29*, 1367–1415.

Chapter 9

"It's Mine!"

Helping a Four-Year-Old Girl Be Autonomous

This chapter presents the case of Chantal (pseudonym), whose challenge was to psychologically separate from her parents and from significant others, individuate, become age-appropriately autonomous, and assert her feelings and needs. The first part presents a brief description of the separation and individuation process. This is followed by a summary of the psychosocial and developmental history of Chantal and the health and relational factors that contributed to her developmental challenges. The third part presents an assessment of Chantal's problems using constructs from Self-in-Relationship Psychotherapy (SIRP) as operationalized by the SIRP Assessment Form (SIRP-AF). This is followed by a conceptualization of her symptoms and the treatment that helped Chantal become assertive, establish boundaries, assert her autonomy, and establish a secure emotional bond, all of which led to greater psychological separation and to individuation.

The Separation and Individuation Process

A primary developmental task for a child is to become "emotionally bonded" with a significant other (e.g., mother) and then in due course to psychologically separate from her, individuate, and become her own person (Mahler, Pine & Bergman, 1975). On a primitive cognitive and emotional level, the infant has an experience of fusion with the mother as well as images of oneness with her. The infant's initial intrapsychic experience is that of being undifferentiated from the mother.

To psychologically separate refers to recognizing that there are persons separate from oneself, that is, to differentiate between the "me" and the "not-me." Psychological separation denotes the child's achievement of an intrapsychic sense of separateness from the mother.

To individuate denotes the evolution of intrapsychic autonomy, that is, the development of psychic structure and personality characteristics. It means to develop a sense of selfhood and identity and to assert one's own preferences, values, dreams, ambitions, and needs (Masterson, 1993). It implies the ability to function in an autonomous and self-directed manner without being controlled and impaired or feeling unduly responsible for significant others (Bowen, 1978).

DOI: 10.4324/9781032655291-13

It is within the context of psychologically separating and individuating that the child constructs her inner world that comprises psychic structure, self-structure, defensive capacities, and relational patterns. In other words, the child lays down the foundation for his personality and for the person that he is to become.

A significant point in the separation and individuation process is the Rapprochement Subphase, during which, if it is successful, the child acquires the skills to regulate emotions and impulses, acquires the capacity to self-comfort and self-soothe, to see self and others as persons, to establish personal boundaries, to integrate impulses and yearnings with a positive sense of self, to achieve object constancy, and to replace the defense of splitting with the defense of repression (Mahler et al., 1975). A failure to achieve this developmental task can lead to deficiencies in these capacities.

Parental nurturing and nudging are necessary to help a child individuate, achieve autonomy, and develop a sense of self (Mahler et al., 1975). Parental indulgence and inadequate nudging may lead to a failure to individuate and to an ill-defined sense of self. The task of the child is to reach a comfortable position in being one's own person and at the same remain connected to the loved object, such as the mother.

An individual works through the separation and individuation processes several times in her lifetime. The first time is as a child, the second time is in becoming an adolescent where she asserts her preferences and choices, and the third time is when she leaves home.

Psychosocial and Developmental History

The parents sought help for their four-year old daughter, Chantal, because they feared that she would not be ready for pre-kindergarten as she was shy and unable to assert herself with other children. They also were concerned about Chantal's delay in speech and language development.

Chantal is the eldest child in a family of three children. She has two younger brothers. Chantal's birth and nursing went well. The mother stated that she foresaw the daughter's needs and she took her with her everywhere that she went. When Chantal cried, the mother cuddled and rocked her or distracted her from what was annoying. Chantal crawled at the age of 15 months, began to walk at about 16 to 17 months, and was potty-trained at the age of two and a half years.

The parents stated that they have a family routine that is characterized by family interactions and activities such as doing crafts and visiting relatives. The parents described Chantal as not being fussy; never throwing temper tantrums; being reasonable, shy, quiet, and soft spoken; and as getting along well with her brothers. She can ask her parents for what she wants. It was also noted that Chantal has a rich imagination and likes to create stories from pictures that she looks at.

The parents valued sharing, which they encouraged by having the children share toys. This encouragement to share toys was to the point that a child did not possess a toy of his/her own. The toys, in fact, belonged to everyone.

At the age of one, Chantal began to attend a family daycare, which she went to until the age of three years. In Chantal's group there were two children who were deaf and one child who had Down syndrome. Chantal did not have the opportunity to speak and to develop language. The babysitter taught the children sign language. Chantal was delayed in language development, used sign language, and had difficulty hearing. Chantal, at the age of three, was not able to speak nor compose sentences. The only words that she knew were daddy and mommy. This was a shock to the parents, who had no reference point to assess the progress of their child.

Chantal underwent tests for audition and vision. It was discovered that she had an inner ear problem that made it difficult to hear high pitch sounds and affected her hearing in a group or in a room with music or a loud television. Her hearing problem was corrected and she made progress both at the level of language and socially. As for the results from the vision tests, it was discovered that she suffered from astigmatism, which had caused her not to see things well from a distance since birth. This condition was corrected by Chantal wearing eyeglasses.

Chantal is described as shy, lacking self-confidence, and feeling not good enough and incapable. She does not assert her needs, thoughts, and feelings. She has difficulty separating, individuating, establishing boundaries, and developing trusting relationships with non-relatives. Chantal allowed others to impose themselves on her, to push her around, and to take things from her without protest. At one time Chantal returned home from the daycare wearing a coat that was not hers. She explained that the educator dressed another girl with Chantal's coat. Chantal observed this and said nothing. She does not initiate play but waits for others to take the initiative before playing with them.

Assessment

The assessment utilizes Chantal's psychosocial and developmental history to explain her presenting personal and relational problems. The assessment is complemented by information from the therapy sessions. Chantal's problems are seen through the lens of the constructs taken from Self-in-Relationship Psychotherapy (SIRP). These constructs are presented in Chapter 7 and their operational definitions are presented in Appendices B and C. The following constructs are relevant to explain Chantal's symptoms. The significance of the relevant constructs is assessed according to the norms for children who are of Chantal's age.

Psychic Structure

The psychic structure (i.e., inner world) according to Freud comprises three agencies, namely, the id, ego, and superego. SIRP has replaced the instincts of the id by core needs that consist of relational, self, and physical intimacy needs. The relational needs are the need for emotional bonding and the need for autonomy; the self needs include the needs for significance and competency; and the physical intimacy needs consist of the need for sensual contact and the need for sexual intimacy. The superego consists of internalized acceptable, and unacceptable behaviors. The ego, as one of its functions, mediates the demands of the superego and the pressure of the core needs.

With regard to the structure of Chantal's inner world, it is characterized by the internalization of parental expectations, the suppression of her own needs, and her incapacity to assert her innate needs. She is quiet, well behaved, reasonable, regulates her behaviors in not throwing temper tantrums, shares toys with her brothers, and suppresses her need to assert her need for autonomy and to say "It is mine." Although she does not express anger outwardly such as in temper tantrums, in her sand play stories she describes characters as being angry to the point of killing them. In brief, her inner world is dominated by a severe superego, an unmet and repressed need for autonomy, and a weakened ego that allies itself with the superego demands.

Self-Structure

The self-structure, according to SIRP, comprises two core needs, namely the need to feel competent and the need to feel significant. In her relationship with significant others, particularly with her parents and peers, Chantal developed a sense of who she is as perceived and treated by others. Chantal perceives herself to be not good enough and incapable, particularly when she attends daycare and school and compares herself to other children. She thinks and/or feels that what she has to say is not important. Her desire that her brothers not enter her room and take things that belong to her did not matter. Her desire to have her own toys did not matter. In summary, Chantal's perception is that she is incompetent when compared to her peers, and she says to herself that what she desires does not matter. That is, her needs are not significant. These two unmet needs impacted her self-confidence and self-esteem.

Characteristic Emotional State

Behaviorally, Chantal is described as quiet, shy, reasonable, and as getting along well with her brothers, yet there is an undercurrent of controlled and/or repressed anger as manifested in her characterization of figures in her sand play creations. Her need to be loved by her parents inhibits the expression of her anger toward them and her brothers and it impedes her assertiveness in her relationships. It is assumed that her anger is related to the unmet need to have a say in things that matter to her, that is, to the unmet needs for autonomy and significance. The combination of being in a daycare with children who were deaf, and with her visual and auditory problems may have contributed to her failure to achieve the needs for autonomy and significance.

True Self

To live from a true self implies that one engages in social interactions that are based on one's core needs, preferences, ideals, and values and at the same time respects the same in others. When Chantal's behaviors are compared to the behaviors of children of her age, she is less able to be true to herself as she lets others push her around and take her things, such as her coat. At the same time, she is not able to tell her parents that she does not want her brothers to come to her room and take her toys. She is not able to assert herself and to say, "It is mine." In brief, when compared to children of her age, she lives more from the expectations of others, including her parents and daycare provider, than from her own needs and preferences. Children of her age, when they do not get their way, will often throw temper tantrums. This is not the case for Chantal as she complies with the wishes of the significant adults in her life.

Defense Mechanisms

Defense mechanisms operate unconsciously and have as their goal to resolve internal conflicts, manage anxieties, and protect one's self-esteem. These mechanisms are often portrayed in a person's behavior, such as in dissociation and rationalization. Technically, they differ from coping strategies, which are consciously motivated and/or selected, such as suppression, negotiation, and compromise.

Chantal tends to engage in the defense mechanisms of repression, rationalization, and reaction formation and suppression as a coping mechanism. She represses and/or suppresses her own feelings, as shown in not throwing temper tantrums, which would be a normal expression of her need for autonomy. She represses her core need for autonomy by not asserting herself and saying, "It is mine." She used rationalization to explain when she did not want her brother to join her in the sand tray. She said that he would get his fingers dirty rather than directly state that she wanted to play alone. At her young age, one can see that she is beginning to use reaction formation as defense mechanism. She portrays herself as quiet, reasonable, and as getting along well with her brothers and peers. Yet in her sand play creations, she characterizes the figures as angry, hurtful, and harmful. Behaviorally, she shows herself to be well behaved and as getting along well with her brothers and peers. This behavior might be motivated by the fact that Chantal does not want to lose the love of her parents, particularly that of her mother. Chantal therefore complies and behaves differently in her relationships than what she feels internally.

Projective Identification

Projective identification refers to a pattern of relating with others where one tries to draw the other into their way of relating. Three patterns of relating are dependency, power, and ingratiation (Cashdan, 1988). The pattern of dependency entails relying on others to take care of them, to make decisions for them, to take the initiative in planning activities and events, and to be included socially and relationally. Power, as a relational pattern, refers to a person who thinks that he knows better than others, including his partner and family members, and who takes charge of specific tasks such as finances, planning vacations, and parenting. Ingratiation is a relational pattern in which one begins and maintains a relationship by laying guilt trips on another person, such as a parent on a child.

With regard to Chantal, she manifests a relational pattern of dependency not only regarding her relationship with her parents but also regarding her peers. She lets others take the initiative when it comes to the nature of their interaction. It has been mentioned that she waits to see how her peers want to play before she joins them. Her dependency is manifested in her tendency to let others take the lead and thereby draw the others into her way of relating, which is that of dependency.

Chantal's dependency on others has broad ramifications. She fails to establish personal and physical boundaries and to set limits as to what she is ready to give to others. These failures result in her not being able to assert that "It is mine" in terms of it is my place, my turn, and my belonging. Children of her age are more vocal about establishing boundaries and setting limits, which they manifest through acting-out behaviors such as crying and throwing temper tantrums. Chantal is rational and does not show anger, which is unusual for a girl of her age.

Developmental Phase

The child's first four to five years of development have been defined as the symbiotic and the separation and individuation phases (Mahler et al., 1975). The separation and individuation phase has four subphases, namely: differentiation, practicing, rapprochement, and consolidation/object constancy. The developmental tasks for each phase and subphase are summarized in Chapter 7. The symbiotic phase and the first three subphases are pertinent regarding Chantal's developmental history.

Symbiotic phase

Symbiosis, which extends from zero to four months, represents a state of inter- mittent fusion with the mother, a state of undifferentiation in which the "I" is not yet differentiated from the "Not-I," and the inside and outside are only gradually coming to be sensed as different (Mahler et al., 1975, p. 8). The major tasks of this phase are the achievement of "safe-anchorage" with the caregiver, the devel- opment of "confident expectation" that its needs will be met, the formation of an inner core and bodily self, and the formation of representations of other and self (Mahler & Furer, 1968, p. 17). The infant's inner body experiences contribute to the development of the body ego and body self and form the very core of the self. These experiences are the crystallization point around which a sense of identity will become established (p. 11).

Chantal did not complete the developmental tasks of this phase as she remained emotionally dependent on others and she did trust that others would respond to her needs and feelings. She also lacked a core self. The failure to complete the developmental task, particularly to become "emotionally anchored," appears to be related to being overstimulated as the mother would respond to her when she cried and carried her wherever the mother went. Chantal appears not to have had sufficient quiet time where she and her mother enjoyed sensual and emotional contact, such as in nursing, which are essential for the development of "safe-anchorage" and "confident expectation" that her needs would be met. Chantal was left with a yearning for emotional bonding that was stronger than her need for individuation.

Differentiation subphase

Differentiation refers to the process of emerging from the "symbiotic state of oneness with the mother, in the intrapsychic sense" (Mahler et al., 1975, p. 290). It is outward and goal directed and occurs between four and ten months (p. 54). A major task of this subphase is for the child to separate psychologically from the caregiver and to develop a sense of identity, that is, a sense of being. It is not "a sense of who I am" but a sense "that I am" (p. 8). The child is helped to differentiate in a timely fashion when her movements toward psychological separation are supported and validated, and when the caregiver is available to her when she returns for emotional closeness.

It appears that Chantal did not achieve an age-appropriate level of differentiation nor a sense of identity. She was delayed in separating intrapsychically from her mother and establishing the "I" and the "Not I." The parents did not validate Chantal to differentiate or to psychically separate her from themselves and from her siblings. Chantal was shy, complacent, and did not throw temper tantrums. She was not encouraged to say "It's mine" and "You can't take it." She was not permitted to own a toy of her own; the toys belonged to all the children.

Likewise, Chantal did not achieve a sense of identity. She was shy, did not assert herself, and let others take things from her without protesting. She did not let others know who she was and did not stand up for who she was. Because she did not achieve a sense of identity, she failed to establish personal and physical boundaries and to develop assertiveness skills. She was outwardly pleasant and yet within she was resentful, which was revealed in the characterization of sand play and play-dough figures (See treatment).

Practicing subphase

The practicing subphase, which is typically achieved between 10 and 14 months, represents the child's movement from the "maternal nest" to exploring the expanding world that lies beyond the relationship with the caregiver; the child begins a "love-affair" with the world (Mahler et al., 1975, p. 70). The child exercises her developing motor capacities (e.g., crawling, walking) and cognitive capacities (e.g., manipulating objects, language), and reality tests her sense of omnipotence. The child feels elated with her own faculties, with the greatness of her own world, and in using her body to explore and master the "other-than-mother" environment and to "escape from fusion with, from engulfment by mother" (Mahler et al., 1975; p. 71).

The toddler learns how to deal with anxiety when the mother is away for a significant period by developing "object constancy" (Mahler et al., 1975, p. 48). This entails having formed a cognitive-affective representation of her mother, to which she turns to comfort herself when the mother is absent. She acquires the capacity to self-soothe, first by internalizing the maternal functions that originally served to soothe, calm, and regulate affect, and later by creating a transitional object (e.g., blanket) that is invested with the mother's tension-relieving and soothing functions. For the child to negotiate this subphase, it is important that the caregiver validate the toddler's efforts toward separation and her strivings toward mastery of her world and be emotionally available when the toddler feels anxious in his separation experiences.

As for Chantal, she did not complete the developmental tasks of this subphase. She was socially shy, quiet, and did not assert herself. Although by the age of four she had developed cognitive skills and language, she did not use these new capacities to assert herself, to establish personal and physical boundaries, and to set limits. She let others push her around, impose themselves on her, and take things from her without protesting. For example, one time Chantal returned from daycare wearing a coat that was not hers. She explained to her mother that the educator dressed another girl with Chantal's coat. Chantal observed this and said nothing. It is possible that Chantal was more preoccupied with not losing the love of the caregiver than with asserting herself. For a similar reason, Chantal did not appear free to venture out and explore her expanding world. It is noted that Chantal has a significant imagination and creates stories from seeing pictures. This implies that she has a rich fantasy life, which in turn might mean that she has not reality tested her sense of grandiosity.

Rapprochement subphase

This subphase marks a pivotal developmental point in the child's struggle toward establishing her individuality. During the rapprochement subphase, which extends from 14 to 24 months, the child continues to strive to: (a) become securely emotionally connected; (b) establish a comfort zone between the "need to be emotionally connected" and the "need to be separated/individuated;" (c) establish physical and personal boundaries between herself and others (e.g., establishes "what is mine" from "what is yours"); (d) internalize representation of good persons (e.g., object constancy) to whom he can turn mentally to gain perspective on issues, comfort self, and regulate affect; (e) relate to others empathically as whole-objects; (f) replace splitting with repression; and (g) move toward individuality (Mahler et al., 1975).

The two main achievements of this subphase are the establishment of object constancy and individuality. To help a child achieve these goals, it is important for the caregivers to be sensitive to the child's emotional needs and to validate self-directed movements toward individuality. At this subphase, the child experiences anxiety in being separated from her caregiver and strives to connect with her. She

manifests this by bringing toys and books to the caregiver and invites her to participate in her activities. It is important for the caregivers to provide a structure to help
the child contain her feelings and behaviors and to provide the child with explanations for the limits that are being imposed.

It is quite clear that Chantal has not achieved the developmental tasks of this
subphase. She has not established physical and personal boundaries between
herself and others. That is, she has not established "What is mine" and "What is
yours." She is not moving in a noticeable way toward self-identity and individuality and continues to rely on others for direction and guidance. In her interactions
with her peers, she waits for them to take the lead. Although she is quiet, shy, and
well behaved, this appears to be more a function of being compliant rather than a
learned capacity to regulate affect. That is, she has not asserted herself to the extent
of expressing anger when what she wants is denied and in learning how to regulate
her affects. The failure to achieve the tasks of this subphase are in part due to her
not having significantly achieved the tasks of the previous phase and subphases.
The other factor is that the parents, especially the mother, emphasized the sharing
of toys and doing things together, but did not equally validate the children's move
toward achieving separateness and autonomy, establishing personal boundaries,
and setting limits. It was acceptable, for example, that Chantal's brothers would
enter her room and take her toys.

Case Conceptualization

Chantal's relational and behavioral problems and difficulties as reported by her
parents consist of being shy; having difficulty expressing her needs, thoughts, and
feelings; being unable to defend herself with other children; allowing others to
impose themselves on her; letting others take things from her without protest; and
not setting limits and establishing boundaries. In short, Chantal's difficulties consisted in not asserting her needs, feelings, and thoughts, and not being able to set
limits and establish boundaries.

It is conceivable that her auditory difficulties would have exacerbated her difficulties in being assertive, establishing boundaries, and setting limits with her peers
as she might not have heard what they said and thus she was hesitant to speak and
interact. It is also conceivable that by being in a family daycare with deaf children and with a Down syndrome child, she did not receive sufficient opportunity
to communicate, to socially interact, to deal with conflicts, and to learn how to be
assertive. The combination of her visual and auditory problems and being in a daycare with children who were deaf may have played a significant role in Chantal's
delay in language development and impacted her psycho-emotional development.

It is of equal importance to understand Chantal's behavioral and relational difficulties in terms of her interaction with her parents and of her upbringing. During
her first two months, Chantal appears not to have had the necessary sensual and
emotional contact to become emotionally anchored, which is revealed in her
intense dependency needs. Chantal was also brought up in a family where there was

insufficient differentiation. Chantal, the eldest of the three children, was treated in the same way, in terms of privileges, as her two younger brothers. One expectation of the parents was that the toys be shared; the toys belonged to all of them. It was permissible for the boys to enter Chantal's room and take toys. Chantal was not allowed to say, "It is mine" and "You cannot take it." Differentiation and the establishment of boundaries were not encouraged and validated. These experiences have wide implications for the development of Chantal's inner world, relational patterns, and coping capacities. The question is: how did Chantal internalize these experiences to form her inner world and how has her inner world affected her behaviors and relational interactions?

It has been reported that Chantal was shy, never threw a temper tantrum, was nonassertive, and got along well with her brothers. This implies that she internalized the parents' expectations regarding acceptable behaviors and values to live by, and at the same she repressed her natural inclinations to assert her feelings and relational and self needs. The parental expectations became her own and she regulated her behaviors and interactions by the voice of the internalized parent. Her inner world comprised an internal parent and inner child relationship with the internal parent dominating. In SIRP terms, she developed a strict superego and an ego that aligned itself with the superego, which repressed her need to assert her own needs, feelings, and thoughts, and in place of being assertive, she developed the attitude of being nice and sharing things with others. The external parents became internalized parents. The consequence, in SIRP terminology, was that her relational need for autonomy and her self need for significance were not given full recognition and were not appropriately validated.

A significant aspect of Chantal's relational and behavioral difficulties was that her innate need for having a say in matters that were important to her, was repressed and went unmet. In SIRP language, this is the innate need for autonomy. In her interactions with her parents, Chantal internalized their expectations and values and repressed her own innate need for autonomy.

Based on her childhood interactions, Chantal was predisposed to relate to others in nonassertive ways, repress her feelings and needs, and not set limits and establish boundaries. She did not learn to say, "It's mine." At the same time, she was predisposed to feel not as good as others (i.e., inadequate) and to be dependent on others (i.e., projective identification of dependency) since to differentiate from others and become autonomous was not encouraged.

Treatment: Goals, Process, Therapist Orientation, and Approach

Goals of Treatment

Treatment goals for Chantal

The therapy goals for Chantal were multiple. Fundamentally, they consisted of helping her assert herself (i.e., state "It's mine!"), establish boundaries, express herself with confidence, and progress toward individuation and achievement of a sense of individuality. The goals were worked on according to the issues that Chantal brought up in therapy. The issues emerged and were addressed particularly in play therapy.

Treatment goals for the parents

The general goal for the parents was to help them understand their daughter's emotional and behavioral problems and to provide them with relational skills and tools helpful to validate Chantal's strivings toward psychological separation, differentiation, autonomy, individuation, and toward becoming her own age-appropriate person. The focus with the parents was not to provide them with therapy, but to develop their parental skills to foster the emotional and social development of their children. With regard to Chantal, the mother's task was to create a personal space, develop secure relationships, help her become autonomous and feel competent and lovable, and involve Chantal in making decisions about matters that concerned her, such as choosing clothes to wear to go to the babysitter.

The treatment of Chantal was facilitated by the engagement and the collaboration of the parents. The parents had the same approach toward parenting. The mother was more available to bring Chantal to the therapy sessions. She discussed the sessions with her husband on a regular basis. The mother was open to learning and eager to know how to help her daughter.

Therapy Process

In working with young children, the therapist regularly included the parents in the therapy. Including the parents allowed for a continuation of the child's treatment in the home. The parents made efforts to implement what they learned in watching the therapist's interactions with the child and what they learned when they were asked to engage with the child during the therapy session.

In her treatment of Chantal, the therapist had a total of 30 sessions and seven telephone calls. This comprised the following: *Meetings*: with mother alone (10); with mother and Chantal (11); with Chantal alone (4); with mother, Chantal, and a son (2); with father and Chantal (1); with father alone (1), and with both parents (1). The *telephone calls* were as follows: with mother (5); with father (1); and with Chantal's teacher (1). Chantal was seen in therapy over a 22-month period.

With regard to Chantal, the therapist saw her and the mother together until Chantal felt at ease being alone with the therapist and with leaving her mother in the waiting room. This happened spontaneously for the first time after the 22nd session. After a good number of sessions with her mother, Chantal asked her mother to remain in the waiting room while she followed, without hesitation, the therapist to her office.

The therapist occasionally met with the parents to provide them with feedback regarding Chantal's progress concerning the issues being addressed. The therapist suggested reading material and a videotape to watch (Hanna & Wilford, 1990).

The therapist also provided them with psychological education regarding child development and pointed out developmental tasks to be achieved at various developmental stages. The parents were also given the freedom to ask questions and discuss their concerns about Chantal and the other children.

Therapist's Orientation

The therapist (M.B.), female, Canadian, was a graduate-level trained and experienced psychodynamic/humanistic- and developmental-oriented child psychotherapist who worked in a community clinic. The therapist used a wide variety of play therapy techniques, including sand tray, puppets, feeling cards, drawings, playhouse, storytelling, playdough, and board games. When required, the therapist designed specific exercises and/or techniques to help a child address and resolve specific challenges and difficulties, such as establishing object constancy and naming and articulating feelings. The therapist also modelled behaviors that helped Chantal learn how to be assertive, establish boundaries, and set limits.

The therapist was actively engaged in therapeutic dialogue, worked in the "here-and-now," and constantly checked back with Chantal to assess what she was experiencing and processing, particularly when she demonstrated changes in behavior, tone of voice, and mood. She provided a safe and secure environment, helped the client contain her feelings, and tried to balance nudging and nurturing. The goal of therapy was to provide Chantal with opportunities to experience herself and others in a new and different way and thereby foster self-understanding, a better understanding of the nature and quality of her relationships, to become skilled and empowered, and to become agent of her own person within the context of her relationships.

Therapist's Approach

In providing therapy to children, the therapist included, when appropriate, the significant persons in the child's life. In the case of Chantal, this included her parents, teacher, and medical personnel. The therapist viewed Chantal's problems in relational terms and worked as a team and included the significant professionals and the parents in her treatment.

The therapist was constantly mindful of the special observational and attentive skills, the unique interventions, and the personal and relational qualities that are essential when providing therapy to young children. These unique skills and qualities facilitate understanding of the conditions that trigger the presenting problems, ascertaining of the child's core needs that are not adequately responded to, and understanding of the relational interactions that led to the problems. The therapist looked beyond the presenting problem and searched for their underlying dynamics. She offered material and/or opportunities for Chantal to express herself symbolically and through projections. She provided a warm, friendly, accepting, and permissive relationship so that the child felt free to play with toys and to openly express her feelings and needs to the therapist and/or to project them onto the toys.

The therapist's approach in working with Chantal combined verbal therapy with play therapy. In verbal exchanges, Chantal opened spontaneously and freely on the different areas of her life that upset her or excited her. Through play therapy, Chantal projected her conflicts, feelings, and needs onto the chosen figurines and objects. After Chantal created constructions that consisted of persons and objects, the therapist asked her to tell her what was going on and/or how it would end. Through the storytelling and with the nudging of the therapist, Chantal explored ways to deal with the difficulties in her life, find a resolution of the problem, and experience a transformation of her inner world, which helped her become more assertive.

When appropriate, the therapist designed an exercise that gave Chantal an opportunity to practice a skill being worked on. For example, the therapist designed a game where Chantal could assert herself in saying "It's mine" or "It's yours." (See below for details).

Treatment

Therapy typically begins with the presenting of behavioral problems, such as difficulty in being assertive, in establishing boundaries, and in setting limits. The focus is on the external sources of the problems (e.g., unmet core needs) with reference to the child's interactions with parents, siblings, peers, and so on. As these problems are addressed, therapy gradually gravitates toward working with their internal sources, such as repressed feelings, unmet core needs, lack of confidence, internal conflict, and low self-esteem.

The goals of therapy with Chantal were multiple. Because of limited space in this chapter, four of the treatment goals are presented. These include: developing assertiveness and autonomy; establishing boundaries and setting limits; identifying and naming feelings; and establishing a secure emotional bond. In selecting these goals for presentation, it does not mean that the other goals were less important. Often by paying particular attention to a specific goal, some of the other goals are indirectly addressed.

The presentation begins by describing the issue to be treated. This is followed by interventions used in the treatment, the nature of Chantal's engagement in the treatment, and the outcome. The therapy goals were implemented primarily through theory-guided play.

Developing Assertiveness and Autonomy

Developing assertiveness

Being assertive means feeling confident and having courage to express one's needs, feelings, and thoughts in an affirmative, appropriate, and nonaggressive way. An assertive person is genuine, honest, and direct, and is willing to stand up for her interests and express her needs, feelings, and thoughts. She knows her rights and is also aware of the rights of others and is willing to work with them. The assertive person possesses the ability to compromise rather than always wanting her own way. The training to become assertive consists of learning the skills for how to be assertive and then implementing the skills.

TRAINING TO BE ASSERTIVE

Chantal had difficulty asserting herself and claiming what was hers. That is, she had difficulty saying "It's mine." She let her peers push her around and take things from her without protesting. To help Chantal recognize what belongs to her and learn to assert it, the therapist used *Milton Bradley's Memory Game*, designed for children 3–6 years of age. The game comprises 72 picture cards. To shorten the game, the therapist selected 15 pairs ahead of time. Each of the players – Chantal, the mother, the therapist – were given five different cards, with their matching pair being placed upside down in the pool of cards. The players took turns, going clockwise, picking up a card. If a player picked a card that matched the one in her hand, the player had to say, "It's mine." If the card matched a card of another player, that player had to say, "It's mine." The card was then given to that player. At times the mother made deliberate mistakes to provoke her daughter to say, "No, it's mine." Chantal freely participated in this nonthreatening way to assert herself.

The game had three purposes. First, to help Chantal assert herself when the card belonged to her. Second, to respect the other when the card belonged to someone else and to give it them. Third, to provide modeling for Chantal in hearing others assert themselves in saying "It's mine" when the card picked, matched the card in their hand.

In the memory game, the therapist modeled for Chantal how to be assertive, validated Chantal in being assertive, and encouraged her to continue to be assertive. In the play, Chantal learned how to be assertive and that it was correct to be assertive about what was hers.

The therapist suggested to the mother that she set up a game at home where they would continue to practice saying "It's Mine." At home, the mother asked each child to place some of their belongings and toys in a bag. Each child then took turns to draw something from the bag and when it belonged to them, they were to say "It's mine." The mother reported that the children loved preparing for the game and playing it.

ASSERTING WHAT IS HERS

Chantal was encouraged to apply her ability to assert herself and say "It's mine" in her relationships with her siblings and peers. One situation that was problematic was at the swimming pool where the children lined up to take their turn to be instructed. Chantal was not able to take her place in the group but instead allowed other children to go ahead of her. The therapist asked her to imagine this happening at the swimming pool and she was to say, "It's my turn; it's my place." At first her voice was faint and lacked energy in expressing herself. The therapist asked her to say it louder so that the therapist's "ears could hear." With encouragement and modeling, she was able to say "It's my turn; it's my place." One week later, the mother reported that Chantal had been able to assert herself nonverbally with a girl who attempted to go ahead of her in the line at the swimming pool. Chantal did not let her go through.

Chantal, with the help of her mother, learned how to assert herself with her brothers. Chantal determined which toys she wanted to lend to her brothers and which toys she did not want to share with them. She also expressed that her brothers could not enter her room without her permission.

Chantal was quiet and shy at school and uttered only a few words. Over time, she became more expressive and assertive. She learned to share what was on her mind, that is, her feelings, preferences, and likes and dislikes. In this regard her teacher was of great help as she was understanding, warm, patient, and friendly, and nudged her. On another occasion, Chantal wanted to take her turn on the swing. With the encouragement of the teacher, Chantal was able to assert herself and take her turn on the swing. After a therapy session, the therapist in a teasing fashion took away Chantal's boots. Chantal reacted and assertively took the boots from the therapist saying, "It's mine."

Developing autonomy

A core relational need, according to SIRP, is the striving to become autonomous and self-determining. The emergence of autonomous behavior during the years of childhood is a major development achievement (Goldberg & Lucas-Thompson, 2008).

Being autonomous means engaging in behavior that is consistent with one's intrinsic goals, interests, and values, and emanates from the self. Autonomy is synonymous with freedom and self-determination. More specifically, autonomy is defined as a state of having the ability to make one's own decisions independently of external control. An autonomous person has a sense of self-worth and self-respect. Children who are independent and autonomous feel a strong sense of efficacy and control and exhibit behaviors characterized by activity and initiative.

As Chantal's ability to assert herself grew, her behaviors became greatly influenced by her intrinsic needs, preferences, and feelings. With the guidance of the therapist, the mother gradually played a greater role in Chantal's asserting her autonomy. For example, Chantal's sand play constructions were typically followed by the therapist asking Chantal to tell a story about what was taking place. When the mother was present for such constructions and the storytelling and would impose her idea about the construction, Chantal became tense, and raised her voice and indirectly told the mother that it was her (Chantal's) story.

The mother reported that Chantal chose her own clothes and coordinated them in tones of rose and purple and wore socks of two different colors. The mother accepted and supported the autonomous behaviors of Chantal. At home Chantal expressed more what she wanted and did not want, and when she had to struggle to get what she wanted or was denied, she developed a crisis and began to have small temper tantrums. When the mother spoke about them to the therapist, she was assured that this was a positive sign as they were expressions of Chantal's attempts to be autonomous, that is, to have a say in what was important to her.

Chantal's autonomous behaviors broadened to include non-family members. During therapy, she developed a close relationship with the therapist. On one occasion as she arrived for a session, Chantal moved toward the therapist all happy, and nonverbally requested a hug. The therapist accepted her request for a hug.

In summary, as Chantal became more self-confident and autonomous, she developed the courage to be assertive in expressing her genuine and true needs and feelings in her interactions with others. Being assertive and autonomous served as the foundation to establish personal and physical boundaries, to set limits, and to develop intimate bonds, particularly with her mother.

Establishing Boundaries and Setting Limits

Boundaries are guidelines that individuals establish in their relationships that let others know what behavior they find acceptable and what behavior they will not tolerate. By establishing boundaries, individuals teach other people how to treat them, and they accept that they are only responsible for their own feelings and behaviors and not for the feelings and behaviors of others. Boundaries define what is theirs and what is not theirs. Individuals establish boundaries by the practice of openly communicating and asserting their personal values to preserve and protect them and not to have them compromised or violated.

There are many types of boundaries including personal, physical, emotional, sexual, material, and time boundaries. The boundaries applicable to Chantal are personal and physical boundaries.

Establishing personal boundaries

Personal boundaries are like guidelines that define how individuals would like to be treated by the people around them and how to react when these boundaries are violated. In defining what he likes and dislikes, the individual sets the allowed distance for others around them to approach. The way they build these boundaries stems from their values, beliefs, opinions, and past experiences (Hamdy, 2021; Nash, 2018).

When the psychotherapist began to treat her, Chantal did not have firmly established personal boundaries, particularly with her peers and her two brothers. The parents did not encourage the establishment of boundaries. They emphasized that the children did not have anything that was their own. It was permissible for her brothers to enter her room and to take toys. Chantal was not allowed to say "It's mine" and "You cannot take it." The failure on part of the parents to help the children establish personal boundaries was coupled with a failure on the part of the children to differentiate from the parents and from each other, and to individuate and to assert their autonomy.

In their conjoint session, the therapist helped the mother allow Chantal to assert her personal boundaries. In one of the therapy sessions, the mother also brought her 20-month-old son. In the session, Chantal played in the sand tray and the mother played with her son on the floor. The mother invited her son to play with his sister in the sand tray. The therapist asked Chantal whether she wanted her brother to play with her. Her response was "No, he will dirty his fingers." It was her way of saying that she wanted to play by herself. She asserted her personal boundary. The therapist intervened so that Chantal's space was protected and personal boundaries were established by not imposing the presence of the son on the daughter. The mother understood and resumed her play with her son in order to let her daughter play peacefully.

The therapist, in the game *Milton Bradley's Memory Game*, offered Chantal opportunities to establish personal boundaries. When Chantal – and one of the other players – picked a card that was not hers, she had to say, "It's yours." The idea of saying "It's mine" and "It's yours" had an impact of the mother's parenting of her children. She reported that the parents were moving away from the idea that "all things are shared" to using the expression "It's yours." The mother added that as she and her husband were working to establish personal boundaries among the children, the children on their own were establishing boundaries regarding the sharing of their toys. The therapist encouraged the mother and her husband to continue with their efforts to teach the children how to establish personal boundaries not only among themselves but also with peers and friends.

Establishing physical boundaries

To establish physical boundaries is to create limits on who is allowed into our personal space, how or when we are touched, and to control when we need to eat, sleep, and meet our physiological needs. In establishing physical boundaries, we tell the other person how close they can get to us, the distance that we want them to stand from us, what kind of physical touch is accepted, the amount of privacy that we need, and how to behave in our personal space.

When Chantal first came for therapy, she did not have her own bedroom and her brothers entered her room without her permission and took some of the toys. Chantal did not assert her physical boundaries in asking them not to enter her room. Initially, the parents accepted that the children shared things such as their toys. The parents did not guide the children in establishing personal and physical boundaries. In the mother's meetings with the therapist regarding Chantal establishing her physical boundaries, the therapist suggested that Chantal have her space and her own toys and that she choose which toys she wanted to lend to her brothers. The mother implemented this suggestion, moved Chantal to a room of her own, and asked her to place in her room the toys that she did not want to share with her brothers. At the same time, the brothers were informed of the new rules and the physical boundaries.

Setting limits

Setting limits refers to letting others know what they are allowed to do and what they are not allowed to do in their social interactions and behaviors (MacLaughlin, 2014). Parents set limits on what they want their children to do or not do. A child learns from her parents how to set limits by having experienced how her parents set relational and behavioral limits with her. In using what she learned from her parents, the child too sets limits in what her peers are allowed to do or not to do.

In being present for the therapy sessions with her daughter, the mother observed how the therapist helped Chantal be assertive, establish boundaries, and set limits by setting up games and situations in which these were practiced and modeled by the therapist. The mother applied these learnings in her parenting of her children, notably by encouraging them to be assertive, establish boundaries, and set limits and to respect the same in their siblings. The mother set up rules at home regarding entering the children's bedrooms and sharing toys.

To help Chantal set limits, the therapist designed an exercise in which Chantal imagined being in a line at a swimming pool for her turn to be instructed, and she was not to let others go ahead of her but to take her place. The therapist asked her to say, "It's my turn; it's my place." At first, her response was faint and the therapist encouraged to say it with more energy and determination so that the therapist's "ears could hear." With the therapist's encouragement and modeling, Chantal was able to say with more determination, "It's my turn; it's my place." One week later, the mother reported that Chantal had been able to assert herself nonverbally with a girl who attempted to go ahead of her in the line. She did not let her go through.

Identifying and Expressing Feelings

The behavioral strategies of being assertive, establishing boundaries, and setting limits are implemented, to a large degree, by one's core needs, feelings, thought processes, and preferences and the response of caregivers to these experiences. A goal of therapy was to help Chantal identify her feelings, name them, and learn how to express them. To help Chantal to achieve this goal, the therapist used Feeling Cards (Cartes de sentiments).

On one occasion, when Chantal arrived for a therapy session, she spontaneously picked up the feeling cards and organized them on the floor and accepted the chance to speak about them with the therapist. Chantal tended to: associate feelings of sadness with losing; being proud with winning; anger with being irritated; sorrow with irritating someone; and fear with objects like spiders. Her preference was the feeling of excitement. The therapist asked which of the cards she liked the least, to which she could not give an answer, but she said that she did not like to be angry. She added that one should be happy and then the other person would be happy too (e.g., mother, father).

Chantal then went to the sand tray to illustrate how she felt angry when her girl-friend visited her and wanted to play with her brothers. On the wet sand, Chantal drew a reversed grin, which she later drew on paper. She said that anger can also be drawn as a straight line. She drew a heart that contained her feelings. The heart helped concretize her experience. She then created a story that described the incident with her friend. Chantal wished that her friend had played only with her, and she was hurt and angry that her friend played with her brothers. Chantal screamed, and her feelings were so intense that she did not know how to stop them (possibly abandon-ment rage). Chantal's and her girlfriend's mother spoke with Chantal in the bedroom, consoled her, and helped her manage her feelings. Chantal understood that her friend did not have a brother with whom to play. Chantal accepted that if they did an out-door sport such as skiing, it was OK for her friend to play with her brothers.

Following her description of the scene, the therapist and Chantal worked on the attitude she might take the next time a situation such as this occurred. The sug-gestion was that Chantal would say to her friend that she would like to have play-time alone with her first, and after that she could play with her brothers. Chantal accepted this approach and clearly explained it to her mother after the session.

Establishing a Secure Emotional Bond

Chantal's symptoms, such as being shy, not asserting herself, and establishing bound-aries, suggest that she did not establish a secure emotional bond. That is, she did not complete the symbiotic phase of development (Mahler et al., 1975). The goal was to help Chantal establish a secure emotional bond. This goal emerged toward the end of therapy. Having a secure emotional bond would change the quality of Chantal's sense of self, her social interactions, her coping strategies and adaptive capacities, and her empathic acceptance and tolerance of others. According to SIRCP, the innate craving for a secure emotional bond with a caregiver is a core relational need.

Definition of an emotional bond

The establishment of an emotional bond represents an infant's investment of psy-chic energy from self to a need-gratifying object (i.e., the mother). The develop-ment of an emotional bond indicates that the infant/child has "achieved a specific symbiotic relationship with his mother" (Mahler & Furer, 1968, p. 13). It marks the beginning of the infant's capacity to invest in, relate to, and care about one special person (Mahler et al., 1975, pp. 46, 52). An indicator of the establishment of this bond is the infant's specific smiling response at the peak of the symbiotic phase. The specific smile attests to a special bond between infant and mother and consti-tutes a significant progression toward the capacity for human relatedness. A secure emotional bond is characterized by "safe anchorage" (i.e., being emotionally con-nected to another at the core of one's existence) and "confident expectation" that its needs will be responded to (Mahler & Furer, 1968, p. 17).

Formation of a secure emotional bond

The formation of a secure emotional bond consists of the involvement of both the mother and the infant/child. The involvement consists of maternal care and the infant's innate tendencies toward development (i.e., the processes that lead to maturation).

Maternal care comprises holding, handling, and object presenting (Winnicott, 1965). This combination of ministrations includes the mother's holding environment, her feeding, smiling, talking, eye-to-eye contact, physical closeness, cradling, supporting, and countless other ministrations. These behaviors are the "symbiotic organizers of psychological birth" (Mahler et al., 1975, p. 49) and promote physiological and sociobiological dependency on her and a sense of oneness. These maternal behaviors at the same time promote comfort, safety, a sense of union, and "safe anchorage" (Mahler & Furer, 1968), that is, a secure emotional bond.

The development of a secure emotional bond is dependent on the infant's capacity to extract needed supplies from the mother, that is, the child's capacity to perceive and accept the "mothering agent" (Mahler, 1968, p. 43). The outcome is also partially dependent on the infant's capacity (e.g., cries and smiles) to stimulate the activities of the mother and to guide her attunement. Although the mother must follow the child's needs through the various phases, Mahler and associates (1975) propose that the "lion's part of adaptation must come from the pliable, unformed infant" (p. 63).

In addition to maternal care and the child's capacity to extract the needed supplies from the mother, achieving a secure emotional bond also requires an optimal level of frustration, which leads the child to develop a constant cognitive-affective representation of mother whether she is absent or present. This is referred to as "object constancy" (p. 48).

Interruption in the formation of a secure emotional bond

Chantal's behaviors (e.g., lacking confidence to assert herself, set limits, establish boundaries, be autonomous) suggest that she did not achieve a secure emotional bond and that the bond she did achieve was interrupted by the birth of her brother. The mother reported that when Chantal was fussy, uncomfortable, and about to cry, the mother picked her up, rocked her, cuddled her, and distracted her. The mother carried Chantal to wherever the mother went. These behaviors on part of the mother may have delayed or prevented Chantal from establishing a secure emotional bond. Chantal appears not to have had sufficient quiet time where she and her mother enjoyed sensual and emotional contact, such as in nursing, which are essential for the development of "safe-anchorage" and "confident expectation" that her needs would be met (Mahler & Furer, 1968, pp. 8–9). On the other hand, with the mother consistently responding to Chantal's discomfort, Chantal did not experience an optimal level of frustration to develop object constancy, which is essential for the development of a secure emotional bond. Chantal was left with a yearning for emotional bonding that was stronger than her need for separateness.

Chantal's continued development of a secure emotional bond with her mother appears to have been interrupted by the birth of the second-born child when Chantal was one year and eight months of age. In a therapy session with Chantal manipulating playdough, the therapist suggested that she construct her family. Chantal asked her father, who was present for the session, and the therapist to participate in the construction of the family. She began her construction by creating the father, the pregnant mother, her brothers, herself, and then the baby (i.e., the fourth child). She fixed the three children on her fingers (i.e., like finger puppets) and made them talk, and she placed the baby in the arms of the mother. The therapist asked Chantal how her story would end. She said that the story ended with her dismembering first her oldest brother (i.e., the second-born child), then dismembering her father and youngest brother. Before she dismembered her mother, she removed her big belly. In the end there remained only Chantal, the newborn that she was taking care of, and the mom's big belly. She placed herself and the baby with the mother's belly carefully in the play dough container. Chantal's emotional reaction to the birth of the second-born child was clearly expressed in her construction of her family using playdough.

This is a horrific story! How to make sense of it? It appears that the birth of the second child in the family was traumatic for Chantal. She felt abandoned and developed "abandonment rage" (Masterson, 1976).

As the first-born child, Chantal developed an emotional bond with her mother. She had her mother to herself. When the second child was born, her relationship with her mother significantly changed. Chantal felt pushed aside because the mother paid less attention to her and more attention to the baby. Chantal felt abandoned to the point of abandonment rage. However, Chantal could not express her feelings for fear that in expressing them, she would lose the love of her mother. Therefore, her feelings were repressed and emerged in her story of the family that she constructed in playdough. According to the father, Chantal gave no indication how distressed she was by the birth of her brother. Chantal either deeply repressed her feelings or she used the mechanism of splitting (Klein, 1957) to form an idealized image of her mother so as not lose her love.

Restoration and development of a secure emotional bond

One of the goals for the therapist was to help Chantal develop a deeper emotional bond with her mother. Chantal's insecure emotional bond showed in behaviors such as her intense anxiety in leaving her mother to go school and in her lack of confidence to assert herself, establish boundaries, and set limits. In general, the caring, respectful, and supportive environment created by the therapist and by the mother in therapy with her daughter and at home, were conducive to the development of object constancy and to feeling emotionally secure with both the mother and the therapist. The therapist and the mother worked together to help Chantal develop object constancy and secure emotional bonding.

The mother in many ways helped Chantal develop a secure emotional bond with her. First, by attending ten therapy sessions with Chantal, the mother and

Chantal had great opportunities to bond by being involved in joint activities, with the mother letting Chantal take the lead. In coming to therapy with Chantal, the mother became more sensitive to her daughter. It was like a new start for Chantal to develop a secure emotional bond with her mother.

Second, the mother used a gradual approach in helping Chantal deal with her anxiety in going to school and in taking distance from her. The mother got involved as a volunteer at school for few hours per week, first in her daughter's classroom and then in the library. The mother offered to pick up Chantal for lunch at home. These contacts with the mother lowered Chantal's anxiety and she was able to face new challenges in going to school.

Third, the mother took time at home to play alone with Chantal, who took the lead in their play. The sign that Chantal was developing object constancy and a secure emotional bond with the mother was Chantal being able to manage distance from the mother. Chantal was able to have her lunch at school, she came home from school full of energy, and she developed a relationship with a girl in her class and they held hands and had fun.

Another indicator of Chantal developing a secure emotional relationship with her mother was Chantal asking her mother if they could go together to a movie. It was her way of having her mother to herself. In this sense, she was restoring her lost relationship with her mother.

Chantal developed a relationship with the therapist, who contributed to the development of object constancy and to a secure emotional bond. On one occasion when Chantal and her mother arrived at the clinic for a therapy session, Chantal approached the receptionist and announced that she wanted a meeting alone with the therapist. Chantal, jumping up and down as she approached the therapist, was very happy to see her alone. Without hesitation, she left her mother and brother in the waiting room. On another occasion as she arrived for therapy, Chantal in a non-verbal way asked the therapist for a hug, to which the therapist responded.

Therapeutic Gains

During her months in therapy, Chantal became more assertive, established boundaries, and set limits. She became more communicative, had more energy, and with greater confidence was being herself with her peers, brothers, and parents. She was excited about school and participated in activities such as her graduation from kindergarten. Her relationships with her parents and others improved and she was more positive about herself. She became more differentiated from others including her brothers. That is, she was able to more clearly assert when things were hers and when things belong to someone else.

Three years after the last therapy session with Chantal, the mother called the therapist to provide her with a report regarding her daughter. The mother stated that her daughter was doing "super well," that she enjoyed going to school and had many friends. The mother found her daughter's morale to be good, she was happy, got along with her brothers, and was very attentive toward them and especially toward the youngest brothers. She liked sports and was into synchronized swimming and had taken up karate.

Conclusion

This chapter presented the case of four-year-old girl, Chantal, who was in therapy to help her become assertive, establish boundaries, and set limits with others. Underlying her difficulties was the failure to develop a secure emotional bond with her caregiver, which led to her lack of confidence to be real and genuine in her relationships. Therapy began with a focus on developing effective ways of relating, such as being assertive. Toward the end of therapy, the therapy shifted to working on the development of a secure emotional bond with significant others, including the mother and the therapist. With the development of a secure emotional bond, the client progressed rapidly in becoming assertive, establishing boundaries, and setting limits.

References

Bowen, M. (1978). *Family therapy in clinical practice*. New York: A Jason Aronson Book.

Cashdan, S. (1988). *Object relations therapy: Using the relationship*. New York: Norton.

Goldberg, W.A., & Lucas-Thompson, R. (2008). Maternal and employment. *Effects of Encyclopedia of Infant and Early Childhood Development, 2* (pp.268–279) New York: Elsevier/Academic Press.

Hamdy, R. (2021). *Drawing the line: What personal boundaries are and why you need to set them*. Retrieved from: www.egypttoday.com/Article/6/108803/Drawing-The-Line-What-personal-boundaries-are-and-why-you April, 2023.

Hanna, S., & Wilford, S. (1990). *A professional development program guide. Floor time: Tuning into each child*. New York: Scholastic Inc.

Klein, M. (1957). Envy and gratitude. In Melanie Klein (Ed.) (1975), *Envy and gratitude and other works 1946–1963* (pp. 176–235). London: Delcorte Press/Seymour Lawrence.

MacLaughlin, S. (2014). *How to set limits for kids without harshness, fear or shame*. Retrieved from: www.huffpost.com/entry/how-to-set-limits-for-kids_b_4610102 April, 2023

Mahler, M., & Furer, M. (1968). *On human symbiosis and the vicissitudes of individuation*. New York: International Universities Press.

Mahler, M., Pine, F., & Bergman, A. (1975). *The psychological birth of the human infant*. New York: Basic Books.

Masterson, J.F. (1976). *Psychotherapy of the borderline adult: A developmental approach*. New York: Brunner/Mazel.

Masterson, J.F. (1993). *The search for the real self*. London: Routledge.

Nash, J. (2018). *How to set healthy boundaries & build positive relationships*. Retrieved from: https://positivepsychology.com/great-self-care-setting-healthy-boundaries/ April, 2023

Winnicott, D. (1965). *The family and individual development*. London: Tavistock Publishers.

Part IV

Philosophical Foundations

This chapter presents two branches of philosophy, namely, ontology and epistemology, which lie at the heart of all psychotherapies (Butler, 2002). In our search to understand human nature and the interactions of the cognitive, affective, and motivational systems in human nature, two fundamental questions arise: How do I know that which I think that I know exists? If it does exist, how do I study it? These questions cannot be answered by social scientists, who pay attention to that which is observable. To answer these questions, one must turn to philosophy, which focuses on that which underlies the observable (Piaget, 1977, p. 8). The first question is answered by the branch of philosophy called epistemology, and the second question is answered by the branch of philosophy called ontology.

The chapter begins with a presentation of ontology and epistemology and how they are complementary but different in studying human phenomena. This is followed by the presentation of three epistemologies, namely, modernism/postmodernism, structuralism/poststructuralism, and individualism and systems approach. In presenting these three epistemologies, it will be shown how Self-in-Relationship Psychotherapy (SIRP) positions itself within these epistemologies that define psychotherapy.

Ontology and Epistemology

Ontology

The term "ontology," a branch of metaphysics, comes from two Greek words, *onto*, which means *being*, and *logia*, which means *study* (Jacquette, 2004, p. 59). It is the "theory of being or the study of existence" (Carroll & Markosian, 2010, p. 11). Ontology is concerned with the ultimate nature of reality and its questions are: What is there? What exists? What is it like? (Grayling, 1998; Vanson, 2014). What kind of world are we investigating and what is the structure of reality? (Crotty, 2003, p. 10). Ontology is concerned about what exists in the world and about which humans can acquire knowledge. The ontological assumptions are those that respond to the question "What is there that can be known?" or "What is the nature of reality?" (Guba & Lincoln, 2001, p. 83).

DOI: 10.4324/9781032655291-14

In the study of being and of what exists in the world, four distinct ontological positions have been identified, which are realism, idealism, materialism, and relativism (Snape & Spencer, 2006; Moon & Blackman, 2014, 2017). Realism claims that there is an external reality independent of what people may think or understand it to be; realism relates to the existence of one single reality that can be studied, understood, and experienced as a truth. Idealism maintains that reality can only be understood via the human mind and socially constructed meanings. Materialism claims that there is a real world, but only the material or physical world is real. Relativism asserts that reality is constructed within the human mind, such that no one true reality exists. Instead, reality is relative according to how individuals experience it at any given time and place.

When it comes to the method of studying the *nature of social entities* (e.g., groups, teams, organizations), one can assume the ontological position of positivism or social constructionism. In taking the position of positivism, social entities are real and stable. On the other hand, in taking the position of social constructivism, social phenomena and their meanings are continually being changed and revised through social interaction. For example, the researcher's own accounts of the social world change, and nothing is definitive as new versions evolve with change – truth only happens in the moment.

Vanson (2014) states that in studying the fundamental nature of existence (i.e., continuance in being or life), there is no right or wrong answer as different people view topics differently depending on their set of values or background. Dilts and DeLozier (2000) state that the "map is not the territory" as each person will filter for preferences in her world according to her metaprograms. These metaprograms are derived from guiding principles and belief systems, motives, and constraints, which in turn decide the events to be noticed and the events to be ignored, the evidence to be noticed and the evidence to be set aside in building an argument (Vanson (2014).

In studying an existing entity (i.e., something that has separate and distinct existence and objective or conceptual reality), the researcher establishes the various categories that constitute the entity and describes how the various categories relate to each other. To conduct their study, the researcher can use various methods such as clinical insights, empathic immersion, qualitative methods, and empirical methods, to name a few. For example, Freud (1923) used clinical insights to study a client's inner world, which was thought to be constituted by the id, ego, and superego, and he demonstrated how they relate to each other. In addition to that which exists, the researcher may also study an entity as it is becoming and trace its evolution. Meier and Boivin (2000), in a case study, tracked how the client began with a low sense of self and gradually arrived at a more coherent sense of self.

How has ontology been applied in the study of psychotherapy? Notably, it has been applied in family therapy, which rejected an individualistic approach to therapy and instead adopted a systems approach. With this change in perspective, family therapists were challenged to describe what is a system and how are its constituents related to each other. For this enterprise, they adopted the concept of cybernetics (i.e., self-regulating system) and viewed the family as a self-regulating system. They identified constituents of this system, which included homeostasis, equilibrium, feedback loops, equifinality, and nonsumativity (Moyer, 1994, p. 273).

Epistemology

The term "epistemology" comes from two Greek words, *episteme*, which can be translated as knowledge or understanding, and *logos*, which can be translated as argument, account, or reason. Epistemology is concerned with the questions "What do you know?" and "How do you know that you know it?" (Vanson, 2014). It is "a way of understanding and explaining how we know that we know" (Crotty, 2003, p. 3); it "examines questions about the nature of knowledge and how we get it" (Grayling, 1998. p. 9). It is about "thinking about how we think" (Dickerson, 2010 p. 349). Its concern is to provide a philosophical grounding for deciding what kinds of knowledge are possible and how we can ensure that they are both "adequate and legitimate" (Maynard, 1994, p. 10).

Epistemology

> sets out to delimit what we know and how we can know it; to describe the methods which offer acceptable proof of a thing's existence and that our idea of it corresponds to its reality; and to define the criteria we use in evaluating the certainty of our statements. (Guttman, 1986, p. 14)

It has to do with all aspects of the validity, scope, and methods of acquiring knowledge, such as: (a) what constitutes a knowledge claim; (b) how can knowledge be acquired or produced; and (c) how to assess its transferability. Epistemology is important because it influences how researchers frame their research in their attempts to discover knowledge (Moon & Blackman, 2017).

One's epistemology influences how one views person (personality), problem (psychopathology), and change (treatment approach) (Dickerson, 2010, p. 350). Simmons and Sutton (2018) clearly state that "the therapist's epistemology colors every utterance, movement, action, reaction, thoughts, direction, stance, questions, statements, interpretations, conclusions, understandings, meanings […] that the therapist makes" (p. 1). Napier and Whitaker (1978) believe that the way a therapist views a problem

> determines what he is trying to change. If he sees the problem as primarily within the individual, he will move to help that individual. If he sees the problem as involving a set of relationships, he will likely try to influence that network of people. (p. 270)

Miller (2012) differentiates between an epistemology that is non-self-reflexive and linear, and an epistemology that is self-reflexive and circular. He names the former a first-order epistemology and the latter a second-order epistemology.

First-Order Epistemology

A first-order epistemology, which is non-self-reflexive, is a process of creating knowledge that operates in a linear fashion. The knowledge that it creates is not explicitly related to the process of its generation, and therefore it does not act as a corrective to its method of producing knowledge. This type of epistemology is not open to changing its ways of creating knowledge; it tends to stick rigidly to its process of creating knowledge (e.g., experimentation). Miller (2012) states that "a linear epistemology is resistant to calibration (higher order feedback)" (p. 2). It produces new knowledge that is innovative but not radical. This type of epistemology is well suited to the kinds of knowledge domains that work toward technical advances but not toward paradigmatic (characteristic) advances. The benefit of a first-order epistemology in producing new knowledge is that it minimizes the recursive complexity and is more amenable to simplification. It does not allow for subjectivism to be part of the production of new knowledge. Reductionisms, where all phenomena are explained in simpler entities, are linear epistemologies. Most modern scientific thinking is based on a linear epistemology, for which it is well suited (Miller, 2012, p. 2).

An example of a first-order epistemology is positivism, which deals with verifiable observations and measurable relations between the observations. It assumes that reality exists outside, or independently of the individual's mind (Moon & Blackman, 2017). It does not allow for the subjective opinions of the researcher nor for speculation and conjecture. It is a more scientific perspective with no room for subjective opinions of the researchers; the approach deals with verifiable observations and measurable relations between them, and not with speculation and conjecture (Vanson, 2014).

Second-Order Epistemology

A second-order epistemology, which is self-reflexive, allows itself "to be changed by the content that it produces" (Miller, 2012, p. 2). It is an open epistemology that operates based on a recursion (i.e., circularity) between process and content; it disavows linearity. It is open to calibration, that is, to the act of checking or adjusting itself by comparison with a standard. It seeks calibration of its own process through actively monitoring what it is generating. Unlike linear epistemology, which tends to minimize calibrative influences, a recursive epistemology actively embodies such influences. Miller states that a recursive epistemology is "not merely open to calibration, but is *self-calibrative*" (p. 2, emphasis in original). It is open to self-revision both at the content level and at the process level. The linking of process and content is akin to the creation of a new type of sensitivity in the process of knowing. One reflects on how one is going about to obtain knowledge and adjusts when needed. Miller adds that a "second-order epistemology is sensitive to its sensitivities; it includes processes whose content *is itself*" (p. 3, emphasis in original). The type of newness that a recursive epistemology yields includes "radical, as well as technical shifts. Radical shifts restructure the further possibilities that are available to the knowing system; they are paradigmatic shifts" (p. 3). A non-linear epistemology "emphasizes ecology, relationship, and whole systems. In contrast to linear epistemology, it is attuned to interrelation, complexity, and context" (Keeney, 2017, p. 14). Bateson (1979) advocates for self-reflection in our epistemology to avoid thinking that one's production of knowledge is independent of that which is produced.

Examples of second-order epistemologies are interpretivism, constructionism, and subjectivism. These three epistemologies share that the knowledge they create is related to the process of its generation and therefore the knowledge created has the potential to change the method of creating knowledge. A description of each follows.

The interpretivist approach rejects absolute facts and suggests that facts are based on perception rather than on objective truth. There are no universal laws or experiences as the world is always being developed and redeveloped by reflective, thinking, feeling beings (i.e., persons) who focus on meaning and perceived realities rather than on facts (Vanson, 2014).

Constructionist epistemology rejects the idea that objective "truth" exists and is waiting to be discovered. Instead "truth" or meaning arises in and out of our engagement with realities in our world. That is, a "real world" does not preexist independently of human activity. The term "constructionist" identifies the basic principle that reality is socially constructed (Guba & Lincoln, 2001; Robson, 2002).

A subjectivist epistemology implies that the standards of rational belief are those of the individual believer or those of her community. A subjectivist approach relates to the idea that reality can be stretched and shaped to fit the purpose of individuals such that people impose meaning on the world and interpret it in a way that makes sense to them (Moon & Blackman, 2017).

SIRP's Perspective

A second-order epistemologist does not search for psychological laws (i.e., internal structures), dynamics, and truths that govern and impact the physical and social worlds or realities. Rather, an individual sees reality as what he makes it out to be through the processes of interpretation and social construction. A first-order epistemology searches for laws, dynamics, and truths that govern physical and social realities. Law and lawfulness in this context refer to psychological law, which is "a lawlike universal statement which correlates some psychological state or event" with "other psychological states or events" (Lycan, 1981, p. 9).

SIRP adopts a first-order epistemology more so than a second-order epistemology as it believes that all human behavior and interactions are influenced by "laws," that is by "internal structures" (Thomas, 2002, p. 85) and psychological dynamics. It believes that these laws and dynamics can be partially discovered and brought to light by both quantitative and qualitative research that is inspired by a first-order epistemology. Although it is difficult to discover the laws, dynamics, and structures, it does not mean that they do not exist.

To illustrate the internal structures that underlie human behaviors, one can take the example of Klaus, who returned from a six-month deployment to a hostile country where he experienced three traumatic events. Since his return he has become hypervigilant and constantly checks his environment when in public places to assure that it is safe. The structure underlying his checking behavior is the innate need for self-preservation, which existed prior to his being deployed. However, his being in a hostile country and having experienced traumatic events raised the need for self-preservation to a heightened and problematic level. His current hypervigilant behavior, therefore, is not solely a socially constructed response but an innate need for self-preservation that has been heightened and shaped by a hostile environment. To treat hypervigilance, it is necessary to normalize the need for self-preservation, which for Klaus became problematic because it was shaped by a hostile environment.

Modernism and Postmodernism

The two dominant epistemologies that influence psychotherapy orientations are modernism and postmodernism. The two represent different worldviews, or "metanarratives" (Butler, 2002, p. 13). Associated with modernism are approaches such as linear epistemology, first-order epistemology, non-cursive epistemology, and structuralism. Associated with postmodernism are approaches such as circular epistemology, second-order epistemology, recursive epistemology, and poststructuralism (Dickerson, 2010). This section describes and critiques these two worldviews with reference to the practice of psychotherapy.

Modernism

The hallmarks of modernism are individuality, self-subsistent autonomy, superiority of reason, transcendence, and the superiority of spirit over matter and body. Modernism believes that there is a "givenness" in the world that humans can come to know, although partially (Downey, 1994). It believes that the mind can know some external reality, particularly through experimentation by which the principles and laws of the natural order are uncovered (Held, 1995). Modernism and essentialism go together. Essentialism views certain categories, such as dinosaurs, as having an underlying true nature that one cannot observe directly. Both modernism and essentialism hold that there are "real things, real objects, real goals, and real understanding about how things are" (Dickerson, 2010, p. 351). By the same token, it is believed that therapists can arrive at principles and methods through research that can improve a client's reality contact and foster the actualization of a person's true self.

Modernism initially dominated the mental health field and viewed symptoms and behaviors in terms of cause and effect. The main therapeutic approaches such as psychoanalysis and cognitive behavioral therapy fit into this structural framework.

Postmodernism

The hallmarks of postmodernism are relationality, interdependence, community, and traditions. Postmodernism rejects the idea that there is a "givenness" in the world to be known (Butler, 2002), and that there are principles, dynamics, and forces underlying the "givenness" (e.g., depression) that can be uncovered. It holds that knowing is a subjective phenomenon and that the mind is not capable of knowing anything outside of itself. That is, it is not capable of knowing objective truth (Held, 1995). Postmodernists believe that the theories and models that we have of any human phenomena are simply constructions of the mind and do not correspond to reality; thus, there is no possibility of arriving at the truth of anything. They believe that reality is co-constructed and changes from moment to moment. Postmodernism replaces the idea of a single reality, including the self, with multiple realities conditioned by individual, social, and temporal factors. Postmodernism is not without its critics. Gergen (2001) has been adamant in his criticism of postmodernism stating that it has "been too much content with bashing existing traditions and too little concerned with the repercussions" (p. 807). When applied to mental health, postmodernism views symptoms and behaviors in the context of relationships and systems rather than in terms of cause and effect. At the same time, postmodernism made more precise the concept of epistemology, which it considered in terms of relationships. It also raised questions as to the ability to objectively know outer and inner reality.

Rather than focusing on a person's inner world to understand symptoms, it focused on human interactions and relational patterns. It also challenged the epistemologies that guided the services provided by psychodynamic-oriented psychotherapists and the medical profession.

SIRP's Perspective

When applied to human conditions, it is not a question of modernism or postmodernism; rather, the question is: How do the two views contribute to our understanding of a human condition and its treatment? SIRP, for instance, incorporates aspects from both modernism and postmodernism. Take for example, modernism's concept of "givenness" and postmodernism's concept of "social construction." An example is a child's movement away from the significant parent in order to achieve separation and individuation, a phenomenon observed in children across cultures. This "urge" to move away is innate; it is the "givenness" or the "potential"; it is not socially constructed. However, the unique way this "givenness" or "potential" of a child is realized, is influenced in part by the environmental conditions in which the child was raised and grew up.

Not everything can be reduced to social construction. If everything is socially constructed, if there is no givenness or potential, then the statement itself is socially constructed and not "an accurate reflection of how things really are" (Detmer, 2003, p. 38). SIRP takes the position that humans are endowed with "potentialities" that are shaped, not constructed, by their familial, social, and cultural environments. Thus, the need to "individuate" is a potential, and the way it is shaped is influenced by external factors such as family, culture, and society (Meier & Boivin, 2011 p, 155).

Structuralism and Poststructuralism

Structuralism

Structuralism, as an epistemology, believes that "the universe and everything within it could be comprehended by discovering the laws (structures) governing all physical phenomena" (Thomas, 2002, p. 1). Boston (2000) describes structuralism as "the notion that there are discernible underlying entities that offer principles for organization, and that these structures have a fixed relationship to each other that transcend time and often operate in a duality" such as the mind and body (p. 453). More succinctly, Dickerson (2010) describes structuralism as positing "that every system has a structure that is 'real' and that lies beneath the surface of meaning [...] it emphasizes logical and scientific results" (p. 350). To learn about these unchanging structures, methods of scientific investigation were developed. It was accepted that "scientific objective exploration could provide reliable, valid, and universally applicable knowledge of the physical world" (p. 1).

When applied to psychology, as well as to psychotherapy, structuralism proposes that deep within a person there is an inner structure, such as the "inner self," and the "truth" of the person's identity. The belief is that people's behaviors including their attitudes are due to these fundamental structures. People in the therapy world, for example, developed a wide range of ways to interpret people's behaviors as if they were in some way related to the "workings of this inner-self, inner-psyche, or inner structure" (Thomas, 2002, p. 2).

Thomas (2002) summarizes the thinking of a structuralist in the following way. The structuralist thinks that the aim of investigation is to search for "deep structures" and that this search for deep structures can be objective. Further, the structuralist believes that these "deep structures" shape life and that our ideas, problems, and qualities are linked to an internal self. Last, a structuralist believes that our identities are fixed, consistent, and essential and are found within our inner selves (p. 3).

Poststructuralism

Poststructuralism is not the same as postmodernism; it is more specific. It is a distinct response to and critique of structuralism. It challenges "any framework that posits some kind of structure internal to the entity in question," whether we are talking about an individual or a family (Hoffman, 1992, p. 7).

Poststructuralists argue that the study of structures, be it in persons (e.g., self) or families, is culturally conditioned and therefore subject to historical changes.

They argue that since the study of structures is culturally conditioned, they are subject to historical changes and that historical conditions change how one interprets meaning. It is this interpretive frame that is important to one's understanding. Poststructuralists point out how the sociohistorical forces and the discursive practices within a given sociocultural context constrain and govern behavior. Dickerson (2010) states that

> one of the ways in which poststructural philosophy influences the field of psychology, and by extension family therapy, is to understand meaning as "a variety of local and partisan truths that may be told about every day life" […] Thus, instead of generalizing from individual experience to some larger meaning that underlies it – a structural approach – the therapist co-researches […] with the client what meaning an experience has for that specific person in this particular time. (p. 350)

SIRP's Perspective

SIRP includes epistemological ideas from both structuralism and poststructuralism. It believes that there are enduring deep inner structures, such as the self, that influence behaviors, thoughts, attitude, and feelings. It also believes that the form that these emerging structures take in their development is in part shaped by the social and cultural context in which the person was brought up and within which she continues to live. The individual's genetic inheritance and cultural influences interact to form psychological structures such as the self. SIRP also believes that structures or organizing principles can be transformed within the context of relationships including psychotherapy.

SIRP postulates that the underlying dynamics in the formation of structures are the individual's innate core needs; they serve as forward-moving urges. The way these needs are realized is influenced by the operation of an individual's emotional and cognitive interactive systems.

To illustrate the development, presence, and influence of deep inner structures, we can take the clinical case of James. James sought therapy because of work-related issues. He strongly felt that he was not measuring up to the employer's expectations, although he received very positive performance evaluations. He became a perfectionist, and developed obsessive compulsive disorder (OCD) symptoms that included indecisiveness and reviewing his work countless times before submitting it. When he was asked for how long he had felt that he was not measuring up to expectations of others and for how long he had felt bad about himself, his response was that he had always felt that way. How to make sense of the OCD symptoms and his fear that he was not measuring up? Was there a deep inner structure that was driving them?

With James's consent, a semi-hypnotic technique was designed with the purpose of uncovering "hidden" past experiences and with them their inner structures. As he was in touch with his experiences of the past, he recalled a childhood event that occurred when he was in an orphanage for the first two years of his life. It was not a memory but a "bodily felt feeling" of an event. When he was near two years of age and playing with other children in the playroom, he approached the caregiver for "emotional connection," but as he approached her, she did not pay attention to him and instead picked up another child and held her in her arms. This was a repeated experience. James felt that he did something wrong and that he was a bad person in being denied cuddles and being picked up and held. Repeated experiences confirmed his perception.

After being in the orphanage for two years, James was adopted by a caring family. It was important for him to be liked by his adopting parents; he cherished their love and affection for him. He wanted to keep things "good" between him and his parents and "not make any mistakes." Both in the orphanage and in his new home, there was a similar relational dynamic, which was a fear that if he was a bad person and made a "mistake," he would be deprived of what he craved most, which was the love and affection of his caregivers. His core need for affection and closeness "drove" his behavior to keep things "good" and "not to make any mistakes."

When he was in the orphanage and when he lived with his adoptive parents, he was able to shape his behaviors in accordance with the expectations and the feedback from the caregivers. When he left home and was on his own, however, he no longer had an external source, such as the caregivers, on whom to rely to assess whether his behaviors were acceptable and to give him direction as to what were acceptable behaviors. Therefore, he began to mentally create his own internal expectations and standards that he could use to evaluate his behaviors. However, he had no reference point as to what these expectation and standards might be; they were created more from fantasy (i.e., perception of reality tinged by feeling) than from reality. He struggled with uncertainty about his performance and indecisiveness. Underlying the three situations – being in the orphanage, living with his adoptive parents, and being in the workplace – there was a need for love and affection (i.e., feel significant) and a fear to "make a mistake" and be deprived of a meaningful relationship with a significant other. This combined unit of the "need to be loved" and the "fear to make a mistake" and "be denied the love" was formed while in the orphanage; it became a structure, an organizing principle that influenced his interactions with others at the orphanage and in his adoptive family, and continued to influence his significant relationships. Based on this analysis, it appears that underlying the OCD symptoms is the "need/fear" structure or organizing principle. For James to resolve his OCD symptoms, the "need/fear" structure must be addressed. The healing power comes from the transformation of the "need/fear" structure or organizing principle.

The analysis of James's current work-related problems and OCD symptoms, particularly perfectionism, are influenced by a "need/fear" internal structure. The development of the structure, according to SIRP, is driven by an individual's innate core needs and shaped by the individual's cognitive processing of inner experiences and by the social and cultural environment's responses to the unmet core needs. These internal structures, in turn, influence a person's relational interactions and the continued development of a sense of self and identity.

From Individualism to Systems Theory

This section presents individualizing and systems epistemologies. This is followed by a description of how SIRP positions itself within these two epistemologies.

An Individualizing Epistemology

Individualizing epistemologies view mental illness in linear terms, with historical explanations for the distress (Hoffman, 1981). They are influenced by modernism and they propose that there are "real things, real objects, real goals, and real understandings about how things are" (Dickerson, 2010, p. 351). Medical and psychodynamic models usually explain symptomatic behaviors linearly. The medical model compares emotional and mental distress to an illness or to a biological malfunction. Treatment consists of finding the origin of the so-called illness (a linear construct) and then beginning treatment. As for the psychodynamic model, symptoms are thought to arise from a trauma or conflict that has its origins in the past and has been repressed in the unconscious. Treatment consists in helping the patient recover the memory of the repressed event and reexperience and reprocess the emotions that were buried with it.

In both the medical model and the psychodynamic model, the individual is the locus of the malfunction, and the origin of the symptoms is related to either biological and neurological factors or to intrapsychic development. They disavow the idea that concepts such as self and self-identity are socially constructed. Rather, they assert that self, for example, exists as an innate potential, which is socially and culturally shaped, not constructed as postulated by social constructionists.

A Systems Epistemology

A systems epistemology emerged within couple and family therapy and their search for models other than structural and cybernetic ones. It was influenced by Bertalanffy's (1950) general systems theory, which differentiated among open systems, cybernetics, and closed systems (Moyer, 1994). The early couple and family therapy models were based on a cybernetic and a structural model (Bateson, 1972; Minuchin, 1968), which incorporated modernism's assumptions of linear causality and homeostasis (Hoffman, 1993). These were followed by new models that incorporated the concept of social constructivism and espoused postmodernism and poststructuralism. The earliest models are referred to as first-order cybernetics and the later models as second-order cybernetics (Simmons & Sutton, 2018). The differences between the two models are addressed.

First-Order Cybernetics

Cybernetics refers to a self-regulating system. The metaphor used to picture first-order cybernetics is that of a thermostat which regulates the temperature in the house. In a cybernetic system, the parameters are preestablished, the goal is to maintain equilibrium and homeostasis, causality is linear, the system is closed, and it requires external energy (e.g., a person resetting the thermostat) to function (Moyer, 1994, p. 277).

Using first-order cybernetics as an analogy, systems theorists view the family system in terms of the concepts of homeostasis, equilibrium, feedback loops, equifinality, and nonsummativity (Moyer, 1994, p. 280). Family therapists considered the family a homeostatic mechanism with patterns of communication analogous to those in mechanical information processing systems. They believed that they can know the dynamics underlying negative interactional patterns and are able to rectify them (Hoffman, 1993; Boston, 2000).

A criticism in viewing a family as a first-order cybernetic system is that the family is an open system and not a closed system. As an open system, it

> maintains itself in a continuous inflow and outflow, a building up and a breaking down of components, never being, so long as it is alive, in a state [...] of equilibrium but maintained in a so-called steady state which is distinct from the latter. (Bertalanffy,1968 cited by Moyer, 1994, p. 275)

An open system has two important attributes, namely equifinality and differentiation. Equifinality implies that the same state (e.g., depression) may be reached from different initial conditions (e.g., physical abuse, parental divorce), and differentiation permits dynamic, non-mechanistic interaction among the system's components. An open system has the capacity for expending energy and the intrinsic capacity for change (p. 276).

A problem with the first-order cybernetic system is that it uses mixed metaphors, that of a closed system (e.g., homeostasis and equilibrium) and that of an open system (e.g., equifinality). One cannot use the concepts of a closed system to describe a couple and a family, which are open systems (Moyer, 1994). A second problem is that it fails to consider that members of a family both act and are acted upon simultaneously. That is, the relational dynamic is circular and not linear (Moyer, 1994).

Second-Order Cybernetics

Second-order cybernetics includes the concepts of constructivism and social constructionism. Constructivism postulates that what is known in the external world is determined by our innate mental and sensory structures (Maturana & Varela 1984). Social constructionism, for its part, rejected the idea that objective truth exists and is waiting to be discovered and that a real world preexists independently of human activity (Guba & Lincoln, 2001; Robson, 2002). Social constructionism suggests that reality is co-created through language in an ongoing interactional and relational process. Gergen (1985) stated that discourse about the world is not a reflection of reality but an artifact of communal interchange. Consequently, family therapists "became interested in the active process of meaning-making and the greater variation of possibilities" such as the "inherent assumptions in particular discourses and ideas that had been excluded" (Boston, 2000, p. 451).

In second-order cybernetics, the observer is as important as those who are being observed. Second-order cybernetics studies the relationship between the observer and the observed and recognizes that observations from the observer always include the observer's epistemological premises and the actions based on these premises. From this perspective, therapy is seen as a relational context that can be defined as an "interactional system within which the participants interact with one another for a given purpose" (Simmons & Sutton, 2018, p. 4). In second-order cybernetics, the therapist and the client are seen to be in a reciprocal relationship and to mutually influence each other. Everything that happens in therapy and how each participant thinks, feels, and relates to one another indicates both their own epistemology and the "new shared epistemology about the nature of their relationship" (Simmons & Sutton, 2018, p. 4). In terms of the application of the new epistemology to family therapy, it meant that therapists were "called upon to include their own personal or theoretical bias as part of the observation" (Boston, 2000, p. 450).

SIRP's Perspective

Second-order cybernetics postulates that human behaviors, be they in a family or a workplace setting, are socially constructed and are the outcome of the interactions of the people at a given moment, and are not due to any inherent structure or hidden reality. It postulates that a real world does not preexist independently of human activity. Further, it holds that truth or meaning arise in and out of our engagement with realities in our world (Guba & Lincoln, 2001; Robson, 2002). Thomas (2002) adds that our identities are "always in the process of being created," that identities are "created in relationship with others rather than something internal," and "that our identities are socially created" (p. 18).

When applied to couples and families, second-order cybernetics postulates that relational problems are socially constructed through the members' actions, reactions, and interactions, and are not due to the influence of individual structures or hidden realities. The negative interactional patterns are corrected through a change in behaviors and communication between members, with a focus on the problems that present themselves at that moment.

SIRP argues that human problems and conflicts are not solely socially constructed through the interactions of the members of a couple and a family. Each member brings something very personal to all relationships. She brings innate potentialities and internal structures that account for "sameness across time" and "a sense of change across time." The innate potentialities are the agents of change, which may, when not appropriately responded to, result in conflicts.

A sense of self is experienced both as a "sense of sameness across time" and as a "sense of change across time." (Lichtenstein, 1961, p. 193). To illustrate the "sense of sameness" and a "sense of change" across time, one can use, as an analogy, a maple tree seed. The seed begins as a sprout and then becomes a sapling and eventually matures into a full-grown tree. In the first year the sapling develops a trunk, branches, twigs, and leaves. In the second year it grows taller, and its branches and twigs grow larger and stronger, and at the same time the tree develops new branches, twigs, and leaves. This continues for years as the initial sapling matures into a full-grown tree that beautifully towers into the sky. All through these years, there remains a sameness about the maple tree and yet there are ongoing changes. The emergence and development of the sense of self is similar; there is a "sense of sameness" and a "sense of change across time."

SIRP presents psychological data that refute the notion that identities "are created in relationship with others rather than something internal" and "that our identifies are socially created" (Thomas, 2002, p. 18). In fact, psychologists who have studied the development of the sense of self, hold the opposite opinion (Jacobson, 1968; Mahler et al., 1975; Stern, 1985). The sense of self is potentially and innately present at birth. It begins as a bodily sense of self and emerges through the way the infant is handled, and continues to develop through the interactions with the primary caregivers. These experiences are internalized as representations of the self that take on the characteristics of internal structures. Piaget (1977) states that epistemology is interdisciplinary in nature and relies on facts. In the case of psychological psychotherapy, epistemology relies on psychological facts (pp. 7–8). Thus, the position that our identities are solely "created in relationship with others rather than from something internal" appears to lack empirical support. Each person is born with an innate potential to develop a sense of self, and the form that the self takes is in part shaped, not constructed, by family, culture, and society. In a discussion about constructs such as a self, it is important to distinguish between that which is "socially constructed" and that which is "socially shaped." SIRP's position is that a sense of self begins as an innate potential that is socially shaped, not constructed, by its interactions with others, including the primary caregiver, parents, peers, and persons in authority.

When a couple or a family seeks therapy, all members have already formed their personalities based on their innate potentialities, which were shaped by their interactions with caregivers, family, culture, and society. The members have become individuals with their own values, ideals, struggles, and challenges, which are "powered" by their internal structures. All of these play a role in the formation of their couple and family relationships. At the same time, it is the innate potentials, more specifically, the innate self, relational, and physical intimacy needs, of the members of a couple and a family that provide the energy for its growth and expansion. The couple and the family are in a constant state of change and adaptation.

When an eight-year-old boy, for example, becomes a teenager, his relationship with the other family members changes because his biological, psychological, and social needs are changing. An open family system accepts the challenge and adapts to the needs of its members. With regard to the teenager, the family therapy must focus on his new experiences and on the "push" of his innate relational, self, and physical intimacy needs to differentiate from family members, to individuate, and to develop a sense of selfhood. This innate "push" on the part of a member provides the energy for the family to expand, change, and grow. A system has no energy; it needs to be energized by individuals' internal structures for interactions to occur. Like resetting a thermostat, the "push" of the members' innate needs resets the couple and family relationships. The innate "push" provides the motives for change and if not dealt with, may lead to conflicts. According to SIRP, couple and family therapy must address both the intrapersonal and the interpersonal issues. That is, there is a place for both "individualism" and "systems" (i.e., relationships) in couple and family therapy.

Summary and Conclusion

This chapter presented the position of three paired epistemologies, namely, modernism and postmodernism, structuralism and poststructuralism, and first-order and second-order cybernetics with regard to three epistemological questions: Are physical and psychological realities knowable? Are there real internal structures, be they in individuals, families, and society, that influence behaviors, and if so, are these structures knowable? Do a person's emotional problems originate from some personal biochemical or psychological defect, or are a person's problems socially constructed by the family, culture, or society of which she is a part?

SIRP takes as its starting point that individuals are endowed with "potentialities" (e.g., core needs) that push for realization, and that the form or shape that these "potentialities" take, is shaped by the interactional patterns of the families, cultures, and societies of which individuals are a part. It believes that these "potentialities" become internal structures and that the internal structures are discoverable and knowable. SIRP proposes that all of that which is human, is "driven" by the inner structures and modulated by reality, and by the interaction with the family, culture, and society of which the person is a part.

References

Bateson, G. (1972). *Steps to an ecology of mind*. New York: Ballantine.
Bateson, G. (1979). *Mind and nature: A necessary unity*. New York: E.P. Dutton.
Bertalanffy, von, L. (1950). An outline of general systems theory. *British Journal of Philosophical Science, 1*, 134–165.
Bertalanffy, von, L. (1968). *General system theory: Foundations development, applications* (rev ed.) New York: George Braziller.

Boston, P. (2000). Systemic family therapy and the influence of post-modernism. *Advances in Psychiatric Treatment, 6,* 450–457.

Butler, C. (2002). *Postmodernism: A very short introduction.* Oxford: Oxford University Press.

Carroll, J.W., & Markosian, N. (2010). *An Introduction to Metaphysics.* Cambridge, UK: Cambridge University Press.

Crotty, M. (2003). *The foundations of social research: Meaning and perspectives in the research process,* 3rd Edition. London: Sage Publications.

Detmer, D. (2003). *Challenging postmodernism: Philosophy and the politics of truth.* New York: Humanity Books.

Dickerson, V.C. (2010). Positioning oneself within an epistemology: Refining our thinking about integrative approaches. *Family Process, 49*(3), 349–368.

Dilts, R., & Delozier, J. (2000). *Encyclopedia of NLP.* Santa Cruz: NLP University Press.

Downey, M. (1994). In the ache of absence: Spirituality at the juncture of modernity and postmodernity. *Liturgical Ministry, 3,* 92–99.

Freud, S. (1923). The ego and the id. *Standard Edition, 19,* 12–63.

Gergen, K.J. (1985). The social constructionist movement in modern psychology. *American Psychologist, 49,* 266–275.

Gergen, K.J. (2001). Psychological science in a postmodern context. *American Psychologist, 56*(10), 803–813.

Grayling, A.C. (Ed.) (1998). *Philosophy 1: A guide through the subject.* Oxford, UK: Oxford University Press.

Guba, E.G., & Lincoln, Y.S. (2001). *Guidelines and checklist for constructivist (a.k.a. fourth generation) evaluation.* Retrieved from https://wmich.edu/evalctr/checklists

Guttman, H.A. (1986). Epistemology, systems theories and the theory of family therapy. *The American Journal of Family Therapy, 14*(1), 13–22.

Held, B.S. (1995). *Back to reality: A critique of postmodern theory in psychotherapy.* New York: W.W. Norton & Company.

Hoffman, L. (1981). *Foundations of family therapy: A conceptual framework for systems change.* New York: Basic Books.

Hoffman, L. (1992). A reflexive stance for family therapy. In S. McNamee & K.J. Gergen, (Eds.), *Therapy as a social construction* (pp. 7–24). London: Sage Publications.

Hoffman, L. (1993). *Exchanging voices: A collaborative approach to family therapy.* London: Karnac Books.

Jacobson, E. (1968). *The self and the object world.* New York, NY: International Universities Press.

Jacquette, D. (2004). *Pathways in philosophy.* Oxford, UK: Oxford University Press.

Keeney, B. (2017). *Aesthetics of change.* New York: The Guilford Press.

Lichtenstein, H. (1961). Identity and sexuality: A study of their interrelationships in man. *Journal of American Psychoanalytic Association, 9,* 179–260.

Lycan, W.G. (1981). Psychological laws. *Functionalism and the Philosophy of the Mind, 12*(1), 9–38.

Mahler, M.S., Pine, F., & Bergman, A. (1975). *The psychological birth of the human infant.* New York: Basic Books.

Maturana, H., & Varela, F. (1984). *The tree of knowledge: Biological roots of human understanding.* London, UK: Shambhala.

Maynard, M. (1994). *Researching women's lives from a feminist perspective.* Abingdon, Oxfordshire, UK: Routledge.

Meier, A., & Boivin, M. (2000). The achievement of greater selfhood: The application of theme-analysis to a case study. *Psychotherapy Research, 10*(1), 57–77.

Meier, A., & Boivin, M. (2011). *Counselling and therapy techniques: Theory and Practice.* London, UK: Sage Publishers.

Miller, S. (2012). *It's elemental–First and second order epistemologies. Blog of applied philosophy: Basic concepts in philosophy.* Retrieved from www. spiritalchemy.com/ 1592/first-and-second-order-epistemologies June, 2020.

Minuchin, S. (1968). *Families of the slums.* New York: Basic Books.

Moon, K., & Blackman, D. (2014). A guide to understanding social science research for natural scientists. *Conservation Biology, 28,* 1167–1177.

Moon, K., & Blackman, D. (2017). *A guide to ontology, epistemology, and philosophical perspective for interdisciplinary research.* Retrieved from: https://i2insights.org /2017/ 05/02/philosophy-for-interdisciplinarity/

Moyer, A. (1994). Cybernetic theory does not explain family and couple process: Systems theory and dialectical metatheory. *The American Journal of Family Therapy, 22*(3), 273–281.

Napier, A., & Whitaker, C.A. (1978). *The family crucible.* London: Harper & Row.

Piaget, J. (1977). *Psychology and epistemology: Towards a theory of knowledge.* New York: Penguin Books.

Robson, C. (2002). *Real World Research*, 2nd Edition. Oxford, UK: Blackwell.

Simmons, B., & Sutton, J. (2018). Epistemology in family systems theory. In J.L. Lebow, A. Chambers & D. Breunlin (Eds.), *Encyclopedia of couple and family therapy.* New York: Springer International Publishing.

Snape, D., & Spencer, L. (2006). The foundations of qualitative research. In J. Richie & J. Lewis (Eds.), *Qualitative research practice (Chapter one): A guide for social science students and researchers.* London, UK: Sage.

Stern, D.S. (1985). *The interpersonal world of the infant: A view from psychoanalysis and developmental psychology.* New York: Basic Books.

Thomas, L. (2002). Poststructuralism and therapy–what's it all about? *The International Journal of Narrative Therapy and Community Work, 2,* 85–89. Retrieved from https:// dulwichcentre. com.au/

Vanson, S. (2014). *What on earth are ontology and epistemology? Retrieved* from: https:// theperformancesolution.com/earth-ontology-epistemology/

Epilogue

Self-in-Relationship Psychotherapy (SIRP) proposes that successful psychotherapy involves the inclusion of a person's motivational system and its integration with affective, cognitive, and behavior systems in the understanding and treatment of emotional and behavioral problems and with self and relational issues. This is true for regardless of a person's age, gender, and cultural background. The motivational system is the source of energy that provides the direction for personal growth and healing. The motivational system has been defined in terms of core relational, self, and physical intimacy needs.

This volume illustrates how uncovering and asserting the unmet core needs in individual, couple/family, and child therapy helps persons work through their emotional and behavioral problems and reorient their behaviors and relationships according to the core needs. In becoming aware of, validating, and asserting their mutual needs, individuals overcome their emotional and behavioral problems. When core needs are honored and validated, psychotherapy becomes focused and leads to positive outcome.

SIRP, which makes core relational, self, and physical intimacy needs its centerpiece, has been successfully applied to individual, couple, and child therapy. It seems clear that when core unmet needs are directly or indirectly addressed, the results from treatment tend to endure over time.

The chapters on individual, couple/family, and child therapy provide the theoretical foundation for more comprehensive publications that address each modality of therapy from the perspective of SIRP. This entails not simply adding to existing psychotherapy approaches but also demands revisioning how affect, cognitive processes, and core needs constitute three interdependent systems, how they relate to each other, and how the three systems influence all behaviors and interactions.

It is necessary to apply SIRP to special human problems such as bulimia, anorexia, drug and alcohol addictions, and to emotional problems such as personality disorders, and to assess the effectiveness of SIRP in treating these issues. To assess the significance of including core needs in a psychotherapeutic approach, it is necessary to develop a reliable and valid psychometric instrument that measures core needs and has the capacity to differentiate among the needs.

DOI: 10.4324/9781032655291-15

SIRP is innovative and integrative and offers a promising approach the psycho-therapy. Future applications of this approach will more clearly define its unique characteristics and its capacity to effectively treat human problems.

Semi-Structured Assessment Interview (SIRP-SSAI) 2023

1. **Reason for requesting counselling and the presenting problem:** The client in contacting a therapist for help regarding a personal or interpersonal problem launches the therapeutic process. During the first 10 or 15 minutes, the therapist explores with the client the nature of the problem, its duration, intensity, its extensiveness, how it affects him, when it is more intensive, and so on. Assuming that the client reports being depressed, one might ask the following exploratory and clarifying questions (for other problems, replace "depressed" with that problem).

   1a. For how long have you felt this way?

   1b. When do you feel most depressed? How strongly do you experience this feeling?

   1c. Is there anything going on in your life now that might be related to you being depressed?

   1d. Have you felt depressed in the past? (If yes, explore their precipitating factors).

   1e. Have you seen someone in the past because of your depression? (If yes, explore).

   1f. Are you seeing anyone now for your depression? If so, who? How do you find this experience?

   1g. Have you ever thought it would be better not to be alive? Have you thought of taking your life? (If yes, explore when, where, and how and precipitating factor). (If no, ask, what it is that is keeping you going despite the difficulty.)

2. **Appearance and behavioral observation:** The way a person presents herself and behaves in the therapy session can provide useful information regarding her mental state, coping strategies, relational style, and capacities. Typically, one asks questions about how the person presents herself only when something stands out. How do you experience the client? What do you experience when

with the client? What is the nature of the client's sharing of personal information? Is she open and forthright? Retentive?

3. **Family background:** Information about one's family and childhood would include the relationship of the person to his father, mother, and siblings; the relationship of the parents to each other; the nature of the father's and the mother's work; the quality of the parents' relationship to their own families, their coworkers, friends, relatives, and so forth. The purpose is to gain an understanding as to how the person perceives his parents and himself, and how the person feels about the parents and himself with reference to the parents. Having these goals in mind, one might ask the following questions (interspersed with empathic responding, summaries, etc.).

   3a. When you think of your childhood and teenage years, what stands out most for you? Could you describe or say more?

   3b. What was it like for you to live in and be with your family?

   3c. How would you describe your relationship with your mother when you were a child?
   How is your relationship with your mother today? How would you describe your mother as a person?

   3d. Repeat question 3c for father, sibling, uncle, aunt, grandparent, and any other significant figure in the person's life.

   3e. (If there are siblings). Where are you in the birth order (Obtain names and ages of siblings). How do you get along with your sister (brother)? Say more.

   3f. How did your father (mother, sibling) feel about you? What did they think of you? How did you feel about the way they thought of you and felt about you?

   3g. As a child, who took care of you? If the person was with a caregiver, inquire as to when this began, how often per week, and for how long. Where were the parents? Working? What was it like to be taken care of by others?

   3h. Have there been any deaths in your family? (If yes, could you say more and how this affected you?). Any tragedies? Any serious illnesses? (Ask the person to say more about these and how he was affected by them).

   3i. Have you experienced any abuse in your family? Mental abuse? Physical abuse? Sexual abuse? By whom? Say more about this.

   3j. Is there anything else about your family and your relationships with your father and mother that would be useful for me to know?

4. **Educational background:** In exploring a person's educational background, pay attention to how well the person did in school, her extracurricular activities, friends, peer groups, how well she related with the teacher, to her academic and career goals, and so on. This information helps in understanding how the person

invested her energy; her enthusiasm and zest for life; academic aspirations and goals, and so on. This information is helpful for understanding the perceptions that she developed of others – peers, teachers – and of herself. The following questions may be helpful to obtain information for this domain.

4a. How has school been for you? How well did you do in primary school? High school? College? University? How would you describe yourself as a student? Bright, average?

4b. Did you take part in extracurricular activities? Which ones? How did you get started with them?

4c. What were your favorite subjects?

4d. Did you have friends at school? If yes, what did you do together? How did you get along with them? Do you still have friends from your school days?

4e. How did you get along with your teachers? Tell me more.

4f. Were there any drugs at school? Vaping? Where are you with that?

4g. Do you have future educational plans? What are they?

5. **Occupational background:** The level of the person's satisfaction with his work, the nature of his relationship with coworkers and supervisors, and the quality of his work provide useful information regarding the person's sense of self, competency, adequacy, and quality of relationships. In obtaining information about this area, one might ask the following questions. If the client is still going to school and has a part-time job, adapt the questions to the situation.

5a. What is the nature of your work? For how long have you done this kind of work? How are you enjoying your work?

5b. For how long have you worked at your current place of employment? Have you worked at other places? Where? What made you change places of work?

5c. How would you describe the working atmosphere of your current place of work?

5d. How well do you get along with your coworkers? Do you prefer to work with men or with women? Alone? With others?

5e. How would you describe your relationship with your supervisor?

5f. Have you been promoted at your place of work? If yes, how is that for you? Do you have aspirations for the future? Could say more about this?

6. **Social background:** A history of a person's social background provides information about her ability to relate to others, to get along, and to be in touch with reality. One might ask the following questions.

6a. How is your social life? Do you have friends? What do you and your friends do when together? Do you like being with people? Are you able to be alone?

6b. (If single) Do you have a girl/boyfriend? Is this your first boy/girlfriend relationship? How is this for you? Is this your first intimate relationship? When did you first date? What was that like for you?

7. **Marital and couple relations background:** Couple relationships are the most challenging of all relationships. Knowledge of this relationship provides information about a person's ability to be intimate, empathic, and accepting; about his ability to integrate sexuality within the context of a set of values and one's own self-identity and self-acceptance; about a person's ability to compromise, collaborate, resolve conflicts, and be altruistic. If the couple have children, how they relate with them, perceive, accept, and discipline them, and so on, provides additional information about the parents. The following questions may be germane in securing information about this domain.

7a. How are things between the two of you? (If they have problems, explore the duration, extent, intensity of the problems). Have you experienced these problems in the past? When? What has brought on the problems?

7b. How would describe your relationship? How do you feel about that?

7c. How do you go about resolving conflicts? Making compromises? Making decisions?

7d. Are you able to count on each other?

7e. How is your love life? Do you have difficulty in being intimate with each other? Do you want to be together? Is there chemistry between the two of you? How often do you make love?

7f. (If they have children) How many children do you have? What are their gender and ages? How would describe your relationship with your children? Their relationship with you?

8. **Health (physical and mental):** Inquire about the person's physical and mental health. If there have been ailments (physical and emotional), determine their duration, seriousness, and what brought them on, and ask if they have received treatment. If yes, what type of treatment and for how long. Are you on medication? (If yes, explore kind, dosage per day). How satisfied were they with the treatment and with those providing the treatment? Has the person struggled with addictions: alcohol, medications, streets drugs, gambling, and so on?

9. **The experience of trauma:** Inquire whether the person has experienced traumas. If so, you can proceed with the following questions.

9a. Tell me more about your experience.
9b. How old were you when you experienced the trauma?
9c. Was the traumatic event physical (e.g., car accident), relational, sexual?

9d. Were you able to talk to someone about your traumatic experience?

9e. Did you consult a professional regarding the trauma?

9f. How is the traumatic experience affecting you today?

10. **The experience of abuse:** Inquire whether the person has experienced emotional, physical, and/or sexual abuse in the past. If so, follow up with these questions.

    10a. Tell me more about your abuse.

    10b. How old were you when the abuse occurred?

    10c. Who was (were) the offender(s) of the abuse?

    10d. Were you able to talk to someone about the abuse? Who?

    10e. How is the abuse affecting you today?

    10f. Have you consulted a professional to talk about the abuse? Who?

11. **Hobbies and leisure:** The ability to relax, play, have fun, and engage in creative projects and activities gives us information about how well the person has integrated external demands, and internal pressures, with the need to respond to one's wishes, desires, interests, and so forth. Leading questions to explore this topic may include:

    11a. How do you spend your free time? For how long have you been spending your free time this way? How do you feel using your time this way? (Notice whether or not she feels guilty, and if so, explore this).

    11b. Are you able to sit down and merely do nothing? Do you have to do this for a purpose?

    11c. How does this hobby help you to take care of yourself, etc.?

12. **Sources of strength:** To assess a person's capacity to deal with current difficulties, that is, her resilience, it is helpful to obtain information as to where she turns in time of difficulties (e.g., to another person, within, to a higher power, etc.). Questions that can be asked about this topic may include:

    12a. To where do you turn in times of difficulty for support and comfort? If the person states several sources, explore each as fully as possible. Be curious.

    12b. What is it about (this source) that helps you feel better? (Explore fully).

In concluding the interview ask the person whether there is anything else that has not been covered, which would be good for the therapist to know to understand her better and be of assistance to her.

Self-in-Relationship Psychotherapy Assessment Form (SIRP-AF)

Augustine Meier, PhD and Micheline Boivin, MA

Name: _____ DOB: _____ Tel: _____

Address: _____ Email: _____

Education _____ Occupation_____

Single ___; Married ___; Widow(er) ___; Separated ___; Divorced ___; Remarried _____

(Place a check mark in appropriate space(s))

Date: _____ Analysis by: _____

The Self-in-Relationship Psychotherapy Assessment Form (SIRP-AF) was designed to code the theoretical constructs of Self-in-Relationship Psychotherapy. Its use, therefore, assumes familiarity with these constructs. The SIRP-AF has been specifically constructed for clinicians to aid them in their understanding of the individual with whom they work and to theoretically guide their assessments, conceptualizations, and treatment.

The SIRP-AF comprises four parts. In Part I, the examiner is asked to provide descriptive data regarding the core self, relational, and physical intimacy needs that influence the person's behaviors and attitudes, the individual's representations of significant others and of self, the affects linking these representations, and the quality of his childhood interactions with his parents. Part II comprises scaled data regarding the manner of relating to others, psychic structure, self-structure, coping strategies, the quality of the emotional bond, object constancy, characteristic emotion, projective identifications, characteristic (developmental) phase, characteristic (development) position, and level of personality organization. In Part III, the examiner is asked to conceptualize the person's current problems with respect to past and current experiences and events, and the constructs from Self-in-Relationship Psychotherapy. The conceptualization typically includes precipitating, predisposing, perpetuating, and protective factors. Part IV presents the issues that need to be addressed in psychotherapy and indicates the form of therapy and possible interventions.

Part I. Descriptive Data: For each of the dimensions presented below, provide descriptive material for the persons (e.g., mother & father) entered in the top row of the table. If other figures were or are important to the client's life (e.g., grandmother, stepfather), additional columns can be created and assessed for each topic under Dimension

Dimension	Father	Mother
1. The striving of self, relational, and physical intimacy needs relative to:		
2. Internal representation of:		
3. Internal representations of self relative to: (How I view myself when with:)		
4. Affect linking representation of other to self: (How I felt my father, mother, etc. felt about me)		
5. Affect linking representation of self to other: (How I felt about my father, mother, etc.)		
6. How I felt/feel about being in the presence of:		
7. Quality or degree of good enough parenting:		

Part II. Scaled Data: Rate dimensions 1, 4, 7, and 11 on a five-point scale. For dimensions 2 and 3, indicate the strength of each component using a five-point scale with 1 = barely and 5 = greatly. For dimension 10, indicate the characteristic phase and the strength of its presence using the five-point scale as indicated above. For the remaining dimensions, check off those that are relevant. See Operational Criteria for more precise instructions. If the dimension is not relevant, leave the space blank. Legend: PO = part object; WO = whole object; PSP = paranoid/schizoid; DP = depressive position; EB = need for emotional bonding; SC = need for sensual contact; AU = need for autonomy; SI = need for sexual intimacy.

| 1. Manner of relating to: | Father: | 1 (PO) | 2 | 3 | 4 | 5 (WO) |
| | Mother: | 1 | 2 | 3 | 4 | 5 |

| 2. Psychic structure | Core Needs: ___ EB ___ SC ___ AU ___ SI | ___ ego | ___ superego |

| 3. Self-structure | ___ striving for competency | ___ striving for significance | ___ capacity to maintain significance and competency |

| 4. True self (Living from) | 1 Minimally | 2 | 3 | 4 | 5 Strongly |

	1	2	3	4	5
5. Coping mechanisms	— repression — denial — dissociation	— splitting — introjection — projection	— idealization — devaluation — sublimation	— regression — other — other	
6. Quality of emotional bond	— emotionally connected	— striving for emotional connection	— avoiding emotional connection	— emotionally disconnected	
7. Object constancy	Not Formed		Partially Formed		Fully Formed
8. Characteristic emotional state	— angry — anxious	— depressed — smothered	— oppressed — abandoned	— sad — other	
9. Projective identifications	— dependency — other	— power	— ingratiation	— sex	
10. Characteristic phase	— symbiosis	— differentiation	— practicing	— rapprochement	— consolidation
11. Characteristic position	(PSP)				(DP)
12. Level of personality	— higher	— intermediate	— lower		

Part III. Conceptualization:

Prepare a conceptualization of the person's current problems using concepts from Self-in-Relationship Psychotherapy. This means, tell the client's story using the language of theory. The conceptualization links how the current problems and symptoms are related to predisposing, precipitating, perpetuating, and protective factors. The conceptualization is by nature abstract and hypothetical and not descriptive.

_____

_____

_____

_____

_____

Part IV. Treatment Aspects: Based on your assessment, indicate the core issues (e.g., splitting, caretaking, separation-individuation, abandonment) that need to be addressed in therapy and indicate primary therapeutic approaches and potential interventions.

_____

_____

_____

_____

_____

_____

Operational Criteria and Coding Procedures (SIRP-OCCP) 2023

Brief conceptual definitions are presented for each of the Self-in-Relationship Psychotherapy (SIRP) constructs. This is followed by operational definitions with examples and coding procedures for each of the constructs. Some constructs are coded on a five-point continuum scale, other constructs are coded on a five-point scale as to the degree of their striving quality, and the remaining constructs are checked off and/or rank ordered.

The Operational Criteria and Coding Procedures for the SIRP constructs (SIRP-OCCP; Meier & Boivin, 2013) have been modified for inclusion in this book. The coding for the conceptual and operational definitions are presented in two parts, one part for the descriptive data and a second part for the scaled data. In using the operational criteria and coding procedures, carefully read the psychosocial history of the client to get a sense of the client.

Part I: Descriptive Data

The client's psychosocial history provides the clinical material for the analysis of his unmet needs, mental representations, and affect. These three classes of data are seen as forming one entity and are not seen in isolation from each other. Although the "other" is often referred to as father or mother, "other" might refer to any significant person in the client's life.

The descriptive data present the client's perception of and feelings about himself and about the significant persons of his childhood. The data provide a picture of the atmosphere of the home environment in which the individual was raised and what it was like to have lived with others in the home of his childhood. These experiences also provide information on how the child might have responded to them and tried to make sense of them all, which is reflected in his perceptions of others and self. It is assumed that the way these experiences were perceived and internalized continue to impact a person's relationships and day-to-day living. In this part, the examiner is asked to describe the unmet needs, mental representations of significant others and of self, the affects linking these representations, and the quality of the person's childhood interactions and experiences with his caregivers.

Organizing Unmet Core Relational, Self, and Physical Intimacy Needs

Definition and description: The term "unmet core needs" refers primarily to those needs not adequately responded to during infancy/childhood and that continue to linger and push for fulfillment in adolescence and adulthood. The core needs are grouped according to core relational, self, and physical intimacy needs. Relational needs refer to the need to be emotionally connected and the need to be autonomous (Mahler, Pine & Bergman, 1975). Self needs refer to the need to be competent and the need to be significant (Kohut, 1977). Physical intimacy needs include the need for sensual contact and for sexual intimacy.

Operational definition and coding procedure: Operational definitions are given for each set of core needs taken separately. With regard to the unmet core needs, code these using, as much as possible, the names of the needs included in the Taxonomy of Needs, namely, emotional connection, autonomy, competency, significance, sensual contact, and sexual intimacy. With reference to needs, one codes for the strength of this striving and not for its state or presence within an individual. Examples are provided for each set of needs.

The first set of unmet core needs are the two relational needs, that is, the need for emotional connection and the need for autonomy. The need for emotional connection can be expressed in terms of words or in terms of a feeling or fear of being abandoned, rejected, cut off, and insignificant. The need for autonomy can be expressed in terms of wanting to have a voice in matters that affect the person.

Examples:

1. I want you to spend more time with me, I am lonely without you, I miss you, I need more quality time together (Need for emotional connection).
2. I need to spend time alone, I need to have time to do my things, you are impinging upon my life and my freedom (Need for autonomy).

The second set of unmet needs are the two self needs, namely, for significance and competency, which are manifested when a person seeks affirmations for them. Examples of these needs are the following.

Examples:

1. I just want to be told that I am OK, that you still care for me, that you accept me for who I am (Need for significance).
2. I do all these things. I run a million-dollar business. I organize charities. I organize all our vacations, and yet I do not hear a word of appreciation from you about how well I am doing (Need for competency).

The third set of unmet core needs are the need for sensual contact and the need for sexual intimacy. The need for sensual contact includes those behaviors that involve touch (e.g., physical closeness, touch, hugging) but not with the intent of sexual intimacy. The need for sensual contact also includes those behaviors where there is no touch but a wanted physical presence (e.g., to be in the same space but not engaged in touch). The need for sexual intimacy includes fondling, intimate touch, hugging, and kissing with the intent of sexual expression.

Examples:

1. I need to be held, touched, and cuddled. We don't do enough of that anymore. We used to do a lot of that when we first dated, but we lost it (Need for sensual contact).
2. The last time that we had sex was three months ago. I need to have sex; a person needs to have sex (Need for sexual intimacy).

When the relational, self, and physical intimacy needs are not adequately satisfied in infancy and early childhood, the person may strive continuously to seek them in adolescence and adulthood. These needs become the organizing principle around which the person might live his life. It is important to differentiate unmet needs of the past from unmet needs appropriate to current relationships. These are referred to as unmet childhood needs and unmet growth needs, respectively.

Internal Representation of Other

Definition and description: The internal representations of the other are cognitive and affective images formed from the infant/child's experience with significant caregivers (Klein, 1959). The representations can bear a positive, negative, or a mixed positive/negative valence. Representations are not to be confused with the feelings that one has for others. It is important to understand that the client's representations of others that were formed in childhood may persist into adult life. The representation that was formed of others is intimately related to having or not having his early core needs positively responded to.

Operational definition and coding procedure: A mental image that a person has of the other might be that he is weak, sad, and sensitive, or that the person is domineering, cruel, strong, and responsible. When identifying a person's internal representations of others, the focus is on the mental and affective image, and not on how the person feels about the other or in the way the other is needed. The mental picture of a person may correspond to how the person is in real life, or it may deviate from this in some dramatic fashion.

Examples:

1. My father was self-centered, controlling; it was always about him and about no one else. He was heartless (Negative internal representation of father).
2. My mother was caring, did crafts with us, took us to the park, she was fair with us, and yet she expected that we participate in household chores (Positive internal representation of mother).

Internal Representation of Self

Definition and description: The internal representation of self is a cognitive and affective image of self formed from the infant/child's interactions with significant caregivers (Klein, 1959). The formation of the mental representation is very much influenced by the quality and nature of the parents' responses to his needs, feelings, and behaviors. These self-representations might include seeing one as lovable, competent, wanted, and intelligent, or their opposites.

Operational definition and coding procedure: The focus when identifying the mental representation of self is on the image or picture that the child has of himself and not on how he feels about himself or on his needs.

Examples:

1. With my father, I was never good enough, was not smart enough, I was the dumb and the clumsy one in the family (Negative internal representation of self with regard to father).
2. My mom helped me realize that I was good at drawing, painting, doing crafts (Positive internal representation of self with regard to mother).

Affect Linking Representation of Other to Self

Definition and description: This refers to the feeling that the individual perceives the other (e.g., parents) to have had toward him when he was an infant/child (Kernberg, 1976; Masterson, 1976).

Operational definition and coding procedure: The linking affect represents the emotional response of the parents toward the client when he was an infant or child, but from the perspective of the client, which might or might not correspond to the way things were. For example, the client might have felt that his parents felt frustrated and angry toward him, but they might not have felt that way.

Examples:

1. My dad was constantly criticizing me, was impatient with me. He did not like me because I was not as smart as my older brother (Father's negative feelings toward child).
2. My mother was affectionate, loving, caring. She would at times become angry with us, but we always knew that she loved us (Mother's positive feelings toward her child).

Affect Linking Representation of Self to Other

Definition and description: This construct describes the feelings that the client, as an infant or child, had toward a significant caregiver and which he might still have today (Kernberg, 1976). Again, this is the client's feeling about the situation.

Operational definition and coding procedure: The linking affect represents how he felt about the significant persons in his infancy/childhood. For example, the client might have been frustrated with and angry toward his parents, or he might have been happy, content, and cheerful when with them. The client might experience the same feelings toward his parents today. It is important to differentiate old (familiar) feelings related to past experiences from new feelings that are associated with current experiences with others.

Examples:

1. My father's criticism hurt me so much that I hated him and I am angry at him and I have no feelings for him (Child's negative feelings toward his father).
2. I love my mother; she has always tried to be helpful and to make things pleasant for the family and for me (Child's positive feelings toward her mother).

How I Feel/Felt When in the Presence of the Other

Definition and description: This dimension assesses how the person felt when in the presence of the significant other such as the father and the mother.

Operational definition and coding procedure: The person as an infant/child might have felt safe and secure, or he might have felt tense, fearful, and insecure when with a significant other such as the father and the mother. The person might still feel this way about being with the other today.

Examples:

1. When I was with my father, I felt very tense and anxious because I didn't know what he was going to criticize me for next. I walked on egg shells when around him (Negative feeling in presence of father).

2. I felt safe and secure and protected when I was with my mother; I also felt proud of myself (Positive feeling in presence of mother).

Quality of Being Parented

Definition and description: This refers to the infant/child's experience of being parented and of being brought up by his parents (Winnicott, 1965).

Operational definition and coding procedure: This construct concerns the nature and quality of parenting, such as: Was there sufficient freedom for the child to be himself and have time for fun and to play? Did the person feel encouraged to develop his abilities and potentialities? Did the person feel that he was a significant part of the family and made a meaningful contribution to the family? Was parenting consistent and free of conflict and violence? Did the person feel safe, secure, and protected?

It is assumed that if these early relationships were satisfying and the infant/child blossomed within context of these relationships, he would have a positive view of himself and of others, and acquire the skills to deal with the day-to-day challenges of life. However, if the infant/child's experiences of others (i.e., caregivers) were more negative in that the caregivers might have been emotionally neglectful and cold, and there was a lack of structure and a lack of love, caring, and support, the individual's experience would have been negative.

Examples:

1. My home life was chaotic; my mother was depressed; my father was on drugs and was unemployed; there was no food in the fridge; they shouted and screamed at each other; we were left to ourselves; my home was oppressive (Depriving and emotionally neglectful parenting).
2. Living with my parents and older sister was OK; my parents were immigrants and worked hard to have money to buy their first house; we often celebrated with my relatives; there was music, singing, and a lot of food (Good enough parenting).

Part II: Scaled Data

The results from the scaled data provide a picture of the person's inner world that was formed in large part through his interactions with significant others. The inner world is composed of memories, affects, motives, image, perceptions, and sensations that influence, to a great extent, how the person processes incoming information and shapes his interactions with others and with the world.

This part consists of the SIRP constructs that are assessed either on a five-point scale or are checked off as being present in the clinical material. The conceptual definitions of these constructs were presented in detail earlier. The operational definitions for these constructs are provided in the Operational Criteria presented below.

When scoring the constructs in terms of the extent to which they describe the client's experience or the strength to which they are present, consider whether the score lies to the left or right of the midpoint on the five-point scale. You can also begin by eliminating categories or ratings that do not fit, and then determine which of the remaining ratings or categories best describe the client's experience and behavior and/or your inference of these. Use as a point of reference clients with whom you have worked. The scores you assign to the various dimensions are based on your inference that is grounded on the material reported in the client's psychosocial history.

Manner of Relating to Significant Others

Definition and description: This construct addresses the way an individual relates to others. When an individual relates to the other as the other is needed (e.g., for advice, emotional support), the other is referred to as a part-object. When the individual relates to the other as someone who has needs, feelings and thoughts, and a life of his own, the other is referred to as a whole-object (Klein, 1952).

Operational definition and coding procedure: In rating the way an individual relates to a significant other (caregiver), take into consideration how the individual generally related to her father, mother, or sibling. Does the person relate to the significant other as he or she is needed (i.e., part-object), or as a differentiated and individuated person (i.e., whole-object)? On the five-point continuum, 1 = part-object and 5 = whole-object, a score of 3 indicates that the person might at one time relate to the other as a part-object and at another time relate to the person as a whole-object.

Examples:

1. My mom and I always got along well; when I came home from kindergarten, she made lunch for us and asked about my day; today we are like friends (Relates to her mother as whole-object).
2. My mother was an alcoholic; when I came home from kindergarten and grade school, she was lying on the floor drunk; I had to prepare the meals for her; today I still crave the love that she never gave me and I also hate her for not having been a mother to me; I need a mother (Relates to her mother as a part-object).

Psychic Structure

Definition and description: The construct, psychic structure, comprises the internalized demands and expectations of others and the world, an individual's own innate needs, and an agent (reason) to negotiate these needs. Freud's (1923) concept of the psychic structure includes the concepts of the id, ego, and superego.

The Freudian concept of the psychic structure has been slightly modified. Freud's concept of the id has been expanded. The two instincts, libido and aggression, have been replaced by four core needs, the needs for emotional bonding, sensual contact, autonomy, and sexual intimacy. These four needs are symbolized, respectively, as EB, SC, AU, and SI.

Freud's concept of the superego refers to both acceptable and unacceptable behaviors and to ideals and values to live by. Freud referred to these as the conscience and the ego ideal, respectively. SIRP adopted Freud's notion of the superego; however, the coding is only for the conscience, which is characterized by a sense of duty and obligation and includes social behaviors that are acceptable and/or unacceptable. A sense of duty and obligation are not to be confused with ideals and values to live by. There is a sense of freedom to live by one's ideals and values, whereas there is a sense of "must" and a lack of freedom to live by duties and obligations. The superego can be reasonable, severe, or harsh/punitive.

Freud's concept of ego has been extended to include adaptive functions in addition to defensive functions. The defensive function of the ego has the purpose of protecting the person from anxieties and conflicts, particularly internal conflicts, and of maintaining self-esteem. The adaptive functions of the ego include the capacities to negotiate, compromise, accept, forgive, and repair relationships, to mention a few. The energy of the ego's adaptive functioning is more creative than the energy used in defensive functioning. In coding the ego, one takes into consideration the ego's global capacity to mediate the person's core needs, and the demands of the superego and of the external realities.

The structures of the psyche are in constant interaction with each other, but one structure (e.g., superego) might be dominant at one time and the others latent. The configuration of the psychic structure affects the development of personality and relationships. For example, if an individual's superego dominates, such a person might be demanding of self and might also be demanding and controlling of others.

Operational definition and coding procedure: The task of the coder is to assess the degree to which the ego has integrated the demands of the superego; the relational, self, and physical intimacy needs; and demands of reality. Each part (e.g., superego) of the psychic structure is scored according to a five-point scale, where 1 means that the part (e.g., AU) is minimally striving for satiation, and 5 means that it is actively striving for satiation. The score assigned to a specific aspect is meaningful only when it is considered in relationship to the scores assigned to the other parts.

In the case of an ego organization in which the core needs, the superego, and demands of reality are integrated, scores of 3–5 might be assigned to each of the parts depending upon the level of energy and passion. The greater the energy, the striving, and the passion, the higher the assigned scores. For a psychic structure that is demanding, self-critical, self-punitive, oppressive, and moralistic, and at the same time striving intensely for emotional connection, one might assign a value of 4.5 for superego, of 3.5 for EB, and of 2.5 for ego. In this case the person is characterized as having a domineering superego and a need for emotional connection that is suppressed but is pushing to be realized, and an ego that is weakened. In the case of a psychic structure that results in aggressive, promiscuous, and violent behavior, one might give a score of 4–5 for AU, of 1–2 for superego, and of 2–3 for ego, depending on the ego's ability to regulate affect and impulses. For a psychic structure that is characterized by logical thinking and practical concerns, one might assign a score of 4 to the ego, of 2–3 for EB, and of 2–3 for superego.

Examples:

1. I am in a constant state of conflict with an inner voice telling me to continue to do the right thing and not to give into my craving to take another drink, and at times I find both the voice and my craving overpowering and I want to go to bed (Possible coding: Superego = 4; EB = 4; and Ego = 2.5 since both the demanding voice and the craving are strong and overpowering).
2. I don't give a darn what others think; I am not hurting anyone and I enjoy playing the slot machines; I have tried to stop and it didn't work, I just go back into it, I have given up trying (Possible coding: Superego = 3; AU = 4; Ego = 3).
3. The one time that I can take time to play and try to relax is when I take the dog for a walk (because I should play with the dog); I find it a waste of time to watch television; when I watch television, I am reading for my work (Possible coding: Superego = 4; AU = 2; Ego = 3 because the person is should, ought, and performance driven).

Self-Structure

Conceptual definition and description: Human infants, generally, are born with a "virtual self" already in place (Kohut, 1977, p. 101), that is, with a biologically determined psychological entity (Brinich & Shelley, 2002). The virtual or potential self is shaped by the child's interactions with his caregiver's sense of what self is and by the individual's reflections in the context of the responses of others in his interactions with them. The interactions lead to the organization of a self that comprises: (a) a sense of competency; (b) a sense of self-esteem; and (c) a capacity to maintain a sense of competency and self-esteem at times of anxiety and stress (Kohut, 1977). Kohut's self-structure has been modified in that the sense of competency refers to a striving for competency, and the sense of significance refers to a striving for significance.

Operational definition and coding procedure: Each of the core self needs, need for competency and need for significance, is assessed on a five-point scale as to the degree to which it is pressing to be responded to and is striving for satiation.

A score of 5 means that the core need is greatly seeking to be responded to, and a score of 1 means that it is minimally pressing to be responded to. A score between 2.5 to 3.5 indicates that a person feels relatively competent and significant. With regard to the capacity to regulate competency and significance, which is like ego resources, a score of 1 indicates that the person lacks the capacity to maintain these two core needs, whereas a score of 5 indicates that the person has the capacity to maintain a sense of competency and significance.

Examples:

1. I feel so ashamed, I feel that I cannot do anything right, and when my partner treats me like a kid, I lose it (Possible coding: competency = 3.5; significance = 3.5; and capacity = 2 because the individual strives to be competent and to be significant and has limited resources to maintain a sense of being competent and significance when he receives negative a response from others).
2. I know myself and I try not to let what others think of me affect how I feel about myself and about my work and my importance to the company (Possible coding: significance = 3; competency = 3; capacity to maintain sense of competency and significance = 4 because the person has the resources to maintain his sense of competency and significance despite the opinions of others).

Social Self

Definition and description: This construct refers to the extent to which an individual organizes his life according to that which is integral, genuine, and congruent with his sense of self and self-identity, or whether the person lives from the expectations, values, wishes, and demands of others. The former is referred to as living from the True Self, and the latter is referred to as living from the False Self (Winnicott, 1965).

Operational definition and coding procedure: To simplify the coding on the True Self and False Self continuum, coding will only be for the True Self. From this code one can calculate the code for the False Self. In coding for True Self, use a five-point scale, where 1 indicates that the construct is minimally operative, and 5 indicates that the construct is strongly operative.

Examples:

1. I just became a pleaser, I aimed to please the people around me, to impress people, and it was easier to do it that way than to speak for myself. I don't like it, I want to get out of it, and I keep slipping back into old patterns (Possible score, True Self = 1.5).
2. I just like to be me and not have to worry about what others think (Possible score, True Self = 4)

Coping Mechanisms

The term "coping mechanisms" includes both (unconscious) defense mechanisms and conscious coping strategies.

Definition and description: Defense mechanisms serve the purpose of maintaining and enhancing an individual's self-esteem by managing internal conflicts, anxieties, and tensions (Freud, 1923). Every person uses a variety of defense mechanisms, and the mechanism used depends on the issue dealt with. Persons who struggle with significant emotional problems tend to use a limited number of defenses repeatedly and rigidly. These mechanisms are unconscious and include defenses such as dissociation, splitting, denial, and repression. The pattern of defense mechanisms provides information regarding the nature of an individual's emotional problems and the age of their onset. The use of splitting and dissociation compared to the use of rationalization, indicates an earlier onset of the emotional problem. The brief definitions of the coping mechanisms are taken from White & Watt (1981), Kaplan & Sadock (1991), and Sadock, Sadock & Ruiz (2014).

Coping strategies can be thought of as being conscious, such as negotiation, compromise, endearment, empathy, and problem solving.

1. Repression: the defense by which unwanted thoughts and feelings are kept out of awareness.
2. Dissociation: the inhibition or alteration of some aspect of consciousness or memory, such as observed in amnesias and fugue states.
3. Denial: the blocking out of disagreeable realities or information by ignoring or refusing to acknowledge them
4. Splitting: a developmental and defensive process of keeping incompatible feelings (e.g., love and hate) apart and separate as seen in idealization and devaluation.
5. Idealization: the psychological process of coping with anxiety caused by ambivalent feelings by attributing overly positive and exaggerated qualities to another person or thing, and negating negative qualities.
6. Devaluation: the psychological process of coping with the anxiety caused by ambivalent feelings, by attributing completely flawed, worthless exaggerated negative qualities to another person and discounting positive qualities.
7. Projection: the unconscious tendency to attribute one's own unacceptable feelings, thoughts, and impulses to other persons or objects in the external world.
8. Introjection: the process of incorporating (without scrutiny) the characteristics of a person or object unconsciously into one's own psyche.
9. Displacement: the conscious or unconscious substitution of an object (e.g., dog) for the appropriate object (e.g., person, place, thing) that is missing, toward whom one expresses negative feelings.

10. Sublimation: the channeling of libidinal and aggressive energy into a socially approved mode of behavior.
11. Rationalization: giving a probable reason for one's type of behavior.
12. Regression: behavior where the individual reverts to a behavior more appropriate to an earlier stage of development or to reaction patterns long since outgrown.

Operational definition and coding procedure: Using the above definitions, select the pertinent mechanisms that constitute the person's defensive structure. The cluster of defenses will often comprise the more "primitive" defenses, such as repression, dissociation, denial, splitting, or the more advanced defenses (i.e., secondary defenses), such as rationalization, sublimation, reaction formation, displacement, and so on.

Code the defense mechanisms that are repeatedly and rigidly used to deal with the same or similar issues. Indicate the appropriate defense mechanisms by placing an X in the space preceding the defense mechanism. If one of the defense mechanisms stands out, indicate this by placing the number one ("1") in the space preceding the defense mechanism, and place an X in the space preceding the other defense mechanisms. To assure yourself of the correct selection, determine whether your selection is supported by other concepts or structures, such as the nature of the ego structure, self-structure, and so on. If the client exhibits a defense mechanism not indicated on the form, add it as Other.

Quality of the Emotional Bond

Definition and description: This construct refers to the quality of an infant/child's investment of psychic energy in another person on whom the individual would normally rely for safety, security, nurturance, stability, and comfort (Mahler et al., 1975). It refers to the degree to which an infant/child feels emotionally connected to and emotionally anchored in the significant other. The quality of the emotional bonding reflects the extent to which the caregiver spontaneously responded to the infant/child's feelings and core relational, self, and physical intimacy needs.

The two essential components of an emotional bond are that the person's needs are satisfied and that the person feels comfortable, safe, and secure with that person. The former is referred to as confident expectation and the latter as emotional anchorage (Mahler et al., 1975). Often the quality of the emotional bond manifests itself behaviorally, but the behavior does not define an emotional bond. The satisfaction of needs and positive feelings and living from them define an emotional bond.

Operational definition and coding procedure: The quality of emotional bonding is assessed using the four categories – being emotionally connected, striving for emotional connection, avoiding emotional connection, and being emotionally disconnected.

(1) Being *emotionally connected* means that the infant/child has developed a satisfying, secure, comfortable connection with the caregiver who responded in a satisfying way to the infant/child's needs and feelings.

(2) S*eek emotional connection* refers to eagerly searching for a meaningful, satisfying, and comfortable emotional relationship with a significant other. This form of connection might manifest itself in emotional pursuit and entanglement, with the expression of negative emotions when not achieved. The search for emotional connection often occurs when the caregiver is inconsistent in her responses or does not adequately respond to the infant/child's needs.

(3) *Avoiding emotional connection* refers to keeping emotionally distant from significant others. This might happen when the parent is overbearing and demanding and does not allow the infant/child space to be himself, or when being emotionally close is too painful.

(4) *Being emotionally disconnected* refers to having limited emotional feeling for others and being emotionally cut off from them. This may be due to a child's many failed attempts to emotionally connect. These experiences of continued rejection and hostility bring about feelings of hurt and anger and result in feeling cut off.

In terms of coding, indicate which of the four categories describes the person's emotional bond with significant others. Place an X in the space preceding the category.

Examples:

1. I have no feeling for my mom, I hate her and I do not care if I ever see her again (Emotionally disconnected).
2. I remember when I was very young, I would follow mom around the house, I wanted her to talk to me, play with me, and hold me; I just wanted to be with her but she did not have the time; I still seek her attention (Seeking emotional connection).
3. When I was very young, I did not want anyone to hold me, touch me, or get close to me; when they touched me, I felt violated (Avoiding emotional connection).

Object Constancy

Definition and description: Object constancy refers to a mental representation of a positive libidinally (i.e., affectionate) cathected inner image of the caregiver (Mahler et al., 1975), whether the person is present or absent. From another perspective, object constancy is the "capacity to recognize and tolerate loving and hostile feelings toward the same object; the capacity to keep feelings centered on a specific object; and the capacity to value an object for attributes other than its function of satisfying needs" (Mahler et al., 1975). The presence of object constancy permits the child to function separately in familiar surroundings despite moderate degrees of tension and discomfort, and acts as an agent to self-comfort and self-soothe. Within the context of psychotherapy, one can see the formation of object constancy by the client saying to himself, when troubled, what would my therapist say about the situation or by writing down a therapist's intervention.

Operational definition and coding procedure: Object constancy refers to the formation of an internal representation of a significant other formed from their positive interactions. The internal representation provides an emotional psychological home to which the person can turn to gain a different perspective on an issue, to comfort and soothe himself, and find a way to uplift himself when emotionally challenged or troubled. On the four-point scale, place an X in the space before the appropriate selection.

Examples:

1. When my boyfriend goes out with the guys to watch the Superbowl, and if he does not come home before midnight, I feel lonely, get enraged, want to end the relationship (Object constancy minimally developed and is mostly absent).
2. Even though I cannot see her as often as I would like to because she is busy with schoolwork and family, I know that she loves me and that is reassuring and comforting (Object constancy fully developed and is present).

Characteristic Emotional State

Definition and description: This refers to an individual's characteristic mood or emotional state, which might be that of anger, anxiety, sadness, and/or depression. The telling sign of a characteristic emotion is that it is a familiar emotion and has been part of the person's life since childhood, and it is disproportionate to the event that precipitated it.

Operational definition and coding procedure: When coding for the characteristic emotional state, consider the emotion that a person has carried across time. Differentiate the characteristic emotional state from an emotion triggered by a current event. Code only for one characteristic emotion.

Examples:

1. I have been depressed for the past month; I often felt depressed as a teenager; I think that I have been depressed all my life (Depression is the characteristic feeling).
2. When I play hockey and a guy slashes me on the shins, I become enraged and slash him back twice as hard; I felt the same way toward my dad, when as a child, he forced me and my brother to fight each other until we were hurt (Rage is the characteristic feeling).

Projective Identifications

Definition and description: These are compulsive and repetitive relational patterns, driven by underlying unmet core needs, which have as their purpose to establish, maintain, and influence the nature of the relationship (Klein, 1959). The way clients perceive themselves (e.g., helpless; unlovable) and how they perceive others (e.g., powerful; admirable) influences the nature and quality of their relationships. The common forms of projective identification (PI) include dependency (playing the role of the helpless and dependent person), power (portraying oneself as being more competent than the partner), ingratiation (laying on guilt trips to get the needed response from the other), and sexuality (arousing a sexual experience in the other) (Cashdan, 1988).

Operational definition and coding procedure: Identify the dominant projective identification (PI) and place a check mark in the box next to it. If there are two or more PIs, rank order them with 1= most prominent, 2= second most prominent, and so on.

Examples:

1. She just doesn't get it; the baby was crying for 20 minutes and then she asks me to bring the bottle of milk from the fridge; couldn't she figure it out that maybe the baby was hungry? (Possible coding is PI of Power since he gives the impression that he knows more about childcare than his partner).
2. My daughter is so selfish. When she needs to have something repaired, I do it right away. When I asked her to pick up something at the store – and she was next to it – she said that she had no time. I became angry at her and told her how I gave up my time to do things for her and that she could do something for me (Possible coding PI of Ingratiation as the mother's behavior elicits the feeling that the daughter owes the mother something in return for her deeds).
3. My girlfriend gets angry with me when I ask her to take care of paying the bills because she is good at finance and budgets and I am not; I rely on her. In my home my mother took care of the finances (Possible coding is PI of Dependency because the young man seems to be looking for a caretaker).

Characteristic Developmental Phase

Definition and description: The term "phase" refers to one of the pre-oedipal (sub)phases, of which the Symbiosis, Practicing, Differentiation, Rapprochement, and Consolidation/object constancy subphases are significant (Mahler et al., 1975). Each of the (sub)phases has specific developmental tasks that need to be completed. These tasks are: (1) the symbiotic phase: for the infant/child to emotionally bond with the mother; (2) the differentiation subphase: for the child to psychologically separate and establish "Me" and a "Not-me"; (3) the practicing subphase: for the child to explore the non-mother world, to practice its new cognitive and motor skills, and to make choices as to the toys it likes and dislikes; (4) the rapprochement subphase: for the child to establish boundaries, form object constancy, regulate affect, replace the mechanism of splitting by repression. When the developmental tasks of a subphase are not adequately negotiated (i.e., completed), the person will push to complete them in adolescence and adult relationships.

Failure to complete the developmental tasks of a specific subphase can have significant implications for development in adolescence and adulthood. The failures at the phase or subphase might be: (1) the symbiotic phase: the infant did not become emotionally anchored; (2) differentiation subphase: the infant/child did not psychologically separate and individuate; (3) practicing subphase: the toddler did not have the opportunity to try out his newly acquired cognitive and motor skills and explore his external world; (4) rapprochement subphase: the toddler did not develop object constancy, achieve emotional anchorage, reverse splitting, establish boundaries, differentiate, and individuate; (5) consolidation and object constancy subphase: the individual failed to work out a balance between being connected to the love object and being his/her own person and having internalized good objects to whom to turn to self-comfort.

Operational definition and coding procedure: Identify the developmental tasks that the person has not completed or strives to complete. Indications that an individual has not completed the developmental tasks specific to a phase or subphase are: (1) symbiotic phase: the individual insatiably yearns for emotional connection, for closeness, for intimacy, is dependent upon the other, is not able to move toward psychological separation and autonomy, and is in search of the unreachable; (2) differentiation subphase: the person is enmeshed or seeks a dependent relationship, and the ME and Not-ME are not clearly established; (3) practicing subphase: the individual has no life of his own, does not know what he wants to do, has no practical ambitions in life, is not adventuresome, feels inadequate, and has an insatiable need to prove himself as being competent; (4) rapprochement subphase: the individual has great difficulty negotiating and compromising, throws "adult" temper tantrums when things do not go his way, wants others to take part in his activity but is not ready to participate in the activities of others, has low frustration tolerance, is not able to establish boundaries, and has not developed object constancy and capacity to self-soothe; and (5) consolidation and object constancy subphase: the individual has failed to establish boundaries between self and other, to replace splitting by repression, to achieve libidinal object constancy, and to achieve the ability to regulate affect.

In terms of coding, indicate the phase or subphases for which the developmental tasks were not achieved or are striving to be satiated. Failures to complete the developmental tasks are easily recognized by their striving to be satiated. Use a scale of 1 to 5 to indicate the degree to which the developmental tasks of a specific phase or subphase failed to be completed. On the five-point scale, 1 = minimally achieved and 5 = greatly achieved. It is possible that the developmental tasks of two or more subphases have not been completed and best describe the person's behaviors and relational patterns. For each of the phase or subphases, indicate the degree to which they have not been completed using the five-point scale.

Examples:

1. I don't know what I want to do in life. I don't like my work. I am not too crazy about school. My girlfriend wants me to make up my mind about our relationship. I am not able to commit myself to anything (Possible coding is the practicing subphase because the individual, as a child, did not have opportunity to adequately explore alternatives, to experiment, and to commit).
2. At the restaurant last evening, my boyfriend asked me to be his steady date. I became anxious, fearful, intruded upon, violated. I felt that I was losing myself. I disconnected, became enraged, and ended up lying under the table in a fetal position (Possible coding is the rapprochement subphase).
3. I am not interested in sex. I like to spend time together sitting on the couch, being held, cuddled, being next to each other, and watching television. I don't get enough of him. (Possible coding is the symbiotic phase as there is an insatiable need for emotional closeness and sensual contact).

Characteristic Developmental Position

Definition and description: Position refers to an individual's position on the paranoid-schizoid (PSP) and depressive position (DP). The PSP represents an individual who is angry, uses splitting, sees others as part-objects, relates from self as a part-self, lacks empathy for others, and has not established boundaries between self and other. The DP represents an individual who has developed empathy, fears losing the love of the love object, repairs injuries caused to the person loved, uses repression rather than splitting, is beginning to see others and self as whole persons, and has established boundaries between self and other.

Operational definition and coding procedure: Determine where the client is on the developmental continuum. Use a five-point scale to indicate at which end on the continuum the client is, with 1 = Paranoid Schizoid Position and 5 = Depressive Position. If the client clearly meets the criteria for the PSP, assign a score between 1 and 3. If the client clearly meets the criteria for the DP, assign a score between 4 and 5. If the client manifests characteristics of both the PSP and the DP, or fluctuates between the two positions, assign a value of 3.

Examples:

1. I truly regret the way that I treated the women that I dated in the past. They were good women; I was not ready for a committed relationship. I regret how I hurt them and I wish that I could say that to them (Possible coding is 4 because the

individual expresses compassion for those he hurt and would like to repair the relationship).

2. When my partner asks me to put away my empty coffee mug and plate or to pick up after myself, I feel treated like a kid and I become so enraged. Does she not know that I have bigger things to do than to pick up dishes? She is like a sergeant major (Possible coding is 2 because he is easily triggered to rage, he has not integrated the good and bad representations, and he is short on empathy).

Level of Personality Organization

Definition and description: SIRP views emotional problems in terms of personality organization and its underlying dynamics. It has modified Kernberg's (1976) approach by replacing the concept instinct by the core needs.

The level of personality organization is determined by the manner in which the core needs have been integrated, the quality of the superego (reasonable, severe, harsh), the nature of defenses used to deal with conflicts and anxieties, and by the quality of relationships that have been formed (Kernberg, 1976). Based on these criteria, three levels of personality organization have been identified. Briefly these are: (1) Higher-Level: core needs are integrated with genital primacy; superego is well integrated but severe; defenses are organized around repression; internalized objects are stable; and concept of other and self is well integrated. This level is manifested in neurotics; (2) Intermediate-Level: pre-genital fixation points are present; superego is less developed; defenses are organized around repression but some primitive defenses are present; internal objects are conflicted; ego identity is established; and there is a stable concept of other and self. This level is manifested in passive-aggressive, sado-masochistic, narcissistic personalities; and (3) Lower-Level: there is a pathological condensation of genital and pre-genital strivings; predominance of pre-genital aggression; unintegrated and sadistic superego; primitive defenses that are organized around splitting; internalized part-objects; identity fusion; and lack of object constancy. This level is manifested in borderline, schizoid, pre-psychotic, and antisocial personality disorders.

Operational definition and coding procedure: Using the above criteria, identify the appropriate level of personality organization and place a check mark in the space in front of it.

Index

For Product Safety Concerns and Information please contact our EU
representative GPSR@taylorandfrancis.com
Taylor & Francis Verlag GmbH, Kaufingerstraße 24, 80331 München, Germany

9 7 8 1 0 3 2 6 7 8 7 9 5